'Social science typically studies individual behavior in isolation from the natural, temporal context in which it occurs. What is needed are data from a broader range of mental and somatic states that can be tied directly to the range and content of activities in which normal and abnormal populations engage. Experience Sampling using ambulatory signaling devices represents another important advance in the clinical understanding of the context of an individual's daily behavior.'

J. P. Robinson. Survey Research Center, Maryland, U.S.A.

'The chapters in this volume share a common assumption. It is that whether a person suffers or feels happy does make a difference . . . psychology and psychopathology cannot be fully understood at the level of chemical processes. The entire organism with its subjective states, operating in its real social and cultural context, must be taken into account if we wish to know what is right or wrong with it.'

From the Foreword by M. Csikszentmihalyi

This book is devoted to the Experience Sampling Method (ESM) in psychiatry, and contains contributions from the leading international pioneers of this approach. Experience Sampling is a methodology for collecting reliable and valid data on patterns of behavior, thought and feeling from real-life situations. It thus yields data complementary to those provided by neurobiological approaches to mental illnesses, and is applicable to the study and management of a wide variety of mental disorders in their natural settings.

The editor, who did much to bring ESM to prominence in psychiatry, has assembled a fascinating range of contributions, many of them never before published, dealing with the diagnostic and therapeutic possibilities of this approach. Methodological and practical issues are also addressed for those wishing to use ESM in their own research or practice.

Case studies illustrate the uses of Experience Sampling in schizophrenia, depression, eating disorders and addictions, and there are chapters devoted to its application to the elderly, those under stress, and in normal subjects. This book is therefore a rich source of information and ideas for clinicians and research workers seeking a new and rigorous approach to understanding the experience of the mentally ill.

The Experience of Psychopathology

The Experience of Psychopathology:
Investigating Mental Disorders in their Natural Settings

Edited by

MARTEN W. deVRIES

Professor, Department of Social Psychiatry, University of Limburg, Maastricht, The Netherlands

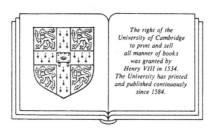

The right of the
University of Cambridge
to print and sell
all manner of books
was granted by
Henry VIII in 1534.
The University has printed
and published continuously
since 1584.

CAMBRIDGE UNIVERSITY PRESS

Cambridge

New York Port Chester Melbourne Sydney

CAMBRIDGE UNIVERSITY PRESS
Cambridge, New York, Melbourne, Madrid, Cape Town, Singapore, São Paulo

Cambridge University Press
The Edinburgh Building, Cambridge CB2 2RU, UK

Published in the United States of America by Cambridge University Press, New York

www.cambridge.org
Information on this title: www.cambridge.org/9780521403399

First published 1992
This digitally printed first paperback version 2006

A catalogue record for this publication is available from the British Library

Library of Congress Cataloguing in Publication data
The Experience of psychopathology : investigating mental disorders in
their natural settings / edited by Marten W. deVries.
p. cm.
Includes bibliographical references and index.
ISBN 0 521 40339 1 (hardback)
1. Psychiatry – Methodology. 2. Mental illness – Case studies.
I. deVries, Marten W.
[DNLM: 1. Data Collection – methods. 2. Life Change Events.
3. Mental Disorders – diagnosis. 4. Mental Disorders – therapy. WM
100 E945]
RC437.5.E97 1992
616.89 – dc20 DNLM/DLC 91–29425 CIP

ISBN-13 978-0-521-40339-9 hardback
ISBN-10 0-521-40339-1 hardback

ISBN-13 978-0-521-03112-7 paperback
ISBN-10 0-521-03112-5 paperback

For Henk and Teuny

Contents

PART III EXPERIENCE SAMPLING STUDIES WITH CLINICAL SAMPLES

Foreword

For one who has been among the pioneers of the systematic study of human experience in natural settings, it is enormously gratifying to greet this distinguished collection on *The Experience of Psychopathology*. My students and I at the University of Chicago began gathering electronic paper-induced responses from everyday life situations some 15 years ago. The Experience Sampling Method – or ESM – has since found numerous research applications. The psychiatric applications reported in this volume by Marten deVries and his colleagues span 10 years of work in the field and are without doubt some of the most important ones.

But, one might ask, how can the study of subjective experience help us understand psychopathology – let alone prevent or alleviate it? After all, now that departments of psychiatry at so many Universities are adopting progressively more molecular approaches, hoping to find mental health in the results of psychopharmacological, neurophysiological, or endocrinological studies, what room is there left for research that tries to understand molar behavior in actual social settings?

The chapters in this volume share a common assumption. It is that whether a person suffers or feels happy does make a difference – in fact, that this difference is the 'bottom line' of mental health research. Psychology and psychopathology cannot be fully understood at the level of chemical processes. The entire organism with its subjective states, operating in its real social and cultural context, must be taken into account if we wish to know what is right or wrong with it.

Naturally such complex information is difficult to get. But the studies reported in this volume are beginning to show the way towards this necessary goal. They describe methods for collecting reliable and valid data on patterns of behavior, thought, and feeling from real-life situations. They suggest how such data can be analyzed and interpreted. They report applications of the method to the study of various impaired populations – depressives, bulimics, schizophrenics, substance abusers, individuals suffering from stress and from multiple personality disorders. In many cases, these investigations of experience reveal important new dimensions of these dysfunctions, and suggest new strategies for intervention.

The flexibility of the method is most apparent in its ability to provide both robust aggregate group profiles that help round out the etiology of mental disease, and at the same time to provide highly specific individual profiles, which makes it possible to tailor clinical intervention to the needs and possibilities of each patient.

These therapeutic applications of the method are probably its most useful feature. On the basis of the studies reported in this volume, there are three ways that the ESM contributes to psychotherapy. First, as a diagnostic tool, it helps uncover the nature of the disturbance, and pinpoints the specific conditions of daily life that exacerbate or relieve it. Secondly, as an adjunct to therapy, it suggests strategies of personalized rehabilitation. And finally, systematic data on daily experience can be used as an outcome measure, to assess therapeutic effectiveness.

It is likely that with time behavioral genetics and psychopharmacology will make it possible for some people to control the behavior of others. But positive mental health involves more than the ability to control or to be controlled. It implies the possibility to use one's capacities to the fullest, relative to the historical period and to the sociocultural milieu.

If psychiatrists and psychologists are to make a contribution to positive mental health, they will have to pay more attention to what people do as they go through their one and only life. They will have to take into account what people think about, how they feel, what they hope to achieve in the future. The present collection is a strong statement, a promising step in this important direction.

Mihaly Csikszentmihalyi,
Vail, Colorado, 1991

Preface

The first Experience Sampling (ESM) studies of psychopathological subjects were undertaken 10 years ago. Enthusiasm was strong and necessary in order to overcome the problems inherent with time sampling of ill individuals as well as technical difficulties. Doubt by the researchers themselves, scepticism by colleagues and critique from grant review committees marked the daily life of these early studies. The critical refrain rang: 'Schizophrenics will not comply, the beep is too startling for anxious people, and heroin addicts are too inaccessible', etc. Gradually, as the data proved worthwhile, confidence grew. ESM was found to work not only across a range of disorders from childhood to old age but also in differing cultural and social settings. As a result, the authors in this volume have created an essentially new data set, that supplements understanding of how psychopathology is actually experienced and lived.

A book about the effect of time and place on mental illness may seem strangely out of place today, a time when psychiatry has placed its hopes almost exclusively on classification and anatomical or physiological explanations of mental phenomena, with the thereby fitting pharmacological interventions. Accordingly, we feel some haste. There is so much to do, so many good arguments must be formulated and tested to shake psychiatry out of its carefully crafted lounge chair of diagnostic comfort, and come again into contact with its patients.

Historically, ESM data are not new. They fit within the integrated biopsychosocial tradition of medical activity where the interdisciplinary contributions of ethology, anthropology, longitudinal life-history studies and, of course, psychology have played an important role. In this sense the studies reported here reintroduce mental health approaches and theories previously formulated. The advantage that ESM introduces is that it is quantitative, replicable and therefore testable. For example, environmental factors that strongly influence the course of schizophrenia in the International Pilot Studies of Schizophrenia may now be better quantified. Vague concepts such as the quality of life, wellbeing and prevention, usually defined by cross-sectional questionnaire methods, may now be better clarified. In the clinic, Experience Sampling reintroduces daily life reality. A reality particularly important today with the changing dynamics of the doctor–patient relationship

xv

and the increasing need to negotiate and reach consensus on treatment. Experience Sampling studies accomplish this by paying more attention to what patients say, expanding the diagnostic profile of patients, for both pharmacological and psychotherapeutic treatments, with experiental variables and by investigating phenomena in the natural environment, generally hidden from the therapist and researcher.

My thanks to many for their help in completing this book. Lyman C. Wynne and Eugene Brody were instrumental, critical reviewers and advisors for the first publication of some of these studies in a special issue of the *Journal of Nervous and Mental Disease* in September of 1987. The diligent editorial efforts of Marylin Mattson were vital to the completion of that international project. This volume serves as an update on that special issue. It includes some of the studies presented in 1987 and a larger number describing continuing work in the field. Norman Sartorius, the Director of the Mental Health Division of the WHO, stimulated the casting of the ESM studies within a larger network of international collaboration that is evident in this volume.

The authors wish to thank the following journals and publishing companies for their permission to republish material that had already appeared in press: the *Journal of Nervous and Mental Disease*, published by Williams & Wilkins; the *American Journal of Psychiatry*, published by the American Psychiatric Association; *Schizophrenia Bulletin*, published by National Institute of Mental Health, the *Journal of Personality*, published by Duke University Press; the *International Journal of Addictions*, published by Marcel Dekker, New York, the *American Journal of Hypertension*, published by Elsevier, New York; *Bulletin de Méthodologie Sociologique*, published by Laboratoire Informatique des Sciences de l'Homme (LISH); Raven Press.

The current collection could not have materialized without the contributions of many scientists and administrative colleagues who have been troubled with the question of how psychopathology is experienced. I would like to mention a few colleagues: at the University of Chicago and Illinois, M. Csikszentmihalyi, R. Larson and associates; at the University of Milano, F. Massimini and A. Delle Fave; at the University of Nevada, R. Hurlburt; at the Center for Study of Man (LISH) in Paris, K. van Meter; at the University of Rotterdam, C. Kaplan; at the University of Liège, M. Ansseau and J. Sulon; and at the University of Liverpool, J. Copeland.

Support in developing ESM in Maastricht was given by the coordinators of the Vijverdal Phobia Ward: E. Griez and M. van den Hout; in Rotterdam by Nico Adriaans, Josien Harms, Gudrun Mühle, Vincent Hendricks, Jean-Paul Grund and Peter Blanken in the drug-craving study and in Heidelberg by M. Galli and A. Enders.

PREFACE

The following members of the Maastricht program investigating the experience of psychopathology in a range of disorders have contributed directly or indirectly to the studies presented here: P. Delespaul, C. Dijkman-Caes, M. Hilwig, N. Nicolson, H. Kraan, E. v.d. Poel, P. Portegijs, L. Meertens, A. Hofman, M. Dormaar, D. Riksen, A. Volovics, Mw. A. Hofman, R. v. Poll, T. Soute, F. van Goethem, Y. Theunissen, R. Rotteveel, M. v.d. Boorn, M. Roosen, M.J. Duchateau and P. Sieben as well as the clinical staff of the CMHC (RIAGG, Director, H. Pomerantz) and the Vijverdal Psychiatric Hospital Maastricht (Dr A.S. Vrijlandt).

Particular gratitude goes to my assistant Carolien Dijkman who worked consistently and critically on the often seemingly endless revisions of the various manuscripts. Without her effort this book would not have been produced. Numerous governmental and private granting agencies have helped with the efforts reported here. The Institute for Psycho-Social and Socio-Ecological Research (IPSER) has provided continual support to the Maastricht program. Warm and special thanks to Dr L. Saugstad of the L.F. Saugstad Foundation in Oslo for providing both personal and financial support at the beginning of the project.

Further, financial support to authors of the chapters in the volume has been granted by: the National Institute of Mental Health U.S.; the U.S. Public Health Service; the German Science Foundation (DFG); the Spencer Foundation; the National Fund for Mental Health in the Netherlands; the University of Limburg; the Netherlands Organization for Scientific Research (NWO); the Letten F. Saugstad Foundation; the Henry Murray Center for the Study of Lives.

Lastly, I would like to thank our research subjects and patients who contributed to the insight into their private lives making the indepth research into experience possible. I hope that in our transformation of their experience into professional communication and data, we have remained true to the reality of their lives. We dedicate any potential influence of this work to the intensity of their effort.

M.W. deVries
Maastricht, The Netherlands, 1991

PART I

Introduction: the experience of psychopathology

I

The experience of psychopathology in natural settings: introduction and illustration of variables[1]

MARTEN W. deVRIES

Over the last decade, psychiatry on an international scale has focused critical attention upon redefining the theoretical and methodological basis of mental health problems. Classification systems firmly anchored in research evidence have been established. Today, psychiatry and psychology have increasingly turned to the empirical findings offered by biological psychiatry. The extent to which situational, social and cultural processes co-determine the appearance of psychiatric symptoms, as well as the subsequent history, continues to merit our attention. There is a growing awareness that life style and stress significantly influence health and disease; diagnosis of itself is insufficient for treatment (Klerman, 1984), and clinical evaluations are incomplete without psychosocial assessments (Engel, 1977; Bronfenbrenner, 1979). Research that adequately describes the person in context, however, has proved difficult, due in part to the lack of readily available and replicable assessment methods with which to describe the places and social contexts of interest to psychiatry. We have thus paid insufficient attention to the variability and patterning of conscious experience over time and may have overlooked important features of psychopathology, just as the endocrinologist once overlooked meaningful within-day variations in the patterning of hormone release.

This volume, *The Experience of Psychopathology*, offers some solutions to the problem of sampling environmental or social situations in relation to psychiatrically disordered behavior. The papers that follow report fundamental research into the nature of psychopathology using new time sampling methods, such as the Experience Sampling Method (ESM), and time-budget or diary methods that have been previously established, but under-utilized.

The methods are quantitative and replicable. They produce a high level of situational and temporal detail, made possible by advances in ambulatory signaling devices, computer science and statistical methods that enable us to acquire, store and analyze vast amounts of useful information about individual subjects. Such advances have allowed time-allocation and time-sampling

[1] This work appeared in the *Journal of Nervous and Mental Disease*, 1987, **175**, 9, 509–14.

techniques to move to the forefront in behavioral science research (Pervin, 1985; Gross, 1984).

Goals and findings

Time budget and Experience Sampling (ESM) approaches in psychiatry have thus far investigated the general issues listed below followed in each case by a brief example of earlier findings:

(1) *Time allocation characteristics of disordered and non-disordered subjects*: variations in the use of time and the selection of places and activities discriminate many diagnostic disorders and developmental stages (Csikszentmihalyi & Larson, 1984; deVries et al., 1986; Delespaul & deVries, 1987).

(2) *Clinically significant within-day variations in experience and symptoms*: the occurrence of symptoms in many disorders is overestimated on global, retrospective reports when compared to actual measures in daily life (Margraf et al., 1987) and variability of mental states is the rule, for example rapid fluctuations in state perception of 'alternates' are found in multiple personality disorder (Loewenstein et al., 1987).

(3) *Patterning of experiences: contributions of context and setting to illness or wellbeing:* mood fluctuates across the menstrual cycle (Hamilton et al., 1984), binge eating as well as anxiety have a dynamic relationship with affect (Johnson & Larson, 1982; deVries et al., 1987), social contexts have a differential impact on symptoms and on the perception of well being of severely ill schizophrenics and chronically-adapted schizophrenics (deVries & Delespaul, 1989), and the recovery from alcoholism demonstrates temporal patterning (Filstead et al., 1985).

(4) *Refinement of current diagnostic categories with time-sampling data:* avoidance behavior appears to be a general characteristic of anxiety disorders and not a behavior that discriminates one class of anxiety from another (Dijkman & deVries, 1987), and experienced autonomic panic symptoms do not provide a basis for classifying panic disorder (Margraf et al., 1987).

(5) *The influence of positive psychological experiences on wellbeing and illness states*; a balance between perceived challenges and skills when a subject is engaged in an activity is related to a self-assessment of general well-being (Massimini et al., 1987).

The above studies illustrate that methods assessing variability and context relatedness of behavior and mental state over time can provide supplementary information that may be as important in psychiatry as the genealogical chart has been to kinship studies and family risk factor research.

4

Temporal approaches in mental health research

Historically, psychiatry has not been blind to the influence of temporal and situational factors on mental disorders. They were recognized in the late 19th century by Kahlbaum, Kraeplin and Bleuler in their detailed descriptions of schizophrenia and today are the focus of study in life history and life event research. The research reported in this issue extends this interest and borrows further from a variety of time sampling approaches that date at least to the ethnographies of Malinowski (1935). Further contributions have been made by the more systematic application of time observation techniques in natural-istic field studies (Chapple, 1970; Munroe & Munroe, 1971a, b; Barker, 1978), by ethological research strategies applied in psychiatry (Reynolds, 1965; McGuire & Polsky, 1979) and by behavior monitoring techniques (Nelson, 1977).

Another important influence has come from research on circadian rhythms. This research has evolved from the early work of Wada (1922), who described rhythmicity in gastric motility, to the discovery and detailed exploration of cyclical rapid eye movements in different stages of sleep (Kleitman, 1963; Kripke, 1983). These investigators have sought a comparable rhythmicity affecting cycles of arousal and behavioral activity in the waking person. This line of research, as yet unsuccessful, has however, highlighted the profound influence of 'zeitgebers' (daily environmental time setters) and setting influences on a variety of biological and behavioral measures (Minors & Waterhouse, 1981; Reynolds, 1965; Monk et al., 1990).

The investigations and research approaches discussed above, except perhaps for behavior monitoring, have had only a modest effect on clinical practice and psychiatric research. For example, in spite of over 30 years of life event research and the inherent validity of life event variables, there is an exhaustive list of non-significant findings from studies that measure the influence of psychosocial factors on psychiatric disorders. One problem may be that until now we have relied on a 'big bang' theory of life events. Although many researchers are interested in intervening conditions and coping style (Bebbington, 1980; Brown, 1974; Sameroff et al., 1982), life event studies have often assumed that the death of a spouse or parent, for example, would necessarily have a predictable impact on psychological outcome measures.

The excessive use of 'events' as salient psychological research variables may be flawed because it implies that development and life can be understood as a series of significant episodes ('events') which, cumulatively and retrospec-tively, yield a valid picture of a person's life. Since life events, while import-ant, are infrequent, they do not capture the routine patterns of life at all. The problem is akin to archaeological findings which are viewed as time signals around which an unseen reality is constructed in retrospect. Life event research similarly manufactures developmental outcomes from life event signals. The most important features of experience, however, may exist in the unmeasured 'space' between events, archaeologically in the historical void that lies between discoveries. At the level of the person, the 'space' between events may best be conceptualized as the ongoing process of daily life. Events are thus only signals and may be construed as 'real life' only when they are matched with data gathered in the day-to-day experiences of individuals.

Gathering data in daily life, while perhaps noble, may to some seem naive, or at least impractical, potentially messy and introducing indecipherable noise. From leaders in the field of biology and ethology, where rich and detailed observations of behavior are the rule, another perspective prevails; we will become hopelessly confused if we deny the complexity of our subject matter. Human beings have 'open behavioral programs' (Mayer, 1974), which are fluid, dynamic and heavily influenced by previous experience. This complexity renders it difficult to categorize behavior without examining the whole situation in depth (Hinde, 1976). Tinbergen (1963) suggests that we should explain the 'why' of any behavior at four levels:

(1) The proximate level: that of external immediate influences on the organism.
(2) The ontogenic level: that of the life history of the organism.
(3) The ultimate level: that of the individual's reproductive success.
(4) The evolutionary level: that of the success of traits in the contexts of the species.

The first two are of particular interest to us. Tinbergen, and later Bronfenbrenner (1979), exhort us not to mix up levels; for instance, the common error of jumping to causal or evolutionary explanations before phenomena are adequately described at the proximate level. The studies in this volume suggest that we must clear our heads, stop and catch our breath, from the rapid movement of behavioral science, at least when humans are the focus of research. Some research should pause at the proximate level, as the clinician generally does, the level of context and experiential meaning providing us with ecologically valid data. Ecological validity is not merely conducting investigations in real life settings, but taking the properties of the environment as experienced by the subject into account and making sure that they are included in our scientific analysis. The range of variables must therefore be increased, not reduced.

Ecological validity may seem an unwantedly large demand, but such factors do reduce. Particularly when social behavior is concerned; social behavior is largely intentional and meant to communicate. In the sense that it must be understood by others; behaviors must be agreed upon for effective social function. Social behavior is thus a priori limited not by the capacity of the actors but by the ability of the audience to understand the behavior. The basic operational taxonomy of behavior is thus already limited, a fact that makes our investigations possible. For example, Whiting (1977) highlighted 12 behavioral styles in children, Sapir (1921) has shown that 12 kin terms sufficed to describe an infinite number of degrees and types of relationships. Furthermore, the infinite variety of sounds that a human can make is usually reduced by the age of four or five to 20–40 phonims that are used in that culture, and most societies use only six words for colour in spite of our infinite rational capacity to perceive colours. Seeking a degree of ecological validity in our explanations of persons and behavior, while difficult, should be possible.

It is, however, not enough to report events and explain them. We must go beyond simply conveying the context of a behavior, but should understand the meaning of the act for the person. This is what Experience Sampling Method (ESM) adds to clinical practice. Since we cannot experimentally manipulate social variables in the natural environment in order to produce human behavior and describe it, we must opportunistically use our available natural experiment, i.e. the context of daily life. Moreover, human beings can, under the right conditions, make their own observations and report them in the flow of time and place. The authors in this volume take these accounts seriously and ask their subjects to self-report (Harré & Secord, 1972). Self-reports are not without problems, methodologically as well as in terms of the data collected. These data introduce personalized illness descriptions, necessarily accompanied by narratives, individual differences and intra-individual variability of state. Such variations bring forth questions about our classification system. This is a necessary perturbation. Psychopathology is not after all static. It is an hour-to-hour and day-to-day affair. The reality of this variability provides us with the opportunity to ask questions about the situations and temporal patterns of illness and wellbeing.

The correct unit of time in which to measure psychological phenomena presents a complex question. Criteria for the frequency and duration of measurement should eventually be derived from empirical descriptions of the specifics of illness course, expected fluctuations in the phenomena under study, or the timing of underlying physiologic processes. Many of the studies reported here, postulate that the 'workshop' of development, health and mental disorder is the day, and that the natural unit for psychological research is diurnal. For this reason, current time assessment studies have increased the frequency of measurement during a standard day period allowing the calculation and comparison of actual time use as well as the assessment of behavior and mental state in different periods of the day.

Methods: general

One of the key ancestors of the studies presented here has been the time-budget survey. Although the scientific study of time-budgets goes back many generations, there has recently been a surge of activity by scientists concerned with a variety of social problems (Michelson, 1978; Robinson, 1985). A good example is the International Time-Budget Study. This was a massive undertaking, which obtained 25,000 24-h diaries in 12 countries and represented more than 640,000 events. Information was gathered on what people did, when and for how long they did it, where it took place and in what social context. This provided information about the frequency duration and sequence of circumstances and events (Szalai et al., 1972; Robinson, 1977; Stone & Nicolson, 1987). The International Time-budget Study ascertained that time use variations differentiated populations on the basis of cultural-political, class, occupational and personal factors (Szalai et al., 1972). This approach might be extended to clinical groups where it could serve a number of psychiatric purposes by broadening the mental status exam, supplementing intake procedures, clarifying points for therapeutic interventions and improving our clinical reasoning and psychosocial formulations.

Two strategies important for mental health research are currently not available in traditional diary approaches, however: a means of obtaining valid subjective reactions to individual experiences as they occur and a means of avoiding distortions inherent in retrospective recall. These additional features are found in the ESM.

ESM provides a representative sample of moments in a person's daily life. It uses an electronic signaling device to alert subjects to fill out self-reports at preselected but randomized time-points, thus providing information about an individual's mental status or symptoms within the context and flow of experience. The method avoids the problem of global and retrospective recall that haunts the one-time sampling procedures of psychiatric research (Lamiell, 1981; Willems, 1969; Yarmey, 1979; Mischel, 1968; Fiske, 1971).

The self-report forms request a range of information about the subject's objective and subjective state 4–20 times per day for one week. Information such as where subjects are, what they are doing and who they are with, as well as information about their thoughts, moods, activities, specific somatic as well as psychological symptoms and specific aspects of their social and environmental context are reported. Responses are noted in small booklets of self-report forms.

One of the earliest lines of investigation at the University of Chicago by Czikszentmihalyi and associates obtained general data on daily activities and experiences which in turn served as a basis for a wide range of studies that followed (for a review see Csikszentmihalyi & Larson, 1987; Hormuth, 1986). Similar techniques were developed by deVries and associates for the study of psychopathology (deVries et al., 1983, 1984, 1985, 1986, 1987, 1988, 1989, 1990), by Hurlburt et al. (1978, 1979, 1980, 1984, 1987, 1989, 1990) for the study of thought content, by Klinger et al. (1980) who studied the stream of conscious thought in daily life, by Massimini et al. (1986, 1987, 1988) for the study of adolescent experience and by Hormuth (1986) for the study of urban uprooting. Many others are today joining this list. In these studies, self-report questionnaires, instructional procedures, coding and data analysis have been developed and validated with a population of more than 1000 subjects. Early research focused on critical aspects of ESM such as reactivity effects, subjects' self-selection biases, missing data, validity of self-reports, comparisons across subjects and the capacity to sample ill individuals.

These studies have relied on self-reports because of the methodological limitation of observing psychiatric phenomena outside the clinic or laboratory. This shortcoming of observational methods (Harré & Secord, 1972) and the apparent strength of verbal self-reports (Simon, 1969; Ericsson & Simon, 1985) support the shift to such methods with human subjects. Self-report measurements have many additional advantages such as transportability, sensitivity in a broad range of environments, and most importantly the ability to test the respondents themselves; on the other hand they also present a number of potential drawbacks such as the unmeasured effects of personal defenses, acquiescence and social desirability. The same problems apply equally, however, to many assessment methods (Rorer, 1965; Norman, 1967; Wiggins, 1964) and self-reports compare favorably with other research procedures that depend on reconstruction and recollection. Of course subject compliance is the key element which can make or break a study of this kind. Procedures that assure a research alliance with subjects have thus been of paramount importance in the investigations reported here.

Measuring mental state and concurrent context frequently, as these studies have done, creates a large data set. Such studies may seem excessive and potentially overwhelming at the data level. Making sense of data collected from different individuals, or from the same individual at different times, with self-reports that are often randomly sampled across contexts requires care with regard both to the coding of data into meaningful categories of experience and the choice of appropriate statistical procedures. Statistical analysis should ensure that the data are not falsely inflated and conversely, safeguard that the very information these methods are meant to uncover is not inadvertently obscured by an overly conservative approach (Margraf et al., 1987; Delespaul & deVries, 1987). Further, the application of time series statistics such as Markov chain models and event history analysis, are already producing promising results (Allison, 1984). New strategies such as ascending cross-classification analysis may also be used empirically to test 'daily life' variables against other diagnostic criteria (van Meter, 1986; Fink, 1986; deVries et al., 1987).

Critical aspects of Experience Sampling: analysis and variables illustrated: an orientation

The theoretical objective of the ESM procedure is to obtain a representative sample of a person's or population's daily experience. The method's usefulness as a research technique depends on how it measures up to this ideal. Since ESM research with psychopathological subjects is still young, it is too soon to make broad claims about its potential. Past research suggests that it can be used with diverse samples of people and that reports can be obtained on nearly all of their experience. These studies also suggest that the effects of the method on what it is measuring are minimal and that the self-reports have construct validity. Nonetheless, more exacting information could be obtained on each of these issues and new studies will be designed to obtain further methodological data. The following questions posed by Larson & Csikszentmihalyi (1983) are answered by the authors in this volume but should continue to be raised:

(1) What types of people are willing to participate in this kind of research? Are there self-selection biases which exclude significant groups of individuals (e.g. antisocial personalities, people under stress, psychotics)?
(2) What parts of people's experience are missed by the sampling procedure? Do participants under-report or hide significant parts of their lives (e.g. sex, illicit drug use)?
(3) What influences does the procedure have on the phenomena being measured? Are there substantial reactive effects on people's experience? Consciousness?
(4) How consistent are ESM findings with those obtainable from observational techniques, portable physiological monitors and cross-sectional assessments?
(5) How valid are self-reports? Do they vary across types of items, situations, and people?
(6) How comparable are data across subjects differing in social class, culture, or diagnostic disorder? Is the meaning of items the same across subjects?

All of these are empirical questions upon which data have been and will continue to be brought to bear particularly as the sample size increases allowing for the applications of appropriate statistical checks in a larger archive of ESM data being developed in Maastricht, The Netherlands.

Research design and analytic hierarchy

In order to facilitate interpretation of the complex data set, a broader frame of reference than a single hypothesis guiding a specific study is necessary. ESM data may be conceptualized hierarchically within a simple design in which diagnosis, group characteristics or severity factors act as independent variables and the ESM data as dependent variables. The ESM variables are further grouped in subsets and ranked by the degree of objectivity. The 'observable' places, persons and activities are on top (see Fig. 1.1). Next to each subset, a reference or comparative data set is offered. These reference data are derived from existing research disciplines concerned with similar information as the ESM subset. For example, the time allocation data gathered with ESM has a reference data set in the international time-budget study. Viewing the data in this way allows one to organize findings step by step without succumbing to the intellectual problem of mixing up levels and types of data. The hierarchy provides a heuristic order descending from the most objective level of the data to a more subjective level or to data that require more speculative, new research or clinical approaches.

Data analysis

The ESM form is organized at three levels of data:

(1) At the **subject level:** independent variables are one-time measures gathered at the start of the study, and include demographic variables, severity ratings, diagnosis and other assessments for each disorder.
(2) At the **day level:** measures repeated once each day, such as the duration and quality of sleep, daily routine information as well as global assessments of the previous day.
(3) At the **beep level:** the 40–60 coded items from the ESM report form, filled in 4–10 times a day.

The computation of results is based on the mean (level), standard deviation (variability) and lag, auto- and cross-correlations (stability, predictability) for data measured on Likert-type scales, and on mode, range, frequency distributions and cross tabulations for ordinal and nominal scaled and coded items. Different analysis can be performed to investigate between and within group differences (see Larson & Delespaul, this volume for details).

ESM results illustrated

The best way to gain insight into ESM is by illustrating how the new variables supplement traditional psychiatric assessments. The data demonstrated here are drawn from schizophrenia, anxiety, drug abusing and pain patients,

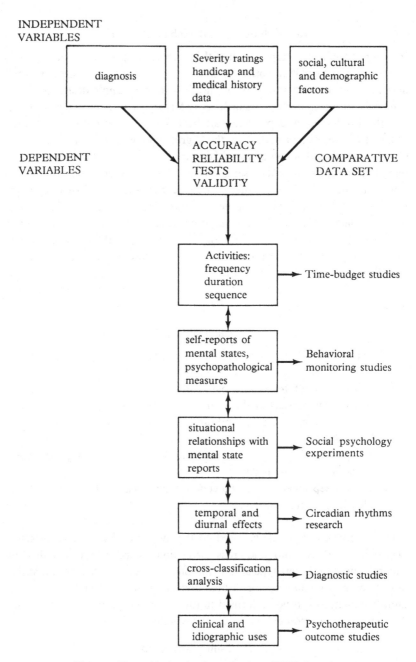

INDEPENDENT
VARIABLES

DEPENDENT
VARIABLES

COMPARATIVE
DATA SET

diagnosis

Severity ratings
handicap and
medical history
data

social, cultural
and demographic
factors

ACCURACY
RELIABILITY
TESTS
VALIDITY

Activities:
frequency
duration
sequence → Time-budget studies

self-reports of
mental states,
psychopathological
measures → Behavioral
monitoring studies

situational
relationships with
mental state
reports → Social psychology
experiments

temporal and
diurnal effects → Circadian rhythms
research

cross-classification
analysis → Diagnostic studies

clinical and
idiographic uses → Psychotherapeutic
outcome studies

Fig. 1.1. Hierarchical order for evaluation of ESM data.

Example depressive patient

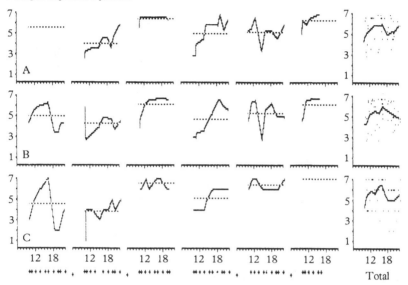

Fig. 1.2. Graphs showing variability of cognitive assessment (A), mood assessment (B), and chief complaint (C) over a 6-d period in a depressive patient.

individuals under stress and normals. We begin by simply inspecting plotted data and then follow the hierarchical model sketched above going from time allocation to mental state reports, and followed by more dynamic and time-based analyses.

Inspection of the plotted data

Since ESM data are gathered sequentially over time, the quantified mental state and experiential variables may be plotted and their variability visualized within the diverse social frames and physical context in which they occur.

(a) In Fig. 1.2 the variability of thoughts, mood and chief complaint per day over a six-day period is shown. The seventh block on the right is a composite day comprised of mean scores of all beeps plotted diurnally. A conclusion drawn from this plot is that mental state variability is the rule, even in the severe and often assumed static mental disorders.

(b) Figure 1.3 depicts contextual relationships and diurnal patterns in psychotic thoughts over three successive days. This graph depicts a constant pattern of afternoon psychoses during which the person was alone at home (deVries & Delespaul, 1987). The hypothesis examined in these early descriptive studies is that psychopathology is significantly,

13

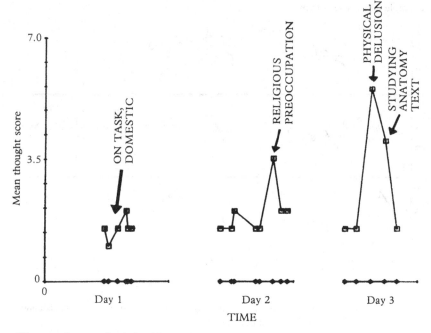

Fig. 1.3. Contextual relationships and diurnal patterns in psychotic thoughts over three successive days.

situation and time bound. Diurnal patterns such as this, while rare in psychosis, are of extraordinary clinical importance when discovered.

Furthermore, we may inspect plots of a number of mental state variables simultaneously in relation to one another, such as mood and anxiety, or physiological data linked with mental state reports. The visualization of these associations over the day is clinically and theoretically useful by providing a direct view of comorbidity; symptom co-variation and the relationship between biological and psychological measures (see Nicolson and Van Egeren et al., this volume).

Time-allocation data

Time-budgets are a concrete representation of the adaptive strategies employed by a subject. They depict the trade-offs and choices made about the places, persons, and activities by subjects. These choices are strongly influenced by culture and mental state, and are an extremely sensitive indicator of behavioral change related to illness particularly when demographic factors such as sex and employment are controlled. Hypothesis: ecological variables such as 'who one is with', 'what one does' and 'where one is' should differentiate the time-budgets of individuals with different mental disorders.

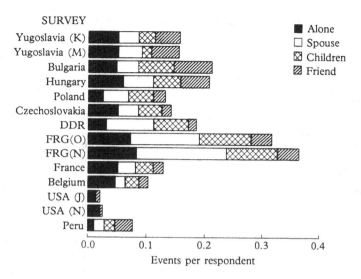

Fig. 1.4. Time budgets showing frequency of walking and its social context in 12 countries. (From Stone & Nicolson, 1987, *Journal of Nervous and Mental Disease*, **175**, 9, 537–45.)

(a) Time-budgets of activities clearly differentiate larger populations from one another as shown in Fig. 1.4. This example shows the frequency of an activity: walking and its social context from the 12 country International Time-Budget Study (Stone & Nicolson, 1987). The report of the activity walking and its social configuration, while a low frequency activity, strongly differentiates nations.

(b) When comparing individuals with diverse mental disorders we observe a similar phenomenon. Groups of 20 chronic schizophrenics, anxiety, pain patients and normals when compared show significant differences in global as well as specific ecological categories. The hypothesis that time-budgets can differentiate psychopathologically defined groups seems to hold (deVries et al., 1988).

(c) The example in Fig. 1.4 demonstrates the sensitivity of time-budgets as a discriminating measure. Examining the difference between two groups of anxiety patients differing only in the degree of depression measured by a standard deviation on the Zung scale, a level barely clinically detectable, time-budget variables still significantly differentiate the two groups (deVries et al., 1987). The discriminating power of the time-budget is present even with only a modest difference in psychopathology. The behavioral consequences of mental state as a useful measure of psychopathology may thus be underestimated.

(d) Alterations in time allocation over a year is also a sensitive indicator of change within an individual. It may thus be used as a measure of clinical

Table 1.1. *Frequency contextual variables per group*

%	Chronic patients	Anxiety patients	Pain patients	Normal group
(a) where am I?				
at home	78.3	75.1	64.5	47.2
with family/friends	4.1	4.9	2.4	6.1
at work	5.3	5.5	20.2	28.9
health care setting	4.6	1.5	0.2	0.2
public places	4.3	5.3	3.8	8.8
transport	2.3	5.3	8.5	8.1
other	1.1	2.3	0.4	0.8
(b) what am I doing?				
nothing	8.3	2.4	2.0	3.5
self care	15.0	17.2	12.3	12.6
care for others	20.1	14.0	12.3	12.6
working	18.5	11.6	16.3	24.6
leisure	29.4	44.1	44.0	37.7
transport	3.5	3.4	5.2	4.9
other	5.1	7.3	7.9	7.9
(c) who am I with?				
alone	35.4	30.1	23.0	24.6
with family	39.8	51.9	55.8	43.2
with friends	13.0	10.2	0.6	2.6
with colleagues	4.2	6.5	19.2	26.7
with strangers	7.6	1.3	1.4	2.9

Table 1.2. *Difference in frequency distribution of nominal variables between groups; high anxiety/medium depression vs. high anxiety/high depression*

	χ^2 of frequency distributions	Significance
Thought/activity congruence	$\chi^2(2) = 4.111$	n.s.
Thought content	$\chi^2(16) = 57.787$	$P < 0.001$
Psychopathology	$\chi^2(5) = 31.475$	$P < 0.001$
Where	$\chi^2(6) = 13.063$	$P < 0.05$
What	$\chi^2(6) = 31.840$	$P < 0.001$
Who	$\chi^2(6) = 54.425$	$P < 0.001$

n.s. = not significant.

change or improvement. In Fig. 1.5, the activity of a chronic mental patient was sampled three times over the course of a year. In these 'pie' plots of relative frequencies, we see changes in the patient's social field over time that were related to changes in psychopathology and treatment interventions (Van de Poel & Delespaul, Delle Fave and Massimini, this volume).

(e) It should be possible to manufacture time allocation 'maps' for specific disorders, individuals or families. 'Time space maps' plot changes in physical and social context for a day or week period. The example in Fig. 1.6 depicts the interaction pattern for a Swedish family in one typical day (Carlstein, 1978). Data such as these may serve as an ethogram or socio-gram for research and clinical purposes that may illuminate hidden aspects of social life and individual adaptation. For example in this case, the amount of time the family actually spends interacting together is limited. Sleeping and eating together is their striking common feature.

Time-budget data thus provide a sensitive indicator of behavioral change, social activities and the influence of psychopathology. Since behavioral adjustments often precede a person's awareness of psychological change, time-budget can become an important aid in the early detection of mental disorders. The evaluation of changes in time use over time offers a potentially powerful therapeutic and research tool. The theoretical underpinnings of many psychopathological hypotheses may be ecologically examined, such as the 'actual' nature of schizophrenic isolation and the 'actual' avoidance behavior demonstrated by agoraphobics.

Mental state comparisons

The ESM self-report form used in most psychiatric studies reported here is derived from time-budget diaries and is based on the Mental Status Examination. The mental state items are organized in clusters that evaluate cognition, mood, motivation and psychopathology. The form further includes a diagnostic module derived from validated cross-sectional tests. Questions are often formulated in collaboration with the subject groups under study. The form thus provides a means of carrying out repeated diagnosis or 'deviance counts' of a given disorder. The presence or degree of pain, panic, depression or psychosis at a given moment may be quantitatively assessed in a Likert-scale format. The diagnostic modules are then factor analyzed and scaled, they generally explain significant amounts of the variance and demonstrate construct validity with cross-sectional diagnostic assessments (see Kraan et al., this volume). In Table 1.3 the anxiety-panic factor and its factor loadings are shown (Dijkman & deVries, 1987).

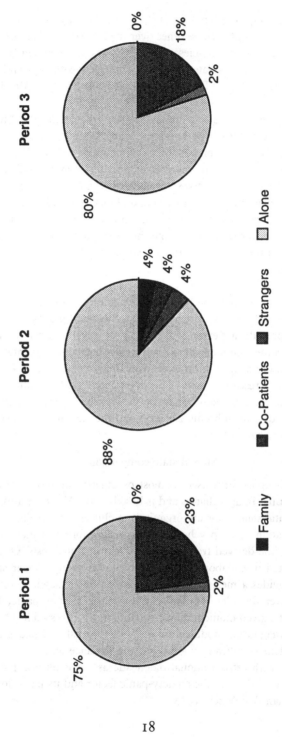

Fig. 1.5. Changes in the social field of a chronic mental patient sampled three times in a year.

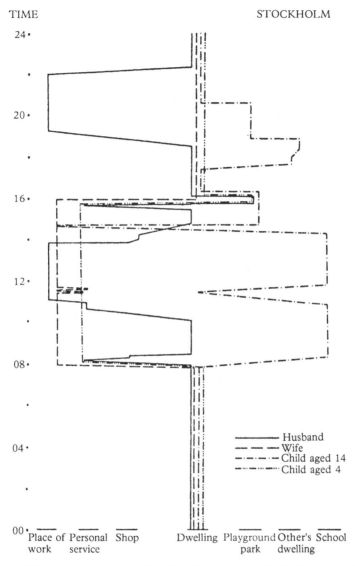

Fig. 1.6. The interaction pattern within a Swedish four-person family during one day.

In preliminary samples, ESM reports of mental state have been able to differentiate diagnostic groups. This is a rather rigid criterion since the expected individual variability of self-reports between subjects is great, one would not necessarily expect this. Any differentiation found, then adds to the construct validity of the method. Indeed, depressives have lower mood, anxious individuals more anxiety and so on. Table 1.4 below shows that mental state

Table 1.3. *Factor loadings of anxiety variables:*
an anxiety factor

anxious mood	0.72
feeling short of breath, suffocating	0.66
having palpitations, pain on the chest	0.66
feeling weak, dizzy or unstable	0.66
feeling unreal	0.66
fear of dying, going mad or losing control	0.66

Eigen value = 6.50
% of VAR = 33%

Table 1.4. *Mean scores and standard deviations for the different modules per group*

Module range 1–7	Chronic patients		Anxiety patients		Pain patients		Normals		One-way ANOVA
	$\bar{x}$	SD	$\bar{x}$	SD	$\bar{x}$	SD	$\bar{x}$	SD	$F_{(3)}$
thoughts (7 = positive)	4.51	1.45	4.51	1.67	4.94	1.38	5.23	1.16	28.80 ***
mood (7 = positive)	4.78	1.36	5.01	1.11	5.86	0.82	6.27	0.67	223.91 ***
mental complaint (7 = strongly present)	3.81	2.16	2.75	1.78	3.24	1.67	1.54	0.84	152.96 ***
somatic complaint (7 = strongly present)	3.78	2.05	2.40	1.67	3.39	1.13	1.61	1.03	204.25 ***
activities (7 = positive)	4.19	1.10	4.76	1.21	4.96	1.11	5.37	0.89	89.05 ***

*** $P < 0.001$.

categories significantly differentiate the diagnostic groups investigated
(deVries et al., 1988).

Going one step further and looking at the results of open-ended cognitive
questions coded into categories of thought, we again find the same significant
overall differences are found (Table 1.5).

A number of other aspects of the mental state report are also of interest. For
example:

(a) When comparing reported panic on cross-sectional or retrospective
reports, to a prospective six-day time sampling period, individuals tend

Table 1.5. *Differences between research groups relating to thoughts*

	Chronic patients	Anxiety patients	Pain patients	Normal control group
(a) % 'online' (congruency between thoughts and activities)				
on-line	37.4	31.1	43.7	42.7
off-line	62.6	68.9	56.3	57.3
(b) % 'goofs' (quality of thoughts)				
specific thoughts	69.7	83.0	79.9	93.9
daydreaming	11.5	4.8	11.7	6.1
worrying (with fear)	14.2	8.9	3.5	0.0
preoccupation	2.7	3.4	4.9	0.0
thought disorder	2.0	0.0	0.0	0.0
(c) % thought content				
nothing	5.4	3.6	8.3	9.5
leisure/travelling	16.2	19.2	20.4	19.3
maintenance/money	11.3	4.0	10.1	10.3
family	13.2	8.5	3.0	2.2
environment	2.6	2.9	4.9	6.3
work	7.1	10.7	13.4	18.3
past	4.7	0.9	1.0	1.4
planning	3.5	6.7	1.4	6.9
physical	9.9	24.3	18.2	5.5
ES-method	4.7	3.3	1.6	2.2
abstract	12.9	2.7	1.0	1.4
other	8.5	13.4	16.6	16.8

to over-report in retrospect the number of panic attacks that they experience (Margraf et al., 1987). The subjects in Fig. 1.7 below had reported six to ten episodes of panic per week. On actual measurement the mean was slightly over two. ESM thus corrects retrospectively reported illness occurrence.

(b) Intra-mental state relationships may also examine. For example, in Table 1.6, when exploring the congruency of mood and thought in schizophrenic subjects, the range of correlations between mood and thought varies significantly more for the schizophrenics than for the non-schizophrenics. The negative correlation as well as the range further supports the hypotheses that schizophrenics indeed are more often mood and thought incongruent than normals (deVries et al., 1984).

Table 1.6. *Integration of thought and mood*

Thought/mood correlations range by group (Pearson)	
	R
Non-schizophrenic	0.65–0.99
Schizophrenic	−0.49–0.76 (0.37)

The range is greater across the schizophrenic population; there was less integration of mood and thought by schizophrenics.

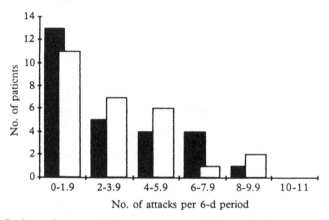

Fig. 1.7. Panic attacks reported by patients over a 7-d time period. ■, spontaneous; □, situational. (From Margraf et al., 1987, *Journal of Nervous and Mental Disease*, **175**, 9, 558–65.)

(c) Since pathological moments can be validly isolated, the recovery from various mental states or pathological conditions, such as panic, high anxiety or depression may be calculated. For example, in Fig. 1.8, the recovery from anxiety and depressive episodes in normals differ. Normals recover almost instantaneously from anxiety and somewhat more slowly from depression.

In Fig. 1.9 a group of anxious depressive patients who vary on the degree of depression, but not anxiety is examined. The group with more depression recovers more slowly from a high anxiety episode than the less depressed group (deVries et al., this volume).

The presence of a comorbid condition such as depression or the severity of the illness itself, may change the recovery slope. Hypothetically, we assume that such slopes (or area under the curve), calculable

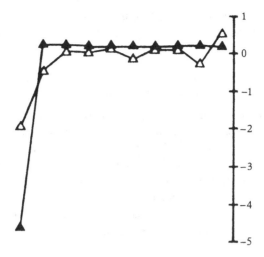

Fig. 1.8. Recovery from anxious (▲) and depressive (△) episodes in normal subjects.

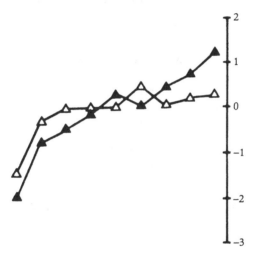

Fig. 1.9. Recovery from an anxious episode in medium (△) and highly depressed (▲) anxiety subjects.

from time data, may be a good indicator of illness severity. The change in slope is a potentially useful indicator of treatment effectiveness (deVries et al., 1987).

In short, mental state comparisons using ESM variables, validly differentiate disorders. They are thus useful for evaluating the recovery from 'pathological' moments, the interrelationships between aspects of mental state and in determining the actual frequency of occurrence of psychopathology, as a check on traditionally gathered cross-sectional psychiatric assessments.

The mental status in situations

Perhaps the most unique contribution that the ESM makes to psychiatric research is the possibility of locating pathological phenomena or mental states in naturally occurring contexts. We hypothesize that much of psychopathology could be behaviorally and contextually explained if the situations were adequately examined. At the idiographic or person level, this may be demonstrated by means of the inspection of plotted variables. But does this hold true for diagnostic categories as well? Do certain situations present a higher probability of risk for the experience of psychopathology. In Table 1.7, we com-

Table 1.7. *Group differences in reactivity to the social environment (absolute differences between alone/not alone)*

	Chronics			Controls			Test
	Mean	SD	n	Mean	SD	n	t(. . .)
Thoughts	0.456	0.134	9	0.301	0.237	11	t(18) = 1.74 P <0.05
Mood	0.530	0.442	9	0.085	0.069	11	t(18) = 3.31 P <0.005
Psychopathology	0.366	0.337	9	0.153	0.265	9	t(16) = 1.49 n.s.
Activity-motivation	0.535	0.386	9	0.231	0.162	11	t(18) = 2.30 P <0.025
Psychological complaint	0.458	0.464	9	0.240	0.240	11	t(18) = 1.19 n.s.
Somatic complaint	0.516	0.433	10	0.291	0.291	8	t(16) = 1.35 n.s.
ITEMS							
Hunger	0.689	0.661	8	0.368	0.321	11	t(17) = 1.41 n.s.
Tired	0.746	0.782	10	0.474	0.320	11	t(19) = 1.06 n.s.
Not feeling well	0.345	0.461	9	0.415	0.535	8	t(15) = −0.29 n.s.

n.s. = not significant.

24

pared normal people and chronic schizophrenics in solitary and social situations (Delespaul & deVries, 1987).

The mood, thought and motivation report of schizophrenics seems to be significantly influenced by social circumstances. This Table demonstrates that the strong effect found at the person level is also evident, although somewhat attenuated, at the group level. Next a group of schizophrenic subjects are compared with normals, regarding the effect of increasing the numbers of individuals in the environment as measured by mood and thought responses. In Fig. 1.10 it can be seen that when the number of individuals in the environment increases, negative feelings arise in schizophrenics, particularly when the number exceeds two or more people; in normals this is not the case (deVries & Delespaul, 1989).

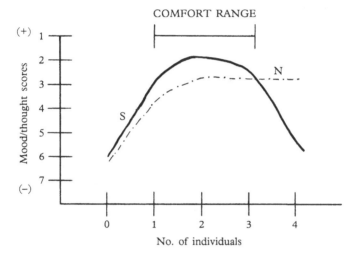

Fig. 1.10. The relationship between mood/thought scores and the number of people in a group of (S) schizophrenics and (N) normal subjects. Being alone or with too many people appears to present a problematic situation for schizophrenics; a comfort range of one to three people is suggestive of an optimal living context.

This is of practical interest because we generally treat these individuals in group settings of four or more. ESM data suggest that such typical treatment situations are an unexpected stressful social setting for the patient group.

Conclusion

The inspection of raw data plots, time-budgets, mental state and situational self-reports illustrated in this Introduction demonstrate ESM's power as a descriptive, clinical and hypothesis testing instrument. The data illustrated in this introduction are but a tiny sampling meant to orient the reader. In the studies that follow the utility of ESM research in psychiatry is discussed in greater detail, by the authors who reason from data gathered across a range of mental disorders. Perhaps a more important use of ESM is in the treatment of individuals. Here, ESM can provide the clinician with a detailed report of the patient's daily life and experience that goes beyond the interconnections that the patient is ordinarily able to provide. ESM then functions as the Holter Monitor does in medicine to assess cardiac functioning outside of the laboratory. Clinical applications have thus far provided promising results (Part IV). The potential range and extent of these therapeutic applications await further systematic research. The studies reported in this volume have responded to the challenge that psychiatric research should provide a more precise description of health and disease as it occurs in its natural setting. The contributors hope that their data are of use to the clinician and behavioral scientist alike.

2

Microbehavioral approaches to monitoring human experience[1]

JOHN P. ROBINSON

Social science typically studies individual behavior in isolation from the natural temporal context in which it occurs. Survey questions ask people to compress their actual experiences by indicating whether they 'often' or 'usually' do something or feel a certain way, rather than examining these experiences as they occur in daily life. Studies of the actual use of time provide an opportunity to study human experience in 'real time', i.e., as individuals are actually involved in daily behavior. This is especially important in identifying and understanding the life experiences of people who undergo periods of stress or mental dysfunction. How do their life experiences in such periods differ from those under more 'normal' conditions and from those of people who do not experience such severe stress or dysfunction?

The most common technique for the study of time use patterns is the 'time diary', a prime example of the 'microbehavioral' approach to survey research. Recognizing the limited ability of respondents to report complex behavior in a survey context requires questions to be limited to elementary experiences. A microbehavioral approach asks about the details of a recent unhappy episode at work or in marriage, rather than posing a global question on job or marital dissatisfaction; it asks for accounts of activities that happened yesterday, not in general or typically, or it combines direct questions about a respondent's specific information on a topic with questions about his or her specific mass media usage over a short time period, rather than expecting a meaningful response to a simple question about 'main sources' of information. It thus provides a more basic and flexible data base from which to draw conclusions about human experience.

The time diary

The time diary is an open-ended, activity-by-activity technique for collecting self-reports of an individual's daily behavior. Such activity accounts are kept for a short period such as a day or week, usually over the 24 h of a single day.

[1] This work appeared in the *Journal of Nervous and Mental Disease*, 1987, **175**, 9, 514–18.

TIME	WHAT DID YOU DO?	TIME BEGAN	TIME ENDED	WHERE?	LIST OTHER PEOPLE WITH YOU	WAS THIS AN ACTIVITY THAT YOU:		ENJOY-MENT SCALE:	DOING ANYTHING ELSE?	CHECK USING		
						HAD TO DO	PLANNED AHEAD	0 = DISLIKE TO 10 = LIKE		P H O N E	T V	R A D I O
MIDNIGHT		12:00										
1 a.m.												
2 a.m.												
3 a.m.												
4 a.m.												
5 a.m.												
6 a.m.												
7 a.m.												
8 a.m.												

Table heading: **WHAT YOU DID FROM MIDNIGHT UNTIL 9 IN THE MORNING**

Fig. 2.1. Sample time-diary page (from 1985 study of Americans' use of time).

In that way, they capitalize on the most attractive measurement properties of the time variable: (a) All daily activity is potentially recorded (including that which occurs in early morning hours when most 'normal' people may be asleep). (b) Each respondent records activities over all 1440 minutes of the day (thus allowing 'trade-offs' between certain activities to be examined). (c) Respondents are allowed to use a time frame and accounting variable that is maximally understandable to them and accessible to memory. The open-ended nature of the time diary makes possible the reporting of types of activity not anticipated by the researcher (e.g., aerobic exercise, illness) and provides a naturalistic framework for capturing the flavor of daily life.

A typical diary page leaves room for respondents to report each activity engaged in, where they were so engaged, with whom, and what other activities they were involved in at the same time. A sample diary page from a recent national time use study (Robinson, 1985) is shown in Fig. 2.1.

Data from open-ended diaries can be coded and organized in a variety of ways. The most widely used activity coding scheme (developed for the 1965 Multinational Time Budget Study, described in Szalai et al., 1972) divides activities into non-free-time and free-time categories. Non-free-time activities are further subdivided into paid work, family care, and personal care; free-time activities are subdivided under headings of adult education, organizational activity, social life, recreation, and communication. Under these broad headings, more fine-grained distinctions are captured in nearly 250 categories of activity. Activities can also be easily recoded or recombined depending on the analyst's assumptions or purposes.

Several methodological studies support the reliability and validity of this approach, both in the United States and in other countries (Juster, 1985; Robinson, 1977, 1985; Szalai et al., 1972). Reliability studies (using the Fig. 2.1 diary approach) have reported correlations of over 0.90 at the aggregate level between time estimates using different approaches: by telephone vs. personal vs. mail interviewing mode, by same-day vs. day-after recall methods, or by studying one community vs. another community in the same society.

Validity studies have involved 'outside' observational techniques, such as participant observation (Chapin, 1974), reports of other household members (Juster, 1985), and placing television cameras in the home (Bechtel et al., 1972). Diary reports have been validated by comparing them to 'instant activity' reports prompted by electronic beepers alerting respondents to report their activities at specific random moments during the day (Robinson, 1985). Correlations of time expenditures between observational measures and time-diary estimates have usually been over 0.80 and often over 0.90.

Such diary data, when aggregated, can provide generalizable national estimates of the full range of alternative daily activities in a society, including: 'contracted' time (e.g., work or travel to work), 'committed' time (e.g., family care), personal care (e.g., sleeping, eating, hygiene), and all other activities that occur in free time. Comparable national time diary data have been collected in more than 25 countries over the last two decades, including virtually all Eastern and Western European countries.

Time-diary data have been especially useful in identifying societal trends in time expenditures. Increased time spent on one activity means time on some other activity must decrease. Data on time use from two American time diary studies done in 1965 and 1975 (Robinson, 1976), for example, indicate certain structural changes in the nature of daily life in America over that decade: declines in paid work time (mainly for men) and in family care activities (mainly for women) left more time available, not only for free-time activities (particularly television and rest) but for personal care (e.g., sleep and grooming). Along with the increase in personal discretionary time, activities such as television watching, perhaps less conducive to mental activity, became more common and less deviant for all individuals in society.

The time diary method provides a systematic, normative framework for inter-individual comparison. For the exploration of mental health issues, the more interesting and useful comparisons may concern how activities are **experienced** by individuals. For example, people with high and low life satisfaction differed little in reports of the activities that they enjoyed (Robinson, 1977). Television viewing was mentioned as a favorite activity just as often by those with high life satisfaction as those with less satisfaction; however, low satisfaction respondents included a high proportion who could not mention **any** enjoyable activities. Additional clinically relevant information can be gained by combining data on how individuals subjectively experience a specific activity with how much time they spend on it.

The subjective experience of daily activities

As can be seen in the Enjoyment column of Fig. 2.1, our 1985 project has begun to collect information on the psychological meaning of each reported activity, especially on the fluctuations in affective or emotional states in terms of respondents' level of enjoyment in various activities. In the first large national study of these affective aspects (Robinson, 1977), respondents reported greatest satisfaction from child-related and social activities and least from housework and organized activities. These results have been generally replicated in smaller samples and community studies, with the additional finding that sleeping, eating, and other personal care activities, along with reading books and magazines, were ranked above average in satisfaction level. These activity-affect rankings also held true for scales of activity enjoyment as well as of activity satisfaction. They indicate a certain commonality across extrinsic and intrinsic sources of affective response, i.e., whether people feel positively about the (external) **results** of the activity or about simply participating in the activity itself.

More recently, Juster (1985) reported 1975 data from a nationally representative sample of more than 1500 respondents, who were asked to rate a list of daily activities on an enjoyment scale running from 0 (dislike a great deal) through 10 (enjoy a great deal). Because respondents were instructed to rate these activities in terms of enjoyment **during** the activity, and not in terms of the **result** of the activity or how they felt afterwards, these ratings should primarily reflect the intrinsic aspects of activities. The average ratings for 20 activities on the scale from 0 to 10 are shown graphically in Fig. 2.2.

Of what relevance are these data for the clinical practitioner? First, they can serve as national norms to identify individuals with abnormally high or low ratings. Second, they can be matched with an individual's time-use patterns. This permits identification of activities to which too much or too little time is devoted relative to the mood elevation or depression that they bring (Dimsdale, 1984).

30

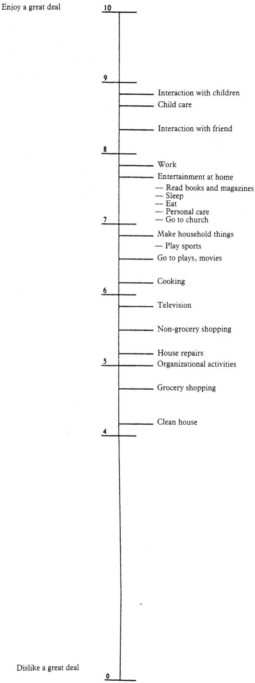

Fig. 2.2. Average enjoyment level, respondent for specific activities 1975–81. U.S. National Data (from Juster, 1985).

The data in Fig. 2.2 suffer from being 'timeless' in the sense of their detachment from actual experience. It is important, therefore, to compare these general affect ratings with what people report in affect rating columns in their diaries (as in Fig. 2.1). In a small-scale study in which both methods were used, Robinson (1977) found a tendency for diary affect ratings to be lower than the general activity ratings (as in Fig. 2.2) using the same scale. This was particularly true for women and for the activities of work, child care, and travel – which, it would appear, can be occasions of considerable unpleasantness, despite their overall aura of positivity in Fig. 2.2. At the other end of the scale, television viewing was rated more positively as experienced in the diary than in general. Data on variations in affect ratings revealed about twice as much variance in diary reports as in general reports, indicating that people experience more high points and low points across the day than one would surmise from the data in Fig. 2.2

Other microbehavioral methods

The time diary provides an indicator of the normal context of daily life. It can be used by clinical observers to identify variations in daily experience; like any single-focus instrument, it may miss or gloss over certain significant aspects of daily experience. Its data should be supplemented or validated with data at an even more microbehavioral level, such as in the electronic paging study noted above.

The Experience Sampling Method (ESM) featured in this volume, collects data on mood and mental states in daily life, using a beeper signaling technique. In contrast to the three subjective variables noted in Fig. 2.1, the ESM records data on a range of mental states (affect, thoughts, motivation and intensity) at particular moments during the day. An ESM study of television viewing indicated that it was not markedly lower than other activities in terms of associated affect ratings (Kubey & Csikszentmihalyi, 1990). In other words, the ESM results support the diary affect ratings for TV viewing obtained by Robinson (1977), as noted above, rather than the below-average ratings for TV viewing as compared with other activities shown in Fig. 2.2. This suggests that TV viewing is experienced as a more positive activity at the time it occurs than viewers generally rate it. The same beeper study also corroborated diary affect ratings for work that are lower than suggested in Fig. 2.2 (i.e., work is associated with about average affect ratings in Kubey & Csikszentmihalyi's study) and relatively high ratings for eating meals, as experienced on a daily basis.

There is an encouraging correspondence in the general affect ratings for certain activities using both diary and beeper methodologies. More exact comparative work of this sort is required. We may find under closer scrutiny that the 'average' rating for a daily entry may differ in important respects from ratings obtained at the particular moment in time; that is, one may rate a particular hour's TV viewing (or work or social interaction) as generally enjoyable, even though one found the program (activity) unpleasant or boring at particular moments during that hour. Such findings can provide insight into individual patients who are undergoing mental stress, as well as to practitioners hoping to help them.

Experience Sampling using ambulatory signaling devices represents another important advance in the clinical understanding of the context of an individual's daily behavior. To learn more about the short-term dynamics of mood swings, however, we need to time-sample more extensively than the 10 to 25 times per day done to date. More elaborate 'objective' data on physical health and psychological characteristics of people who are being time-sampled are also needed. The development of less-invasive monitoring techniques has begun to allow study of physiological correlates of behavior in real-life situations (e.g. Van Egeren & Madarasmi, 1988; Nicolson, this volume). In short, what are needed are data from a broader range of mental and somatic states that can be tied directly to the range and content of activities in which normal and abnormal populations engage. This requires a commitment to synthesize our diverse research interests, needs and conceptual frameworks into a workable whole. The other articles in this volume demonstrate that we are moving in that direction.

3

Experience Sampling and personality psychology: concepts and applications[1]

STEFAN E. HORMUTH

Over the past decade and a half, a number of psychologists and behavioral scientists have felt the need for a method that allows the study of the ongoing everyday behavior and the experiences of people in their normal life and environments. For this purpose, investigators have sampled thoughts and experiences at random points in time over several days in a person's life. Typically, subjects in these investigations carry electronic beeping devices and report or rate their experiences by filling out questionnaires at the time of a signal. This methodological need arose from different sources, for instance, the call for ecological validity of behaviors studied, the attempt to understand behavior as being embedded in an ongoing context and sequence, the increased interest in the interaction of situation and person variables, the study of situations as individuals seek them out, the necessity to generalize from laboratory settings to the real world, the wish for extensive study of single individuals, or the attempt to study processes that are difficult to create in a laboratory setting. Developments toward the ESM originated in one form or another in the 1960s as behavioral observation gained a foothold in psychology and medicine. Several researchers often simultaneously in different places around the globe, and without, until recently, being aware of (or citing) each other's work have developed this approach (DeVries, 1987; Hormuth, 1990; Csikszentmihalyi & Larson, 1987; Hurlburt, 1987a). Instead of trying to trace these influences historically, this paper will describe the theoretical and methodological needs of psychological research in general and personality psychology in particular that can at least to some degree be met by using ES designs.

Conceptual bases and areas of application

Ecological validity. Ecological validity is a concept introduced by Brunswick (1949). It refers to the occurrence and distribution of stimulus variables in the natural or customary habitat of an individual. A psychological method is ecologically valid to the extent that its stimulus variables are a representative

---

[1] Part of this work appeared in the *Journal of Personality*, 1986, **54**, 1, 262–93. Copyright 1986 Duke University Press, Durham, NC. Reprinted with permission of the publisher.

sample of those in the individual's habitat. This principle, when combined with the call for the study of functional organism–environment relationships (Brunswick, 1952), requires that '. . . situational circumstances should be made to represent, by sampling or related devices, the general or specific conditions under which the organism studied has to function' (p. 30). Brunswick went on to point out that the extension of the sampling requirement from persons to situations has methodological implications especially as far as the number of variables included in a research design is concerned. Brunswick did not necessarily suggest that his thinking would lead to the study of behavior *in situ*, that is, in the actual situation. Rather, the way he conceived representative designs assumes a prior knowledge of the population of stimuli. The random sampling *in* rather than *from* situations, as it is practised with ESM, is one response to the request for the ecological validity of the study of personality.

Studying behavior in the actual situation to obtain data on the distribution of psychological phenomena was the concern of Barker (1968). As an operationalization of Lewin's (1943) concept of psychological ecology, he studied the 'behavior setting' as an ecological situational unit. The method developed for that purpose was painstaking, close observation over long periods of time (e.g., Barker & Wright, 1951). His observations included longer periods of time and thus led to increased understanding of specific behaviors as part of an ongoing 'stream of behavior' (Barker, 1963). This metaphor, in turn, is already known from James (1890) who wrote about the 'stream of thought'. The conceptualization of thinking or behavior as an ongoing stream requires a method that is able to follow a person over a longer time period rather than creating or observing only short isolated episodes. However, a method such as Barker's that tries to assess the totality of behavior is for most purposes inappropriate. While the method requires one to follow the stream of behavior, it is, however, almost impossible to follow a person consistently and record behavior in a wide variety of situations through observational methods. Indeed, the need for the reduction of information led Barker to concentrate on observation within geographical units, or settings. These observations contributed to understanding of the degree to which behavior can be accounted for by the setting in which it takes place. However, the approach seems inadequate to understand a person's ongoing behavior in and between different settings and situations. Any method trying to capture behavior as an ongoing activity must be able to follow a person through different situations and therefore must reduce the information already at the point of sampling.

Theoretical and methodological needs of personality psychology

The major source of several theoretical and methodological developments in personality psychology within the last 15 years was the apparent failure of the field to predict behavior adequately from personality variables. This was pointed out by a number of critiques, for instance, Mischel (1968). The failure was attributed by some to the overpowering effect of situational variables over personality variables. Others argued that development of new theoretical models emphasizing interaction between the person and the environment would improve the prediction of behavior. Still others have attributed the lack of predictive success to a variety of methodological inadequacies.

The study of individuals As a further result of the discussion whether personality psychology is able to predict behavior from traits, another question has received renewed attention, namely, achieving the right balance between a methodological approach that studies many individuals on one trait or many traits on one individual (as Stern, 1921, described it), or the idiographic versus nomotheic approach (as Allport, 1937, called it).

Lamiell (1981) refutes personality psychology's individual differences paradigm as being irrelevant to the description of the personality of individuals. Instead, he proposes what he calls an *idiothetic* approach in which personality is described 'in terms of information of what that person tends to do – not in direct contrast with what others tend to do, but in direct contrast with what that person tends not to do but could do' (Lamiell, 1981, p. 281). Methodologically, he exemplifies the idiothetic approach through the behavioral alternatives and stability in the face of these alternatives of behavior and attributes recorded from individuals over a period of several days. These and similar critical evaluations (e.g., Runyan, 1982) of the dominant approaches in personality and differential psychology contributed to the need for methods that allow one to capture the behavior of individuals over time in different situations. A more recent reviewer (Pervin, 1985) could already point to some adjustment that personality psychologists have made, among them examples of the application of the ESM.

Experience Sampling yields large amounts of data on individual subjects. However, it is used only rarely in single-case designs even though it may be usefully applied there. Rather, because the method collects large amounts of data on several individual subjects, it allows for extended analyses of individual cases as well as for useful aggregation over cases (Epstein, 1983), thus possibly bridging a gap between the two methodological approaches of personality psychology. Csikszentmihalyi & Larson (1984) demonstrate the dual use of one Experience Sampling data set to describe days or weeks in the life of an individual adolescent as well as a 'topography of daily experience' (p. 33) of adolescents across a large sample of people.

The study of situations If personality traits are defined as theoretical constructs that account for the stability of behavior over situations, and are then found to be of low predictive value, one possible response is a greater concern with the heretofore unquestioned part of the definition, that is, the situational variable. When traits were found to be of low predictive value, investigators turned to the study of situational variables (e.g., Mischel, 1968). This approach, situationism, was criticized by Bowers (1973) on a variety of theoretical and methodological grounds. Methodologically, he argued that situationism's emphasis on the experimental method, where a specific treatment is induced, favors the investigation of change and thus reduces the chance of finding stabilities in behavior. The empirical evidence obtained in favour of situationism lacks ecological validity because situations as studied are experimentally created. An ecologically valid study of personality would, according to Bowers, necessarily have to turn toward the study of naturalistic situations because situations, in turn, are 'as much a function of the person as the person's behavior is a function of the situation' (Bowers, 1973, p. 326).

An alternative approach to the lack of success of traits in predicting behavior has been the renewed interest in interactionism (Endler, 1983). Here, traits and situations are assumed to produce behavior only in combination with each other. Interactionist approaches study then how different traits or different dimensions of a trait are cognitively or behaviorally expressed in certain classes of prototypical situations.

Typical situations selected by the investigator to study the interaction between personality traits and situations can reduce the possible range of situations to a large degree. But the description or creation of situations by the researchers also reduces ecological validity. The question of whether the situations or classes of situations selected are relevant to the trait investigated is not answered by using such a design. In addition, it may be not only the behavior *in* a situation, but also the selection *of* a situation that is determined by a given trait, as has been suggested by Snyder (1981) and discussed, for instance, by Diener, Larsen & Emmons (1984). If situations are selected or created by the researcher they cannot be selected or avoided by the person being studied. Finally, situations arise from the interaction of a multiplicity of variables and thus present constantly changing degrees of novelty. Again, this aspect of situations can be created only to a limited degree by the researcher investigating the effects of situations on the stability and expression of traits.

Several researchers considered the study of behavior in situations as they occur, naturally the appropriate approach in face of the theoretical postulate of person–situation interaction. For instance, Pawlik & Buse (1982) and Buse & Pawlik (1984) were critical of methods that symbolically presented situations verbally and assessed the reaction to them by using questionnaires when actually the registration of behavior and the access to natural situations is required. Desirable are, according to Buse & Pawlik (1984) 'ecologically valid studies, based on a representative sample of situations from the everyday life of subjects' (p. 47, translated by the author). To this end, they developed a technique that allowed behavior to be recorded by research participants in everyday situations. In a similar vein, Schuster, Murrell & Cook (1980) were interested in an exploratory answer to the question 'What are the relative contributions of individual traits versus situations in predicting behavior?' To answer this question, they considered a 'knowledge base of established relative person/setting/interaction predictive strengths for different categories of behaviors' (p. 27) in certain environments necessary. To determine the situational and personality components of behavior and their interaction, the ESM or closely related approaches have also been employed by Diener, Larsen & Emmons (1984), Kirchler (1984), and Savin-Williams & Demo (1983). More than any other interactionist approaches, such studies seem to take Bowers' (1973) criticism of the study of situations in personality psychology seriously. Situations are studied as selected by an individual under ecologically valid conditions, thereby allowing assessment of the psychological importance of the relevant findings on the basis of naturalistic studies and correlational analyses of data. Yet these are desirable goals not only for the study of interactionist models of personality but for other problems of psychology as well.

Other applications of ESM

Naturalistic extensions of laboratory findings Naturalistic methods are frequently used to test results that have been obtained under controlled laboratory conditions in the real world and to extend the realm of these findings. After a psychological phenomenon has been established under controlled conditions, the validation of its relevance in the everyday life of people becomes of interest. ESM has been found useful for this purpose, for instance, in the area of self-awareness research (Duval & Wicklund, 1972). Csikszentmihalyi & Figurski (1982) analyzed the direction of subjects' attention using ESM and could relate it to mood as reported at the same time. Their findings provided not only an extension of existing findings into the real world but contributed to theoretical discussion as well. Franzoi & Brewer (1984) also used the method to determine the occurrence of self-awareness, its affective concomitants in real-life situations, and its relationship to the trait of self-consciousness.

The study of the stream of behavior A different point of departure, namely to capture the ongoing stream of behavior or thought in its natural sequence and occurrence motivated, for instance, Hurlburt (1979) to develop and McAdams & Constantian (1983) to use methods that allowed one to conduct investigations concerning 'sampling of ongoing thought in subjects over an entire day' (Singer, 1975, p. 734). McAdams & Constantian (1983) specifically used the Experience Sampling analysis to study the realization of specific motives, namely intimacy and affiliation, in everyday life. The research interests of

38

Klinger, Barta & Maxeimer (1980) were similar. They studied the motivational correlates of thought content in a questionnaire study and used thought sampling as a validity check. Klinger had initially employed random thought sampling in 1978.

The study of naturally occurring events   Under other circumstances, researchers wish to study events that are difficult to create under experimental or quasi-experimental conditions but involve naturally occurring events that can only be studied by using records of subjects' everyday lives. For instance, Reis, Wheeler, Spiegel, Kernis, Nezlek & Perri (1982) were interested in how a person's physical attractiveness determines that person's participation in everyday social life. Hormuth's (1983, 1990; cf., Hormuth, 1984) research on relocation as an opportunity for self-concept change involves the study of people's social behavior in a new environment and their adaptation over a period of several months. Both the long-term nature of the change process and the variety of novel situations encountered resulted in methodological requirements that seemed best fulfilled by experiential sampling.

Outlook

ESM has established itself as a tool for collecting psychological data that may be inaccessible through other methods. It is especially useful for addressing some questions of great relevance to personality research, for instance, the interaction of person and situation variables, the conditions for the actualization of traits and motives in everyday behavior, the validation of questionnaires on ecologically valid data, and the choice of situations. While ESM has already been employed for a great variety of research issues in personality and other areas of psychology and psychopathology, far more use seems possible, for instance, in the investigation of complex social behaviors, or the succession and dependence of situations over time. In idiography and clinical psychology, the establishment of base rates and behavioral changes through ESM can greatly enhance the usefulness of single-case designs. In behavior therapy, random sampling may even prompt other behaviors besides the response to a questionnaire.

Investigators have not yet explored fully the possibilities of different types of sampling schedules. Schedules can be devised to concentrate on particular types of experiences or times in a person's day through changes in frequency. Short-term sampling studies can concentrate on a specific situation (for instance, on an examination: Klinger, 1984; Nicolson, this volume). Studies of interactions may be possible when two partners are equipped with beepers having identical schedules for the study of marital interaction (Donner, 1985). Times series analyses may require one to deviate from the random timing in favor of an equal or mixed interval schedule.

The current methodological weakness lies mainly in the responsibility that is given to the research subject in collecting not only subjective data, like thoughts and feelings, but also objective ones, like the description of situations. Being left alone for long periods of time, and being untrained raters, makes the reliability of responses difficult to determine. Investigators may want to obtain different kinds of data in addition to Experience Sampling, like observational, peer ratings, retrospective, or through questionnaire. Also, controls and checks on the subject should be built into ES designs. Checking on the timeliness of responses is only one such check, others will have to be devised. Collection of objective data and the use of coding systems require careful training of research participants.

Most difficult is the assessment of the validity of the information obtained through the ESM. Almost by definition, a comparison with one set of data collected through another psychological method cannot provide this information. The collection of physiological data, such as heart rate, blood pressure and saliva cortisol at the time of the self-report (Donner, 1985; Van Egeren, 1988; Nicolson, this volume) are promising new developments.

No one method in psychology is able to capture a particular phenomenon in a perfectly valid way. To overcome the weaknesses that always lie in the ascertainment of validity and reliability of data provided and rated by research participants, the strongest approach that can be chosen by an investigator is a multiple-method approach rather than reliance upon one specific method, no matter how appealing. Quasi-experimental designs should be explored to compare experience and behavior in experimental and various control groups. Short-term and longitudinal ESM designs may be combined with longitudinal studies through mail surveys. Comparative studies use various populations, non-students as well as students, healthy and ill populations, and different sampling procedures. Only after a combination of various methods, designs, and samples may the ESM results be interpreted in terms of the full promise of this methodological advance.

40

PART II

The Experience Sampling Method: procedures and analyses

4

Validity and reliability of the Experience Sampling Method[1]

MIHALY CSIKSZENTMIHALYI
and REED LARSON

Sampling of experience

In recent years a growing number of investigators have sought information on the daily events and experiences that make up people's lives. Pervin (1985) identified the 'increasing use of beeper technology' as a research methodology in which signaling devices carried by respondents are used to elicit self-report data at randomized points in time. One of the earliest lines of investigation using pagers to stimulate self-reports began at the University of Chicago in 1975, under the name of 'Experience Sampling Method' (Csikszentmihalyi et al., 1977). The general purpose of this methodology is to study the subjective experience of persons interacting in natural environments, as advocated by Lewin (1936) and Murray (1938), in a way that ensures ecological validity (Brunswick, 1952). The need for this kind of approach arises from research demonstrating the inability of people to provide accurate retrospective information on their daily activities (Bernard et al., 1984; Juster, 1985; Yarmey, 1979) and emotional experience (Thomas & Diener, 1989). Its goal is similar to the one Fiske (1971, p. 179) set out for psychology as a whole: 'to measure . . . the ways a person usually behaves, the regularities in perceptions, feelings and actions.'

The objective of the research described in this chapter is to sample experience systematically, hence the name Experience Sampling Method (ESM). The present article describes ESM and reports on its reliability and validity, using findings from a number of studies. (The history and context of the development of the ESM, as well as recent applications, are chronicled in Csikszentmihalyi & Csikszentmihalyi, 1988; readers may also wish to refer to two earlier and more restricted reviews of the methodology, i.e. Hormuth, 1986; Larson & Csikszentmihalyi, 1983.)

The development of experience sampling responds to a number of currents within psychology and the social sciences. Two methodological traditions are the most direct ancestors of the present approach: first, research in the alloca-

[1] This work appeared in: *Journal of Nervous and Mental Disease*, 1987, **175** (9), 526–37.

tion of time to everyday activities (time budgets); and second, research measuring psychological reactions to everyday activities and experiences. Time budget studies have typically assessed time investment in different activities by different categories of persons (Altschuller, 1923; Bevans, 1913; Robinson, 1977; Sorokin & Berger, 1939; Szalai, 1972; Thorndike, 1937; Zuzanek, 1980). Another approach has been that of the Kansas School of Ecological Psychology, which observationally investigated behavioral settings and focused on time use in the socialization of children (Barker, 1968; Barker & Wright, 1955; Barker et al., 1961). These studies were later extended cross-culturally (Johnson, 1973; Munroe & Munroe, 1971a, b; Rogoff, 1978).

A second tradition of research focused on the impact of everyday life situations on psychological states, such as 'psychopathology and coping' (Gurin et al., 1960); and 'well-being' (Bradburn, 1969). These studies provided data on global psychological states in representative populations. Researchers in the field of social psychology, on the other hand, performed experimental studies in which respondents were asked to imagine themselves in various life situations and then to report their psychological reactions (Endler & Magnusson, 1976; Magnusson & Endler, 1977).

Although these methods have enriched our understanding of individual lives, they have several shortcomings: Imagery evoked in laboratory studies is not necessarily typical of experience encountered in real-life situations. In quality-of-life studies, only global assessments of extremely complex phenomena are presented. The data are gathered in retrospect, outside the context of the situation, thus permitting distortions and rationalizations to become important. Time budget studies have been obtained from observer data or from diaries that do not provide direct access to the subjects' internal states. Nor in these studies is it clear what the link is between behavior and psychological states or between time use and experience. The ESM, which assesses subjects in real time and context, attempts to overcome some of these shortcomings.

Conceptually, the ESM 'exposes' regularities in the stream of consciousness, such as states of heightened happiness or self-awareness, concentration experienced at work, and symptoms of illness. The research aim is to relate these regularities to characteristics of the person (e.g., age, aptitude, physiological arousal, medical diagnosis), of the situation (e.g., the challenges of a job, the content of a TV show) or of the interaction between person and situation (e.g., the dynamics of a conversation with a friend, the circumstances that lead to a specific event). The objective is to identify and analyze how patterns in people's subjective experience relate to the wider conditions of their lives. The purpose of using this method is to be as 'objective' about subjective phenomena as possible without compromising the essential personal meaning of the experience.

44

Methods

Instruments

Signaling device To obtain representative self-reports of experiential states, the ESM relies on an electronic instrument that emits stimulus signals according to a random schedule. Different sound or vibration signalling devices have been used by different research groups: pagers such as those used to page doctors in the hospital (e.g., Csikszentmihalyi & Graef, 1980; Csikszentmihalyi & Figurski, 1982; Larson & Csikszentmihalyi, 1983), programmed pocket calculators (e.g., Massimini, 1989; Schifman, this issue), programmed wrist watch terminals (e.g., deVries, 1983; Brandstatter, 1983), and other devices that signal at random intervals, such as those used in thought-sampling research (Hurlburt, 1979; Klinger et al., 1980) and occupational studies (Divilbiss & Self, 1978; Spencer, 1971). Some studies have had the subjects themselves set watches according to predetermined timetables (Brandstatter, 1983; Diener et al., 1984), but most program the signal devices for the respondents. The signal devices can also be programmed simultaneously and this provides special opportunities for analysis of the interdependence of experience in studies of couples, families, or friendship groups. Pawlik & Buse (1982) have pioneered data-recording units that, in addition to signalling, are also able to record coded responses directly on tape. At the University of Heidelberg, Hormuth (1985, 1986) built a device that can be programmed from a portable Epson computer to signal 128 times over a period of eight days. Different devices have different advantages and disadvantages. The choice also depends on the groups of subjects under investigation (e.g., the vibration option is more practical for research with adolescents, who spend part of their day at school; the sound of wrist watch terminals can be too soft to page the elderly, etc.). The function of the signaling device is always to cue respondents to report their activities, thoughts, and inner states at unexpected random times in natural settings. Any technique providing this function is adequate.

Experience Sampling Form (ESF)

At the signal, the respondent writes down information about his or her momentary situation and psychological state on the ESF self-report questionnaire (see Appendix). This record becomes the basic datum of the ESM. The ESF is typically designed so that it will take no more than two minutes to complete. Respondents usually carry a full packet of the forms in a booklet.

Items contained in the form vary depending on the investigator's goals. In the authors' research, the objective has been to seek comprehensive coverage of the respondent's external and internal situation at the time of the signal. Hence, the ESF includes open questions about location, social context, primary and secondary activity, content of thought, time at which the ESF is filled out, and a number of Likert scales measuring several dimensions of the respondent's perceived situation including affect (happy, cheerful, sociable, and friendly), activation (alert, active, strong, excited), cognitive efficiency (concentration, ease of concentration, self-consciousness, clear mood), and motivation (wish to do the activity, control, feeling involved). The sample ESF used in a study of adolescents is reproduced in the Appendix.

Variants of this form have been used with other samples. Some researchers have focused exclusively on thought content (Hurlburt, 1979; Klinger et al., 1980) or emotional experience (Diener et al., 1984). Other investigators have developed specialized item sets on self-image and self-awareness (Franzoi & Brewer, 1984; Savin-Williams & Demo, 1983), adjustments to changes in residence (Hormuth, 1986), intervening daily events (Greene, 1985), binge eating (Johnson & Larson, 1982), alcohol and drug consumption (Filstead et al., 1985), thought disorders (deVries, 1983; deVries et al., 1986) and the special problems of physically disabled children and adolescents[2], among others.

Procedures

Scheduling of signals   In the majority of ESM studies respondents received 7 to 10 signals per day for seven consecutive days. Usually the scheduling of signals is a variant of what Cochran (1953) describes as 'systematic sampling', a procedure that typically obtains more precise estimates of population characteristics than a purely random sample. Within the 15 to 18 target hours each day, one signaling time is selected for every block of 90 to 120 min, using a table of random numbers, with the provision that no signals should occur within 15 min of each other. The length of the reporting period and the timing of reports again depend on the scope and aims of the investigation. Filstead and colleagues (1985) asked alcoholics coming out of treatment to respond to a schedule of four signals per day for three months. In a study of the menstrual cycle, LeFevre et al. (1985) signaled married couples three times a day for one month. At the other extreme, studies of thought content have had signals with a mean delay of only 30 min for three days (Hurlburt, 1979). A concentration of signals during crucial points of the day or in different situations has also been used (deVries, 1983). However, the more that researchers have demanded of respondents, the fewer people have been willing to take part in the research. Generally, when frequency has increased, shortening the duration of the total sampling period gives augmented compliance.

Before beginning Experience Sampling, respondents receive instructions on

---

[2] Marta Wenger and colleagues of the Collaborative Study of Children with Special Needs at the Children's Hospital Medical Center in Boston have used ESM with several samples of physically disabled children.

the use of the signaling device and are instructed on how to fill out the ESF. They are told that they should fill out the form as soon as possible after each signal; typical situations in which this might be difficult (driving car, playing sports) are discussed. Subjects are asked to keep the pager turned on and to respond to all signals received, unless they go to bed or they 'really need privacy'. The general purposes of the research are described, and the necessity for the respondents to report their life as it actually is – with all its joys and problems – is stressed.

Respondents should be given a chance to fill out a practice ESF. Subsequently, each subject is provided with a bound booklet of about 40 to 60 ESFs and a telephone number where someone can be reached in case any question or complication arises. When the week is completed, each subject is debriefed and the ESF booklets are collected. Additional interview or questionnaire data may be obtained before or after the test week.

Coding

Most of the data consists of self-scoring rating scales. The open-ended items may be coded in different ways, depending on the goals of the study. In some studies (Buse & Pawlik, 1984; Hormuth, 1984a, b), activity and thought categories are provided on each ESF for the respondent to check, thus eliminating the need for the researchers to code open-ended responses. In the Chicago research each variable was coded in fine detail, although codes in most analyses are aggregated in larger categories.

Activity codes   For the adult sample studied by the authors, the answers to the item 'What was the main thing you were doing?' were initially coded in one of 154 activity categories (e.g., 'operating a typewriter', 'playing with a child', 'planning a meal'). In most analyses, however, activities were combined into 16 larger groups (e.g., 'working at work', 'other at work', 'transportation'). Sometimes only three global activity areas are contrasted: work, maintenance, and leisure. Agreement between two coders at the level of the 154 categories was 88%; at the level of the 16 variable grouping it was 96%.

Of course, subjects may vary in how they report an activity. The same activity can be described by one person as 'I was typing at my desk', by another as 'I was helping out my boss', and by still another as 'I was waiting for 5 o'clock to come so I could leave the office'. Action identification theorists (Harré & Secord, 1972; Vallacher & Wegner, 1985; Wegner & Vallacher, 1977) find important differences associated with different ways of segmenting and labeling behavior. In our studies activity reports were collapsed into functional categories (e.g., work or leisure) without concern for structural characteristics such as the 'level of identity' of the response, although such coding could also be attempted.

47

Thoughts We used the same codes as for activities to code the content of thought, with only a few additions. The categories were then aggregated into fewer functionally equivalent groups (e.g., thoughts about work, family, or self). Other researchers have developed schemes for coding thoughts that are specifically designed to study the stream of consciousness and psychopathology (deVries et al., 1986; Hurlburt, 1979; Klinger et al., 1980).

Data structure

Data are typically stored in two major computer files: a 'beeper' and a 'person' file. The first contains the data from each separate ESF in its entirety. The second contains percentages, means, standard deviations, and other aggregate scores for different variables, compiled by respondent, as well as information from interviews and questionnaires (see Larson & Delespaul, in this issue).

Because the ESM obtains random samples of daily experience, the data base in these files is a representative record that can be accessed over and over again, to test any number of hypotheses formulated at the time of collection or 20 years later. One can think of the data base as a permanent laboratory in which an almost unlimited number of relationships may be tested (e.g., Graef et al., 1983). To the extent that new records are continuously being added and the number of observations in each cell increases, ever more refined questions can be asked of the data.

Compliance

Volunteer rates The ESM can be used with a variety of populations, provided that they can write and that a viable research alliance can be established. To date the youngest respondents have been 10 years old (Larson, 1989), and the oldest 85. ESM research has been carried out on people with schizophrenia (Delespaul & deVries, 1987; deVries et al., 1986), anxiety disorders (Dijkman & deVries, 1987), multiple personality disorders (Loewenstein et al., 1987), bulimia (Johnson & Larson, 1982), alcoholism (Filstead et al., 1985) and paraplegia[2]. In our studies we have been able to include adults who spoke little English and had only a few years of grammar school education, but the rate of volunteering from unskilled blue-collar workers was extremely low (12% of the target sample), and of those who volunteered only half completed 30 ESFs or more. It was clear that for them the task was unusual and difficult to handle. At the other extreme, among clerical workers and technicians, 75% of the eligible population volunteered and completed the study. Among randomly selected fifth and ninth graders the rate was 75% and the researchers found no differences between participants and refusers in age, sex, self-esteem, or peer population, but did find lower participation among depressed boys and among youth in families with remarried parents (Larson, 1989). Among high school students and adults, females have been more willing participants than males (Larson, 1979).

Response frequency Respondents varied in their rate of compliance with the method. Blue-collar workers have responded to 73% of the signals on the average, clerical and managerial workers to 85% and 92%, respectively, for an overall average of 80%. High school students had a median response rate of 70%. Pawlik & Buse (1982) and deVries et al. (1986) reported an 86% completion rate, and Hormuth's study (1985) had a median completion rate of 82%.

Missing signals occur for a variety of reasons. From the debriefing interviews these appear to be due primarily to technical problems such as beeper malfunction or reception difficulties. The second most frequent source of attrition was forgetting the pager or the ESFs at home. A third source was related to the nature of the activity at the time the signal was transmitted, such as being in church, in the swimming pool, or in bed. Larson (1989) demonstrates that since missed reports are spread across a wide range of contexts, they have relatively little effect on the representativeness of the sample of experience.

The frequency of delay in response to the pager is typically quite small. In our study of 75 adolescents (Csikszentmihalyi & Larson, 1984), 64% responded immediately when they were signaled and 87% responded within 10 min. In Hormuth's (1985) study of 101 adult Germans ($N = 5145$ observations), 50% of the signals were responded to immediately, 80% within 5 min of the signal, and 90% within 18 min. Similar results were obtained in other studies. Delays are usually due to being engaged in activities that cannot be interrupted, for example, taking a test in school, driving a car, or talking to a customer. In most studies, ESFs filled out more than 20 min after the signal were discarded.

Experimental effects Analyses of debriefing responses suggest that the intrusiveness of the method is not felt to be excessive. Among U.S. adults, 32% said that the beeper was getting disruptive or annoying by the end of the week; 22% of the German adults complained that it disrupted daily routine (Hormuth, 1985). Ninety percent of the Americans and 80% of the Germans felt that the reports captured their week well. When asked whether they would participate again in such a study, 75% of Hormuth's subjects answered yes.

Reliability of ESM measures

Sampling accuracy

Because the ESM obtains a systematic random sample of daily life, it provides a measure of how people spend their time during a typical week. This measure is important both in its own right, indicating the frequency of different activities, and as a means for determining sampling accuracy of the ESM reports. A comparison with diary records from time budget studies (Robinson, 1977; Szalai et al., 1972) shows that the frequency of activities measured with the

ESM correlates well with the rank of time budget activity frequencies ($r = 0.93$). Although diaries and the ESM provide very similar measures of activity frequency, a few discrepancies between the two are worth mentioning because they seem to be exceptions that prove the accuracy of the ESM. Respondents report to be 'idling' over 5% of the time, while this category does not appear in the time budgets. Idling was coded when the respondents reported staring out of the window or standing about without doing or thinking anything. Apparently this type of behavior is drastically under-represented in retrospective reports. On the other hand, the ESM appears to slightly underestimate time away from home, because participants occasionally forget the pager (Robinson, 1985). Overall, however, the two measures produce almost identical values of time allocation for different daily activities. The duration and sequence of activities, however, are more clearly calculated with diary approaches.

Stability of activity estimates

How stable are these measures over time? To answer this question, the week has been divided into two halves, and the frequency of activities for the group was computed within each period. By and large, activities are reported with the same frequency in the two halves of the reporting period. For a sample of 107 adults the difference was not significant ($x^2[15] = 8.1$), in spite of the enormous number. For a sample of 75 students on the other hand, the differences were significant ($x^2[13] = 3.4; P < 0.01$). The primary difference was the greater percentage of time at work during the second half of the week, and it is attributable to the fact that more people, especially in the adolescent sample, started the experiment toward the end of the week (Thursday and Friday), so that the first half included more weekend self-reports.

Stability of psychological states

Another issue is whether self-reports of affect, activation, motivation, and cognitive efficiency are stable over the testing period, or whether the pattern of responses changes over time as a result of the measurement procedure. To answer this question the mean scores for each individual from the first half of the week were compared with those from the second half.

None of the averaged individual mean response variables showed a substantial change from the week's beginning to its end. It should be added that for both adolescents ($N = 75$) and adults ($N = 107$) the most extreme change was on the variable free vs. constrained: adolescents (difference=0.26, $P = 0.002$) and adults (difference = 0.16, $P = 0.006$) felt more constrained in the second half of the week, probably in reaction to the method itself.

The variance in responses around an individual's mean diminished by 5 to 15% from the first to the second half of the week. This shrinkage was less for

Table 4.1. *Proportion variance in psychological states accounted for by persons and activities in the first and second half of the week of ESM self-reporting*

Item	Adolescents				Adults			
	Persons (N = 75)		Activities (N = 14)		Persons (N = 107)		Activities (N = 16)	
	1st	2nd	1st	2nd	1st	2nd	1st	2nd
Affect								
Happy	0.18	0.23	0.05	0.05	0.25	0.34	0.04	0.04
Arousal								
Active	0.15	0.20	0.10	0.10	0.16	0.29	0.11	0.07
Cognitive efficiency								
Concentration	0.18	0.28	0.07	0.07	0.32	0.41	0.07	0.06
Motivation								
Wish to be doing	0.16	0.24	0.13	0.13	0.20	0.25	0.05	0.09

adolescents than adults and less for 7-point semantic differential items dealing with affect and arousal than for 10-point scales dealing with cognition and motivation.

Does this mean that in the course of the reporting period people become stereotyped in their responses and fail to differentiate between situations? To answer that question, we compared the first and the second halves of the week to determine whether the amount of variance accounted for by activities diminished with time, by calculating the variance attributable to the person's own response pattern and that to his or her activities (see Table 4.1).

To save space, only one variable for each of the four dimensions is presented here. Person effects were in general more powerful, accounting for between one fifth and one third of the variance, whereas activity effects explained only about 5%. In the second half of the week all the person effects increased, indicating that with time individual responses became more predictable. However, activity effects did not show a comparable decline over time for either adolescents or adults. Thus the reduction in variance does not imply a lessened sensitivity to environmental effects, but a more precise self-anchoring on the response scales.

Individual consistency over the week

Contrary to a one-time measure, the ESM is not based on the assumption that people are going to be entirely consistent in their responses. Person A might be happier than person B on Monday, but on Thursday B could be happier than A, depending on intervening experiences. Because the technique was devised to measure the effects of life situations on psychological states, perfect reliability would in fact defeat its purpose. In general, however, it was expected that relative differences between respondents would tend to persist over time. To check on individual response consistency, each subject's means and standard deviations in the first half of the week were correlated with the means and standard deviations in the second half.

All correlations were significant, for the means as well as for the standard deviations, indicating that levels of both response and variability are fairly stable individual characteristics. The median correlation coefficient on the eight variables was 0.60 for the adolescents and 0.74 for the adults, suggesting that better anchored psychological states develop with age.

One investigator (Wells, 1985) added five items intended to measure self-esteem to each ESF and collected 2287 observations from 49 mothers of small children. The Cronbach alpha for the set of items was 0.94, and coefficient of the correlation between the mean self-esteem scores in the first half of the week and the second half was 0.86 ($P = 0.0001$).

Pawlik & Buse (1982), studying 135 high school students in Hamburg, also correlated the frequency of responses between the 3651 protocols in the first half of the week and the 3729 protocols in the second half. Their subjects reported only the presence or absence of various subjective states, instead of using Likert scales. The correlation coefficients were 0.57 for locations, 0.76 for moods, and 0.80 for motives, quite similar to the ones reported above despite the difference in methods.

Individual consistency over two years

Test-retest data are available for 28 adolescents (Freeman et al., 1986) who took part in ESM for a week first in their freshman or sophomore years in high school, and again, two years later, in their junior or senior years. The stability in their responses ranged from $r = 0.45$ ($P = 0.05$) for the variables active and concentration, to $r = 0.75$ ($P = 0.001$) for control.

Validity of ESM measures

The reliability data on the convergence of diary and ESM measures also provide information on the validity of the ESM for measuring time usage. Here we will focus on its use for assessing internal states.

In general, the data suggest that: (a) ESM reports of psychological states covary in expected ways with the values for physical conditions and with situational factors such as activity, location, and social context; (b) measures of individual differences based on the ESM correlate with independent measures of similar constructs; and (c) the ESM differentiates between groups *expected* to be different, e.g., patient and nonpatient groups or gifted and average mathematics students.

Situational validity

Eight subjects wearing heart rate and activity monitors as well as ESM pagers were asked to supplement each self-report with a rating on a 10-point scale on 'How physically active have you been in the past 3 minutes?' (Hoover, 1983). This self-reported item predicted heart rate as well as readings from the ankle and wrist activity monitors: the correlation of self-ratings with heart rate was $r = 0.41$ ($P < 0.0001$), and with monitor readings, $r = 0.36$ ($P < 0.0001$). Substantial individual differences in this relationship, ranging from $r = 0.61$ to $r = 0.16$, were significantly correlated with other personality variables that suggested important individual differences in how physically aware the subjects were.

In addition, the physical activity self-ratings differentiated very highly between four body positions. When respondents were lying down, the mean z-score for self-reported physical activity was -1.47, when sitting it was 0.34, when standing it was 0.43, and when walking it was 1.03 (analysis of variance, $F[3,268] = 41.7$, $P < 0.0001$). Heart rate also varied in relation to body position ($F[3,268] = 6.95$, $P < 0.0001$).

Another example of an expected relationship between activity and experience is the association between what people do and their level of motivation. When activity categories are arranged on an obligatory-discretionary axis, the productive ones (work) are rated as obligatory 80% of the time. Maintenance activities are obligatory less often, from cleaning house (54%) to shopping (37%), and leisure is rarely seen as obligatory, from socializing (15%) to watching TV (3%).

In the study of working women with small children mentioned above, it was found that the self-esteem of mothers was much higher when they were working or involved in leisure than when they were taking care of the house or of their children (analysis of variance, $F[1,46] = 13.77$, $P < 0.0005$) (Wells, 1985). Additional expected relationships between activity and experience can be found over a wide range from states related to drug and alcohol use to binge eating (Johnson & Larson, 1982; Larson et al., 1984) to emotions when alone on Friday or Saturday night (Larson et al., 1982), or to stress experienced in anxiety-provoking situations (Dijkman & deVries, 1987; Margraf et al., 1987).

Individual characteristics and variation in experience

In addition to using ESM data to assess regularities in how people experience different daily situations, they may also be useful when the *person* is the unit of analysis. For example, a number of researchers have found correlations between participants' responses on the ESM and their scores on other psychometric instruments.

Giannino et al. (1979) entered ESM scores of a workers' sample into a regression analysis with 27 predictor items. The variable that accounted for the largest proportion of variance in the affect dimension (13%, P <0.0001) was the alienation-from-self subscale of Maddi's Alienation Test (Maddi et al., 1979). In other words, the best predictor of positive affect on the ESM was the absence of alienation from the self. Moreover, workers who scored high on a work satisfaction test scored much higher on the item 'involved' when they were alone and actually working on their jobs than did subjects who scored low on work satisfaction. Satisfied workers had higher scores on concentration, skills, alertness, and motivation (in each case, P <0.0001).

The strength of the need for intimacy was measured by McAdams & Constantian (1983) using projective techniques and comparing them with ESM measures. People with a high need for intimacy reported more thoughts about people and relationships ($r = 0.52$, P <0.001), more conversation with others ($r = 0.40$, P <0.01), higher affect when with others (P <0.001), and a lower rate of wishing to be alone when with others ($r = -0.32$, P <0.05).

Hamilton et al. (1984) developed a questionnaire scale for measuring the amount of enjoyment subjects report in their daily lives. The amount of intrinsic enjoyment was related to several ESM variables such as motivation, wish to be doing the activity (P <0.001), concentration, ease of concentration, control, and activity/potency (P <0.05 in each case).

One-time assessments on the Rosenberg Self-Esteem Scale (RSES) were compared with the average of a repeated self-esteem scale (four items from the RSES included in the ESF) and with the average of five ESM items related to self-esteem (Wells, 1985). The one-time RSES correlated with the repeated RSES items $r = 0.62$ ($N = 49$, P <0.0001) and with the ESM self-esteem items $r = 0.42$ (P <0.002). This latter correlation varied considerably depending on the social context: When alone, subjects' responses on the ESM self-esteem items correlated with the one-time RSES at only $r = 0.26$ (NS), when only children were present at $r = 0.36$ (P <0.05), and when adults were also present at $r = 0.50$ (P <0.001). In other words, self-esteem as measured by a one-time traditional test corresponds to the self-esteem people report when they are in public.

Clinically, Loewenstein et al. (1987) reported the use of ESM with a woman with a multiple personality disorder. They found that the alternates displayed quantitative differences on the affect and motivational scales comparable to those observed between separate individuals.

Differences in experience between groups

The ESM has also differentiated well between the responses of groups with distinctive behavioral patterns and groups with psychopathology. For example, deVries and associates (deVries, 1983; deVries et al., 1986) coded the thoughts reported on the ESFs of Dutch schizophrenic and nonschizophrenic mental patients; the schizophrenics generally suffered more severe thought disorders, whereas the other patients suffered mainly from affective disorders.

He found that nonschizophrenic patients evidenced congruence between thoughts and actions 75% of the time, whereas the schizophrenics did the same only half of the time ($t = 2.82$, $P < 0.005$). The thoughts reported by the schizophrenics were also coded as disordered much more often than were those of the control group ($t = 9.13$, $P < 0.005$). On the other hand, the schizophrenics reported a more positive average affect ($t = 1.78$, $P < 0.05$).

In their investigation of women with eating disorders, Johnson & Larson (1982) found that bulimic women were involved in food-related behavior or thought on the average of 38% of their waking time, as opposed to the 14% average for a comparison group of women. They also found that the overall level of positive affect was lower for bulimics than for normal women (happy, $t = 4.66$, $P < 0.001$; cheerful, $t = 4.14$, $P < 0.001$; sociable, $t = 4.12$, $P < 0.001$).

Overview

Since its introduction 15 years ago, the ESM has proved to be a useful tool for psychological research. Its main contribution has been to make the variations of daily experience, long outside the domain of objectivity, available for analysis, replication, and falsifiability, thus opening up a whole range of phenomena to systematic observation.

The most heuristic usefulness of the ESM lies in its *description of the patterns of an individual's daily experience*. Because the method yields repeated measurements of a person's activities, feelings, thoughts, motivations, and medical symptoms over time, questions such as the following can be answered: How much of the person's variation in happiness (or any other state) is related to what the person does; to the company he or she keeps; to the time of day; to intervening events? By the same token, the ESM can reveal subjective effects of major life changes that might otherwise be hidden from consciousness by distortion or inaccurate recollection. The comparison of responses before and after a job or family change, a clinical intervention, or other changes in life situations can reveal what impact such transitions have on a person's daily life.

Adding up patterns within a person, it becomes possible to use ESM *to evaluate the common experience of situations*. For instance, is solitude, housework, or marijuana smoking experienced similarly by different individuals? It follows that the ESM can be used to compare the subjective experience of different events. Do men and women differ in their daily emotions? What states, feelings, attitudes differentiate talented achievers from talented nonachievers? How can we compare the experience of physically handicapped children with that of other children? Likewise, ESM data can reveal whether changes in life situations elicit consistent changes in experiences of people in general.

A final use of ESM is *to study the dynamics of emotions and other subjective states*. The study of consciousness has lagged behind other fields of psychology. We know little about the structure of emotions and less about how other dimensions of our psychological state (e.g., concentration, involvement, motivation) ebb and flow in daily experience. ESM data allow examination of the magnitude, duration, and sequences of states, as well as an investigation of correlations between the occurrences of different experiences. For example, one can examine whether concentration is typically associated with positive affect, how long it lasts, and what factors are related to its ending.

The major limitation of the ESM is the obvious one: its dependence on respondents' self-reports. This limitation becomes a concern in situations in which it is conceivable that a large segment of one's sample provided inaccurate or distorted data. For example, if an employer used the method to study his employees' productivity, the accuracy of self-reports related to working would be suspect, as would the ESM results in an investigation of private, sensitive, or illegal activities.

When self-reports deal with the immediate, however, they have been found to be a very useful source of data (Ericsson & Simon, 1980; Mischel, 1981). In this chapter we have presented ample evidence indicating that they typically provide a plausible representation of reality.

Appendix to Chapter 4: Experience Sampling Form

Date: _____ Time Beeped: _____ am/pm   Time Filled out____am/pm

as you were beeped . . .

What were you thinking about? _____

_____

Where were you? _____

What was the MAIN thing you were doing? _____

_____

What other things were you doing? _____

_____

WHY were you doing this particular activity?

☐ I had to   ☐ I wanted to do it   ☐ I had nothing else to do

	not at all		some what		quite			very
How well were you concentrating	0	1	2	3	4	5	6	7	8	9
Was it hard to concentrate?	0	1	2	3	4	5	6	7	8	9
How self-conscious were you?	0	1	2	3	4	5	6	7	8	9
Did you feel good about yourself?	0	1	2	3	4	5	6	7	8	9
Were you in control of the situation?	0	1	2	3	4	5	6	7	8	9
Were you living up to your own expectations?	0	1	2	3	4	5	6	7	8	9
Were you living up to the expectations of others?	0	1	2	3	4	5	6	7	8	9

Describe your mood as you were beeped:

	very	quite	some	neither	some	quite	very	
alert	0	o	.	–	.	o	0	drowsy
happy	0	o	.	–	.	o	0	sad
irritable	0	o	.	–	.	o	0	cheerful
strong	0	o	.	–	.	o	0	weak
active	0	o	.	–	.	o	0	passive
lonely	0	o	.	–	.	o	0	sociable
ashamed	0	o	.	–	.	o	0	proud
involved	0	o	.	–	.	o	0	detached
excited	0	o	.	–	.	o	0	bored
closed	0	o	.	–	.	o	0	open
clear	0	o	.	–	.	o	0	confused
tense	0	o	.	–	.	o	0	relaxed
competitive	0	o	.	–	.	o	0	cooperative

Did you feel any physical discomfort as you were beeped:
Overall pain or discomfort none slight bothersome severe
0 1 2 3 4 5 6 7 8 9
Please specify: _____

Who were you with?
(☐) alone   (☐) friend(s)   How many?
(☐) mother
                   female (☐)   male (☐)
(☐) father   (☐) strangers
(☐) sister(s) or brother(s)   (☐) other _____

Indicate how you felt about your activity:

	low								high
Challenges of the activity	0	1	2	3	4	5	6	7	8 9
Your skills in the activity	0	1	2	3	4	5	6	7	8 9

	not at all								very much
Was this activity important to you?	0	1	2	3	4	5	6	7	8 9
Was this activity important to others?	0	1	2	3	4	5	6	7	8 9
Were you succeeding at what you were doing?	0	1	2	3	4	5	6	7	8 9
Do you wish you had been doing something else?	0	1	2	3	4	5	6	7	8 9
Were you satisfied with how you were doing	0	1	2	3	4	5	6	7	8 9
How important was this activity in relation to your overall goals	0	1	2	3	4	5	6	7	8 9

If you had a choice . . .
Who would you be with? _____
What would you be doing? _____

Since you were last beeped has anything happened or have you done anything
which could have an effect on the way you feel?
Nasty cracks, comments, etc. *****************

5

Analyzing Experience Sampling data: a guidebook for the perplexed

REED LARSON
and PHILIPPE A.E.G. DELESPAUL

This chapter provides a guidebook for doing simple analysis with the complex-data obtained by experience sampling. We describe the basic types of questions investigators may ask, and discuss the strength and limitations associated with different approaches to testing these questions. Because ESM data reflect the complexities of everyday life, no analysis can fully capture the underlying trends, and few analyses will fully meet the assumptions of statistical tests. Nonetheless, we argue that careful and creative analysis of ESM data can provide provocative information about the daily lives of a research population.

'Danger, lives have been lost!' reads a sign on the rocks by a raging cascade near one of the authors' places of birth. A similar warning should accompany Experience Sampling data, for a novice could easily squander many years on the slippery terrain of ESM data analysis. Such a warning should be in bright neon for students trained in the positivist framework of experimental science; like the daily experience they attempt to mirror, ESM data have a complexity which defies traditional textbook analysis. Rarely do they fully oblige the stringent assumptions of inferential statistical tests. The many factors imping-ing on daily life, and thus upon these data, demand a constant vigilance to statistical artifact and possible confounds. Therefore, even the seasoned ESM researcher takes many trips back to the computer before finalizing an analysis in a way that most clearly expresses the relationship he or she wishes to capture.

Having issued this Surgeon General's warning, we can now go on to say that, given the right frame of mind, ESM data analyses can be rich, rewarding, and fun. This article is intended as a kind of *Joy of Cooking* for the uninitiated. It lays out basic approaches to statistical analysis of ESM data, identifying the potentials and shortcomings of each. Our underlying philosophy is that the study of daily lives is an interpretive science – there are many valid and interesting ways to address the same question and no final or 'correct' answers.

The goal is not prediction and control, but description and deeper levels of understanding. The process of analyzing ESM data, therefore, is a process of continual rethinking what findings mean, what factors might be influencing an apparent relationship, and how an analysis might be redone to represent the phenomenon of interest better. It involves a kind of 'creative worry', which, given a sufficient computer budget and some capacity for humour, can be highly engaging and enjoyable.

At heart most statistical issues are conceptual issues, thus in this article we first talk about the clarification of research questions. One of the most frequent problems of ESM data analysis is confusion about what specifically is being asked. We differentiate between two basic types of questions that can be addressed: (1) *questions about situations*; and (2) *questions about persons*.

In the second section which forms the body of the paper we discuss how these questions about situations and questions about persons can be analyzed using different subsets of the complex ecological data set. The discussion will be illustrated with examples and is written to provide rules of thumb as to when different types of approaches might be appropriate.

We should note that the focus of this guidebook is the design of an analysis that addresses a single question and results in one finding, table or graph. For a paper or article one will want to combine several such analyses, probably synthesizing questions about situations and persons. Indeed the richness of an article often comes from the juxtaposition of findings and the tensions or congruence found between the situational level and the person level. Here, however, we are able to comment little on the aesthetic of bringing together a set of findings, and speak more narrowly to the statistical technique of finalizing one analysis.

Formulation of research questions

Psychological states can be properties of situations and of persons. There are some situations, for example, that create anxiety in most people (e.g. driving in fog) while other situations are specific to groups of subjects (e.g. elevators); and there are some people who experience anxiety in most situations (e.g. anxiety patients). The excitement of the ESM is the potential convergence it offers between these questions about situations and questions about persons: the same data set allows one to consider both. This combined data set contains, however, a major pitfall: we can easily forget the distinction between both sets of questions and carry out analyses that blur person and situation together. Thus, do not mistake a delirious moment with the trait of delirium. Prior to conducting an analysis, it is essential to determine whether it will address a question about one or the other. There are some complex circumstances in which one might want to consider the two within the same analysis, but these are fewer than one would think and the beginner is strongly encouraged to frame the analysis around either the situation or person before going near the computer.

We will present some examples of questions about situations and questions about persons to clarify what each is. Afterwards we will discuss the possible confusion that can arise between the two types of questions when the aim of the analysis is not clearly defined.

Questions about situations

For our purposes here we define 'situation' very broadly. Questions about situations include comparisons between contexts of daily life, as defined by people's activities (e.g., work vs. leisure), companionship (being with family vs. friends), location, or time of day. 'Situations' might also be differentiated by subjective states (e.g., the experience of craving or panic), or by any other criterion one can think of that differentiates moments in time (e.g., the smoking of a cigarette, a stressful event). The independent variable for these questions will most often be a datum recorded on the ESM self-report form, such as a contextual variable or a mood score, but might also be derived from a prior ESM sheet, a daily diary report, or some other criterion that differentiates categories of experience in daily life.

Here are some examples of questions about situations:

Are people more motivated in work or in leisure?
Do drug users experience a greater craving for the drug in the morning or evening?
What psychological states precede an epileptic episode?
How long does a panic attack typically last?
How are patterns of daily moods and time use different before and after a divorce?

Observe that the concern in these questions is not with comparisons between groups of people. Rather they entail comparisons between moments in time, but within individuals. They are concerned with describing or contrasting some pattern of experiences that differ systematically between situations for a target population.

Questions about persons

Now we switch to looking at the other type of question. Questions about persons include comparisons between groups of people, including comparisons between people having different traits. One's independent variable may be a demographic variable (age, sex, SES), a diagnostic category (schizophrenic vs. normal control), a score on a test, or even a score derived from the ESM data (subjects who report frequent panic attacks vs. those who do not). Here are some examples:

60

Are women more emotionally variable than men?

How is the daily experience of handicapped children different from non-handicapped children?

Do patients treated in a hospital experience more social interaction than those treated in the community?

Do the patients' reports of agoraphobia in a clinical interview correspond to greater agitation when they are with people?

Questions apt to create confusion

In some cases researchers may be unclear whether they are interested in situations or persons. Consider the next two questions:

Is TV viewing correlated with depression?

Is frequent hallucination associated with anxiety?

In our experience it is not uncommon for students to get excited about questions phrased like these, without being clear about what they are really asking. The wordings used here leave it unspecified whether the issue being addressed is depressed and hallucinating people or depressed and hallucinatory situations. Thus it is essential to decide whether your questions are about persons:

Is the amount of TV a person watches associated with the severity of that person's depression?

Do psychiatric patients who describe themselves as frequent hallucinators also experience more anxiety [than those hallucinating less]?

Or about situations:

Are [depressive] persons more depressed when watching TV?

Do psychotic patients who describe themselves as frequent hallucinators also experience more anxiety when hallucinating?

Failure to make this differentiation can lead to erroneous conclusions. Two examples illustrate how an ill-defined question can lead to findings which obscure the underlying relationships.

Example 1: A novice investigator might naively ask, 'Is the experience of subjective control correlated with happiness?' This question fails to distinguish between two separate issues: (1) Are happy experiences associated with greater control? (a question about situations), and (2) Are happy people also people who experience more overall control? (a question about persons). Larson

(1989) demonstrates that for normal samples the answers to these two questions are quite different. Happy experiences are not strongly related with subjective control, but happy people *do* experience substantially greater average control. Failing to distinguish the two questions would have resulted in these two separate relations being blurred and probably in the findings being misinterpreted.

Example 2: Larson (1979; see also Csikszentmihalyi & Larson, 1984) provides another example of the difference between these two levels of analysis in his investigation of how time alone is related to affect among adolescents. Across all categories of teenagers in his sample the immediate experience of being alone was one of lower affect: they felt worse alone than at other times. From this finding one might expect that individuals who spent more time alone would report lower overall affect, but this was not the case. Among older adolescents, those who spent an intermediate amount of time alone (25 to 35% of waking hours) reported the highest average affect. Paradoxically, spending time in this *relative* negative context was related to higher, not lower, overall average mood states. Differentiation between the situation of being alone and the personal 'trait' of spending time alone was critical to understanding the underlying relationships.

From these examples it becomes clear that ill-defined questions may become a threat to the internal validity of an analysis. The conclusion that those adolescents who spent much time alone must feel worst because the overall sample shows lower affect when alone cannot be derived from the data and is therefore an error. We will use the term 'perspective fallacy' for the error of mixing up person- and situation-level questions in the wording of the research question, in the setting up of the analysis, or in the formulation of concluding comments. In the next section we will discuss how to analyze both questions about persons and questions about situations and show how the 'perspective fallacy' may easily be introduced in the actual setting up of the analysis.

Analyzing research questions

The research questions in ESM studies, both those about situations and those about persons, can be analyzed using two different configurations of data. One type of analysis uses the individual self-report, the 'beep', as the fundamental unit or case. The other uses the subject (the person) as the unit of analysis. The two types of analyses correspond to two types of datafiles, a beeper file and a subject file, which are described in the Appendix. We will adopt the term 'beep-level' to refer to analyses using the beep as the unit of analysis and 'subject-level' to statistical approaches using scores aggregated for each person or one-time subject measurements (e.g. age, diagnosis, sex ...) as the reference case in the analysis. Readers are warned not to confuse questions about situations and persons with analyses that use the beep or the subject as the unit of analysis. All four combinations of questions and analyses are considered below.

In general, beep-level analyses are simpler, more flexible and easier to understand and communicate than most of the subject level analysis. Subject level analyses are more complex due to both the (unexpected) effects of aggregating variables and the sophistication of the analysis, but typically provide a statistically more conservative test and reduce the probability of Type I errors. In the following section we will discuss and illustrate how we can approach the analysis of questions about situations and questions about persons respectively and show the possible strategies that are available for the most appropriate tests.

Analyzing questions about situations

Are people happier with their friends or families? How long does an anxiety episode last? In the following sections we will discuss how these kinds of questions about situations can be analyzed with a beep and a subject-level approach.

Beep-level analysis *Example 3*: Csikszentmihalyi & Larson (1984) used beep-level analysis to describe first, how normal adolescents, divide their day between different activities and second, how they feel in these activities. In these analyses the activities define the 'situation'. For the first one, the authors computed a frequency distribution on their Beeper-File for the variable 'Activity', which contained codes for what the teens were doing at the time of each signal. The frequency of these codes over all beeps ($N = 2734$) form a 'time-budget' for adolescents as a group and suggests that socializing is the most frequent activity for them. The authors did not compute significance figures for these percentages, but might have done so by computing confidence intervals based on the standard error of a percentage,[1] using analysis of variance on the z-scored version of their beeper file, with mood as the dependent variable and activity as the independent variable.[2] Positive scores point to feelings above the subjective average, while negative scores are below average moods. Because N was large for these analyses, the ANOVAs were

---

[1] $SE_\% = 100 \times (pq/N)^{\frac{1}{2}}$, with p being the proportion, q equal to 1-p and N the sample size. The Normal distribution fits this statistic so the confidence intervals are $p \pm 1.96 \times SE_\%$ (at 5%) or $p \pm 2.58 \times SE_\%$ (1%). The statistic is inadequate for extreme values and specially when N_p or N_q are less than 5 (Ferguson, 1959).

[2] The normalization process which is referred to as z-scoring in this chapter is computed by the formula $z_{ij} = (x_{ij} - X_i)/SD_i$ (with i the subject index, j the beep index within subject, x_{ij} the assessment of subject i at beep j, X_i the mean of subject i over all the beeps j and SD_i the standard deviation of subject i). The process is repeated for each subject and each item independently.

wildly significant. In order to provide a more specific test for each activity they computed whether the average state for each situation was significantly different from zero. These analyses revealed, among other things, that sport was one of the most positive experiences in the adolescents' lives (Table 5.1).

Other similar analyses on the daily experience of enjoyment are provided by Massimini et al. (1987) and on the experience of drug and alcohol use by Larson (1984).

Example 4: deVries et al. (1987) used beep-level analyses to examine the recovery of psychiatric patients from anxiety episodes. In order to do this they identified a subset of occasions in which anxiety was above $+1.00$ SD compared to the subjects' own mean. They then drew curves of the mean levels of anxiety on subsequent self-reports. These analyses demonstrate that the patients had a very slow rate of recovery from anxiety episodes, much slower than that of normal controls and, surprisingly, slower than their recovery from depressive episodes (Fig. 5.1). Procedures for evaluating the significance of these analyses are suggested by similar work carried out by Larson et al. (1980).

The most important criticism of beep-level analysis, particularly as employed in the second part of Example 3, is that it has an inflated N. The significance tests used assumed that all data points were independent, but in this case they were not, since the 2734 observations came from only 75 individuals. If signals occur close together in time, there may also be some interrelationship between adjacent reports (see Larson et al., 1980; Larson, 1987). Nonetheless, in certain circumstances violating this assumption is almost unavoidable and may represent the best possible presentation of the data. In such circumstances it is understood that the significance figures do not represent a strict Baysian test of probability, but rather provide a loose and probably inflated index of confidence. In some instances investigators in this situation will raise their P level to 0.01 to reduce the chance of Type I errors.

A related problem with beep-level analyses is that they give equal weight to all instances of a category of experience; thus those individuals who report that category more often will have more influence on the outcome. People who fill out more ESM sheets (who are in some cases the psychologically healthier subjects; Larson, 1989b) will also carry more weight. It is for this reason that z-scores are preferred for these analyses, because one does not want some small group of people with high or low means on a variable to exert an overwhelming influence (resulting in the perspective fallacy).

Using z-scores, however, can still leave additional problems. For example, if you are examining anxiety episodes, as in Example 4, those people who are anxious most often will contribute the most instances to the pool and thus carry more weight. In some instances this may be conceptually acceptable – we are interested in high anxiety people after all – in other instances it may be unavoidable. It would surely not be the first time that a significant group result

Table 5.1. *Mean z-score data by situation (Csikszentmihalyi & Larson, 1984)*

Activity	Freq.	Affect	Activa-tion	Concen-tration	Motiva-tion
Studying	346	−0.27***	−0.13**	0.49***	−0.44***
Eating	153	0.30***	0.06	−0.29***	0.45***
Rest & Napping	87	−0.59***	−1.37***	−0.94***	0.57***
Sports & Games	93	0.22**	0.80***	0.36***	0.48***
Art & Hobbies	41	−0.01	0.77***	0.61***	0.65***

*$P < 0.05$; **$P < 0.01$; ***$P < 0.001$.

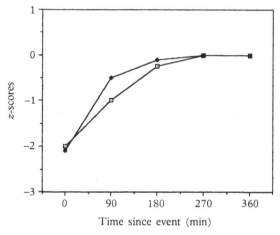

Fig. 5.1. Recovery from anxious (□) and depressive (◆) episodes in highly anxious patients (deVries et al., 1987).

is caused by a small number of subjects. At the least, one should check how many people have provided instances of the focal category, how many each has provided, and whether the number of instances is associated with the dependent variable of interest. Whenever possible, however, we recommend subject-level analysis.

Subject-level analysis In many cases the problems of inflated N, unequal weighting, and the danger of a perspective fallacy can be diminished by employing a subject-level analysis. This involves computing appropriate aggregate scores for each individual and analyzing these scores using the person as the unit of analysis.[3]

---

[3] However, see warning on aggregating data in the appendix.

Table 5.2. *Perceived interaction when with family and friends (Larson, 1983)*

Items	With family (mean mean)	With friends (mean mean)	t ($N = 73$)
Rating of self (1 to 7)			
Clear (vs. confused)	4.65	4.88	2.06*
Open (vs. closed)	4.58	5.13	4.65***
Free (vs. constrained)	4.70	5.14	3.87***
Ratings of the situation (1 to 6)			
Goals same (vs. different)	3.89	4.50	3.25**
Feedback positive (vs. negative)	4.42	4.94	3.57***
Talk joking (vs. serious)	3.34	4.04	5.35***
Mood (−12 to +12)			
Affect score	7.75	9.64	5.57***

*$P<0.05$; **$P<0.01$; ***$P<0.001$ (two tailed test of significance).

Example 5: Larson (1983) used this approach in evaluating whether adolescents' psychological states with friends are different from their states when they are with family members. Nearly all of the 75 subjects in his study reported at least one occasion of being with friends and being with family members. Thus, for each subject he computed a mean for each variable of interest for all times the subject was with each type of companion using the raw data.[4] Matched pair *t*-tests between these means revealed that when adolescents were with their friends they reported higher average ratings of affect, freedom, and openness than with their families (Table 5.2). Larson & Johnson (1985) used a similar approach in testing the moods of bulimics at home vs. at work vs. in public and deVries et al. (1987) did the same (using *z*-scores) for schizophrenics and anxiety subjects.

Example 6: In some cases an investigator develops a single coefficient that tests a specific situational hypothesis within each subject. A significance test is then performed to evaluate whether a significant majority of subjects confirm the hypothesis. Portegijs (1988) used this approach to evaluate whether the intensity of pain in 24 lower back pain subjects was related to time of day. He computed correlations between time of day and ESM reports of pain for each

[4] Larson's approach in this analysis controls for individual differences in the mean (because it used a matched pair *t*-test), but fails to control for individual differences in variance – which would be controlled had *z*-scores been used. The latter approach (norming by variance using *z*-scores), however, is also criticizable because we can prove that: $x_a - x_b \neq z_a - z_b$. As a consequence the choice option is not arbitrary. It is up to the researcher to make this choice consciously.

person. Using a *t*-test he then found that the mean of these 24 correlations was significantly below zero, indicating, contrary to Folkard (1976), that pain diminishes across the day. In another use of this approach Larson et al. (1982) simply counted the number of people showing one trend vs. another (whether a given activity was more frequent when alone or with people) and tested these counts against chance using a sign test. We think these simple descriptors are underused.

Subject-level significance tests are conservative tests and tread on fewer statistical assumptions. Because the individual is used as the unit of analysis, the assumption of independence is not violated, as it is in the beep-level analysis. Therefore, we should try whenever possible to aggregate the situational information to a one score per subject datum. This requires creativity and can cause some consternation before the database is fitted for analysis, but it is worth the trouble because person-level tests that can be used then meet basic statistical assumptions. They will be more persuasive when significance is found.

From this it must be clear that whenever possible, the subject-level analyses are preferred above the beep-level approach.[5] Unfortunately, subject-level significance tests are not foolproof and different possible pitfalls can be discussed for them.

It can be argued that aggregating data to the subject level squanders the repeated measurements, increasing the probability of Type II errors in which a true relationship is not detected. Folkard (1976) showed that the increment of pain by time of day is linked to the diurnal variation in body temperature. This, however, is a correlational observation. Environmental changes with a daily pattern such as 'being alone'-frequencies, which are lower in the evening, may also cause these differences. The adequate analysis of environmental effects on experience must therefore necessarily be conducted on the residual data after fitting a diurnal model upon the data. Techniques for these analyses are described by Gottman (1981).

The next possible problem is related to the actual computing of the aggregated scores at the subject level and here both authors take different stands. The second author and others in the Maastricht group commonly set a minimum limit on the number of data points required to compute a summary score for an individual (e.g., a person must be alone at least five times in order to compute a mean for alone time). The argument is that a mean based on one or two self-reports is not a very reliable estimate of that person's true value. The first author, however, argues that this is not important since the issue of confidence in a relationship is addressed by the significance test. He further

---

[5] cfr. comment on MANOVA's.

points out that setting such a minimum may exclude many individuals and lead to the test being conducted on a biased subsample (e.g., people who are alone more often). In part this difference in opinion reflects our respective research backgrounds. The first author, primarily identified with developmental and social-psychological research, is concerned with revealing trends that characterize broad populations, while the second author, primarily a clinical researcher, must be much more attentive to individual variations that may be of clinical relevance.

This bone of contention identifies the major restriction on use of subject-level analysis – they require that a substantial number of participants have one or preferably more moments where they report the target categories of experience. In an analysis of relatively rare behaviours (e.g., using drugs, riding in a car), this may not be the case and beep-level analysis may be the best you can do. This restriction becomes particularly severe when you are interested in making comparisons across three or more situations using a MANOVA model. These statistical techniques do not tolerate missing data, yet it is likely that few individuals will have enough in each situation to compute a mean.[6] Again, in such circumstances, unless one can invent a plausible algorithm for substituting missing data, one may have to settle for a beep-level analysis, with accompanying exploratory analyses to be certain that differences found are not an artifact of a person-level variable.

It might be noted that subject-level analyses dealing with percentages also run into severe problems if the category of interest is relatively rare (for example if you are interested in the amount of time spent talking to a parent vs. a spouse). Because the great majority of people will have no instances of these categories, the researcher will be left with skewed distributions in which nearly everyone has observed frequencies in those situations of zero per cent. Making things even worse, demographic correlating variables may cause these differences.

This brings us to our final problem, one that applies to all analyses of situation-level questions (and to all ecological research!): the possibility that an apparent relationship is actually the result of some third variable. In particular, it would be embarrassing and unconscionable if that third variable were something that was measured in the study. Hence, in Example 5, one might wonder whether the higher moods reported with friends might really be due to the fact that the subjects play sports more often when with them, which in Example 3 was reported to be a high affect activity. Or perhaps it is due to the time of day or the environments in which interactions with friends take place.

Unfortunately, it is generally not feasible to create an analysis of variance

---

[6] The authors have typically worked with data sets with 30 to 50 time samples per person. Many of the difficulties identified here with subject level analyses of situations would be much less acute were it possible to obtain more data points per person.

that evaluates all of these independent variables simultaneously (because the time samples are not randomly distributed across all combinations of situational variables and the ANOVA is likely to be defeated by many poorly filled and empty cells).

The best one can usually do when confronted with such a complex data base is to design alternative analyses and examine competing explanations for the finding on an ad hoc basis. For example, one could compare states with family members on an activity-by-activity basis, at least for those activities that are done and reported both with family and friends. Csikzentmihalyi & Larson (1984) found that such analyses supported the integrity of the original finding. This is the point at which creative worry and discussion with colleagues is useful and may lead you to a deeper and more complex understanding of the true relationships. It was only after much thought that the second author and colleagues realized that their counterintuitive finding – that agoraphobics feel best outside their homes – may be due to the fact that these patients only leave home when they feel good. To decide how, finally, to present your data, you may end up trying several different approaches, beep-level and person-level analysis, using z-scores and raw scores, splitting up the database to conduct independent analysis, and attempting to control for various variables. Losing significance in seemingly parallel set-ups should always be considered an important signal. The decision rests on which approach most satisfactorily presents the underlying pattern in the data. In some cases one may find it necessary to present the results of two or more different approaches to express the pattern.

Analyzing questions about persons

Questions about persons can also be analyzed using beep- or person-level data. Again we will show that the person-level approach is preferable and provides a more persuasive presentation of the data, but there may be occasions when beep-level analysis is the method of choice, especially whenever low frequency events or situations are the focus.

Beep-level analysis *Example 7*: deVries et al. (1986) compared the psychological states of chronic psychiatric patients and normal controls in relation to the number of persons in the environment at the moment of the beep. They used the z-score Beeper File in order to control for between-subject differences in overall means and standard deviations. Analyses showed that the schizophrenics reported the most positive states when in small company (two persons present), while for normals there was a progressive improvement in state with additional companions up to a maximum of four, with stabilization above this.

deVries & Delespaul (1988) replicated the study at the subject level but encountered difficulties computing mean scores for larger social situations because of the restricted environment in which ambulatory chronic mental patients live. The differentiation of companionship at the moment of the beep was almost impossible at a level higher than three people, because of the small number of observations in each cell.

Example 8: In a special journal issue Larson & Richards (1989), and colleagues, were interested in describing the changing time-use patterns associated with the transition years from childhood into adolescence. Their primary interest was in comparing the percentage of time pre-adolescents and adolescents spend in a variety of contexts. A large sample size ($N = 483$ people, 18,022 time samples) allowed them to look at a wide range of contexts, including contexts that occurred quite rarely, for example, watching different categories of TV shows. The rarity of these contexts, however, made subject-level analyses difficult for reasons discussed above. While some of the analyses might have been performed at a person level, the investigators decided for consistency to do all analyses at the beeper level. Fig. 5.2 shows an analysis from an article by Raffaelli & Duckett (1989) that shows a dramatic increase in the amount of time girls spend talking over this age period.

All of the limitations of beep-level analyses discussed on pp. 64–5 apply here as well, so this discussion is primarily a recapitulation of the previous one. N's are inflated, so statistical tests do not provide a precise representation of probabilities. There is a danger that certain subgroups of individuals may exert unequal weight in determining specific values. Nonetheless, particularly in instances when one is concerned with relatively rarely occurring categories of

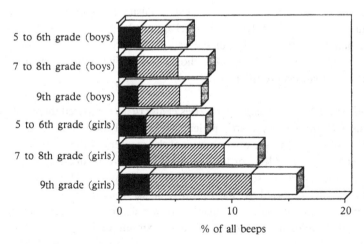

Fig. 5.2. Age differences in 'Who young adolescents talk with' (Raffaelli & Duckett, 1989), ■, family; ▨, friends; □, others.

experience, this approach may be the only possible one. In this situation the data must be analyzed with appropriate extensive checks for possible confounds.

Subject-level analysis   Example 9: The most common type of analysis at this level is comparison of groups in terms of average subjective states, variance in states, or the percentage of time spent in a specific context. Delespaul & deVries (1987) computed the mean mood states for each subject in a sample of chronic psychiatric patients and a sample of normal controls. They then computed a simple *t*-test between the sets of means and found that the psychiatric subjects differed significantly from the normal controls in their average subjective state (Table 5.3).

This procedure was then repeated for the difference of mean *t*-scores across a set of dichotomized situations (alone/not alone and home/not home). Difference scores were not significantly higher in schizophrenics than in normals but the absolute value of this difference was. The authors concluded that patients are more reactive than normals to different aspects of the environment (Table 5.4).

Johnson & Larson (1982) provide a similar comparison of the average and the standard deviations of psychological states experienced by bulimics vs. normals.

One criticism sometimes expressed of these types of comparisons for subjective ratings is that they merely measure differences in response sets – in how different groups use the items. In this case observed differences are considered habitual narratives of individuals. Larson & Lampman-Petraitis (1989) circumvented this criticism by having participants use the ESM scales to rate emotions in a standard set of faces and were able to demonstrate that the group differences they found in the ESM reports were not replicated in the ratings of faces, indicating that response set could not have caused the differences.

The response set issue can also be avoided when one is comparing people in terms of their states in a specific context. By evaluating people's mean *z*-scores in a context (instead of their mean raw scores), one can determine whether states in that context differ between two groups – relative to the subjects' respective normative states. In some cases, however, use of mean raw scores is preferable (see for example, Larson & Asmussen, in this book).

Example 10: In a very creative use of ESM data, Graef, Gianinno & Csikszentmihalyi (1981) used each person's reports on their daily activities to estimate how much energy each person consumed in daily life. Activities such as daydreaming and socializing use little gas and electricity, according to data from other investigators; media use and shopping use more. Their curious finding – one provocative from a philosophical standpoint – is that there was an inverse correlation between this estimate of energy use by women and their

Table 5.3. *Between group statistics (Delespaul & deVries, 1987)*

Item group	Schizophrenia (N = 9)	Normals (N = 11)	t-statistic
Thoughts	4.33 (0.85)	5.14 (0.70)	$t(18) = -3.10$ $P<0.01$
Mood	4.47 (0.95)	6.27 (0.37)	$t(18) = -5.76$ $P<0.001$

Table 5.4. *Difference in alone/not alone mental state (Delespaul & deVries, 1987)*

Item group	Schizophrenia (N = 9)	Normals (N = 11)	t-statistic
Thoughts	0.46 (0.13)	0.30 (0.24)	$t(18) = -1.74$ $P<0.05$
Mood	0.53 (0.44)	0.08 (0.07)	$t(18) = -3.31$ $P<0.005$

average happiness on the ESM sheets. Women who used more energy were less happy.

Clearly these subject level analyses are powerful and convincing in answering questions about persons. Nonetheless, there are potential problems. As we have said before, care should be taken to avoid confounds, and we propose never to carry out subject analysis without concurrent testing of competing hypotheses.

Confound variables are a constant threat to all kinds of studies, even those using control or contrast groups. In studies of the influence of context on psychopathology we are faced with the fact that mental illness is always related with a set of co-occurring life style differences. For example, a higher proportion of sick people are unemployed and unmarried; unemployment has direct repercussion on the time spent at home, and being married influences the alone time significantly; both in turn are likely to be related with average moods. While one cannot separate these variables using the classical experimental approach of random assignment, attempts to decompose these relations are essential to understanding differences in how groups spend their time and how they feel in different contexts. As was illustrated in Example 2, and in the chapter by Larson & Asmussen (this book), an overall pattern of time use of mean moods may mask important situational differences or similarities. The only way to deal with these possible threats is to challenge one's conclusions constantly – think about them in the shower, present them to colleagues, discuss them with your research subjects.

The second limitation is related to the issue of response set discussed under Example 9 above. Data derived from the anxiety research (Dijkman & deVries, 1987) suggest that the way subjects perceive themselves and the surrounding world may influence their responses in clinical interviews and on one-time questionnaires. In these data-collecting situations subjects seem to present their individual 'stories'. We often get other responses when the same questions are asked repeatedly and linked to a real natural situation as in ESM. Another process seems to regulate the formulation by the subjects of ESM answers although it is difficult to understand how this should work, considering that the ESM assessment form often mirrors traditional questionnaires.

No control situation exists to test the validity of experiential assessments in natural environments. Response sets can partly be ruled out by methods as described in Example 9. Other, indirect approaches have to be used but most of them are handicapped by the fundamental difference between moment-to-moment experience and retrospection. In this situation also, the creative design of alternative evaluating strategies and search for confluence of results is the method of choice to circumvent possible pitfalls.

Interpreting results

Good questions and optimal analysis are easily destroyed by poor discussions. A straightforward explanation for the finding in Example 10 is that less-happy people use more energy, perhaps as an attempt to compensate for a lack of personal energy. It is also possible, however, that people who use a lot of energy may have more free time than others, perhaps as a result of lower employment, and this may influence the findings. Hence jumping to the conclusion that energy use does not serve people's happiness may blur the real relationship, an error which these authors carefully avoid.

The discussion part of papers presenting results derived from ecological datasets is usually the moment for free speculation. That is what discussions are for, you may say, but this does not mean that the above-mentioned possible pitfalls should not be considered carefully. As we stated repeatedly ecological datasets can be described, sometimes interpreted but almost never fully understood. We advise some humbleness in summarizing the data and caution in the projection of the utility. We advise authors to carry out an open discussion of rival interpretations, the description of discussions with colleagues, as well as the projection of future research lines with better controls of possible intervening variables.

Final comments

After hearing about all the possible confounds in the ESM analysis, you may easily be seduced into thinking that more advanced statistics might be better for these data – that some complex multivariate design will allow you to control for the whole world of confounding variables at once and test person and situation effects simultaneously. We would like to warn against this fantasy, because even skilled statisticians will probably fall back in lethargy when they have to conclude that most of the premises of the tests they want to use are not met. We advise investigators to start with these basic descriptive statistic techniques, because their robustness is well known and findings closer to the original data are more easily understood. Most ESM questions can be translated into a set of alternative operationalizations, sometimes leading to divergent results. Our advice is to select multiple approaches when possible and look for results that converge upon the same conclusion.

Nothing can replace the basic process, supported with elementary statistics, of looking at the data and getting a feel for it. Writing out and submitting case studies should also not be neglected. After doing these simpler steps it may be possible to explore the new horizons of the sophisticated statistical techniques. Remember though that statistical procedures, after all, are a means not an end.

Appendix to Chapter 5

The fundamental data of the ESM are a set of hundreds (or thousands) of self-reports obtained from participants at random times. For each self-report one will have a small number of variables on context, moods, thoughts – whatever questions have been asked on the ESM self-report form (the ESF). Along with these data one typically has information on the 10, 50, or 200 participants who were in the study. This information will include at least their ages and sexes, but probably also some questionnaire or interview data obtained before or after the period of paging; in some cases one may also have data from school or medical records, from teachers, nurses, parents or other sources. These two types of data, the beeper data and the data on one's subjects, correspond to the two types of computer files one will want to create to store and organize one's data. The first is commonly called a 'Beeper File'; the second is commonly called a 'Subject File'.

The beeper file

In the beeper file the individual self-report or ESF is the unit of organization, what in SPSSX or SAS is referred to as the 'case'. Typically all of the information on the self-report form comprises only 30 to 50 variables and fits on to one 80-character computerline. But since there are hundreds or thousands of self-reports, some dozens for each subject, this file typically contains many, many lines (see Fig. 5.A1).

In this file the person is not the significant unit of organization, but one needs to include the subject ID number as a variable in order to have it available. Note that the number of cases per person will vary, since some people will have responded to the beeper more often than others. We also recommend that you create a variable that identifies the order in which each person filled out his or her beeper sheets – the 'page number' – should you decide to do any sequential analysis. In the Maastricht database the page number is substituted for a day counter and a within-day counter because the night is considered as an important break in the continuity of the data sequence. You may also wish to repeat two or three of the most fundamental subject variables (e.g., sex, age, diagnostic group) on each case.

Typically we create a 'z-score' version of the beeper file. In this file all the continuous variables have been standardized to remove differences between individuals in how they responded to each item. These z-scores are created by subtracting the subject's overall mean for the item and then dividing by the subject's standard deviation. In SAS you use PROC STANDARD; in SPSSX you use CONDESCRIPTIVES (now called DESCRIPTIVES) preceded by SORT CASES BY ID and temporary SPLIT FILE BY ID commands.[7] The

---

[7] Spot-checking these computations is important. The first author has found instances when SPSSX mishandles cases when a person has no variance.

Record j	field 1	..	field 2	...		...	field i	...		...	field n	

with:
    Subject Identification Part
    field 1   Subject ID
    field 2   Subject File data   optional
    ...

    Beep Identification Part
    field ...   Beep Sequence Number (day/beep)
    field   Date
    field   Beep time
    field   Answering time   optional
    Beep Experiential data
    field   e.g. happiness rating   customized to study...
    ...

    Beep Situational data
    field   e.g. activity, companionship,...customized to study...
    ...

Fig. 5.A1. Typical field structure of a beep file record.

z-score file provides a file in which variance due to subject main effects have been removed; thus it allows one to make comparisons *within* individuals on a scale where values are relative to each person's distribution for that particular item. z-scores, however, are no panacea and may be mislead by introducing spurious variability in the data, e.g., when the subject's SD is small, deviation from the mean will be blown out and may cause unwanted significances.

Rarely, if ever, would we recommend that final analysis of mood data be carried out on the raw beeper file alone. The values on this file are affected both by person-level and moment-level sources of variance; thus any simple analysis leads one into the perspective fallacy discussed in Example 1. A common example of this mistake that can be avoided using z-scored data, is the factor analysis of the beeper file with the objective of simplifying a set of mood variables to a smaller number of factors. The problem when done on raw data is that one does not know whether the factors obtained represent qualities of people or qualities of moments or situations.

The subject file

In the subject file the individual subject is the unit of organization or the 'case' (see Fig. 5.A2). Since you probably have relatively few subjects, but much information on each one, this file – in contrast to the beeper file – is likely to be short and fat. In fact we are going to suggest making it a lot fatter in a moment and you may even decide that you need to have several subject files, indexed by subject ID. The initial data on the subject file will include all of your demographic data on the participants, questionnaire and interview data, and information from archives or from other sources. In addition to these you probably want to add various ESM summary variables, computed from the beeper file, that describe the typical experience of each subject.

ESM summary variables can be computed on an ad hoc basis, as needed, but you will find it useful (and cheaper) to generate a standard skeleton of

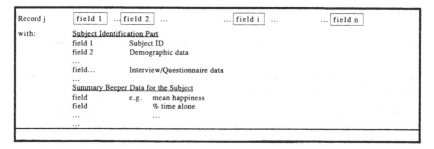

Fig. 5.A2. Typical field structure of a subject file record.

summary variables that you anticipate using again and again. These might include each person's mean score for each ESM scaled item, the standard deviation for these items, the percentage of time the person is alone, with family members, and with friends, and the percentage of time he or she is engaged in various activities, thinks various categories of thought, or experiences various extreme emotional states. These might also include the person's mean states in certain contexts (e.g., alone, with family, with friends); typically the first author stores the raw values of these contextual means, but frequently converts them, when necessary, to mean z-scores by using the overall means and overall standard deviations available on this file.

Basically, you need to decide what the key variables are likely to be for your project – and be prepared to create more as your understanding of the data set matures. We recommend extreme care and ample discussion with colleagues before selecting aggregated data for analysis. Seemingly harmless conversions may have unexpected consequences for the analysis. In this case also we advise not to trust one summary score but design different ones that should give the same results in the analysis. When divergence is found it should be interpreted in relation to the summary procedure used, e.g., summary z-scores of experience in situations will reach 0.00 when the frequency of the situation is high.

These summary scores are computed from your beeper file. In SPSSX one can use the procedure AGGREGATE and in SAS the procedure PROC SUMMARY. Subject ID is used as the BREAK or BY variable. The output file created by these procedures is then merged with your subject file using ID as the matching variable and the enlarged subject file is saved for future use. As with all file manipulations, investigators are warned that they must check and double check all these computations by listing out data before and after the manipulations. Numerous horror stories could be told at this point about people who created files that seemed right, but months later were discovered to be wrong, requiring computer runs to be redone and findings to be rethought.

Additional variations

In addition to a beeper file and a subject file a particular investigator may require a file organized by some other unit. Mayers (1978) was interested in investigating high school students' experience in different school classes, and therefore organized a file in which the classes for each person were the fundamental case – with the ESM data aggregated using ID and class as the break variables. Increasingly investigators are having ESM participants fill out diary reports at the end of each day. This leads to the creation of files in which the day is the case and the unit of analysis. It is also conceivable that investigators may find it useful to create files in which a specific episode (a drinking binge or a stressful event) defines a sequence of ESM sheets and becomes the unit of organization, though often these analyses can be carried out on the beeper file.

The organization of data is the key to analysis of ESM data since the type of analysis follows directly from the file organization. Given a choice between hiring a research assistant with talents in data management or statistical analysis we highly recommend the former.

Table 5.1 is modified from the one appearing in *Being Adolescent: Conflict and Growth in the Teenage Years* by M. Csikszentmihalyi and Reed Larson. Copyright © 1984 by Basic Books, Inc. By permission of Basic Books, Inc., Publishers, New York.

Figure 5.2 appeared in M. Raffeilli & E. Duckett's article in *Journal of Youth and Adolescence*, 1989, **18**, 6, 567–82.

Table 5.2 appeared in R. Larson, Adolescents' daily experience with family and friends: contrasting opportunity systems, *Journal of Marriage and the Family*, 1983, **45**, 739–50.

6

States, syndromes, and polythetic classes: developing a classification system for ESM data using the 'ascending' and cross-classification method[1]

KARL M. VAN METER,
MARTEN W. deVRIES, CHARLES D. KAPLAN
and CHANTAL I.M. DIJKMAN-CAES

Introduction

A universal problem encountered in all social, medical and behavioral science research is the coherent and rational operationalization of the formal and conceptual categories that have been elaborated through previous work. This intrinsic problem is compounded by the equally universal one of the difficulty of communicating and comparing scientific research results from different disciplines, as well as from different cultures, languages or nations. The World Health Organization for instance has clearly stressed the chronic difficulty in securing any common rubric for a disease diagnosis that involves biological, psychological and sociological considerations (WHO, 1981). The universality of these problems implies the corollary that progress in a particular domain may lead to progress in all domains of social and behavioral science research. In this chapter we will illustrate a new cross-classification approach (van Meter, 1986) using psychiatric and drug abuse data obtained by a new method of evaluating illness behavior and experience, the Experience Sampling Method (ESM) (deVries, 1987; Csikszentmihalyi & Larson, 1984).

Syndromes, classifications and models

Today, although recommendations are often made to refine classification and diagnostic systems by including syndromes, patterns and models, it is the underlying difficulty of operationalizing and executing such revisions that often blocks the implementation in research that would lead to the creation of a new system. Much confusion and error are also introduced by the way terms are generally employed. For example, classification and diagnoses are often coupled and presented as interchangeable or equivalent while in fact they are

[1] This work appeared in *Bulletin de Méthodologie Sociologique*, no. 15, 1987, pp. 22–38.

different processes. Further, terms such as syndromes, patterns, models and variables are used loosely, adding to the difficulty in implementing further research. The processes involved and the qualitative aspects of disorders are also often left ill-defined.

For example, clustering entities of different intensities into one or more syndromes by using multiple criteria is obviously a notion that generates operational problems. The definition of a syndrome offered by the WHO is helpful but quite general. It is defined as 'the clustering of phenomena so that not all the components need always be present or not always be present in the same intensity' (WHO, 1981). Although class is not mentioned in the definition of syndrome, the association syndrome-classification permits us to describe a syndrome as a class of entities (separate incidents, individuals, cases, states, etc.) that are described by variables and grouped together in a class on the basis only of the values taken by those variables. This, in turn, allows us to make a clear distinction between a syndrome and a model. A model is an attempt to explain course, initiation, continuation and discontinuation of a phenomenon which must represent the dynamic relationship between sets of variables and their interactions. Thus, a model must furnish an explanatory schema of the intervening factors that generate the perceived syndromes and the distribution of the entire population of entities under consideration.

A syndrome thus necessitates a certain form of classification and can be the embodiment of a model of the phenomena under investigation. The definition of syndrome implies that it would correspond to a class in a classification, instead of corresponding to an entire classification. This, in turn, implies that a model includes several syndromes or classes and that it is compatible with a certain classification of the phenomena. Using these conceptual principles, let us proceed further.

Classifications and models

The analysis and classification of research data need not be carried out without previously formalizing explicitly the relations, functions or operations that we suppose are active in producing and structuring the data. The term 'exploratory data analysis' is the more accentuated form of such analysis. It is usually portrayed as opposed to 'confirmatory data analysis', though both these terms are vague enough that they generate many problems when one attempts to apply them concretely.

The result of data analysis is a certain form of organization that is equivalent to a certain form of concentration or condensation of the original data. The form of organization can be, for example, a collection of polythetic classes, as described below, or a log-linear equation. The former provides a schema and the latter a mechanism. Inversely, the polythetic class does not provide a mechanism that can be 'fitted' to the data and the latter does not provide a schema for organizing the data. Both analyze the data but the former attempts to provide a pertinent or even essential organization of the data, while the latter attempts to provide a pertinent or even essential mechanism for generating the data.

Therefore, we can define a model as a formalized and coherent mechanism, precise enough to imply unambiguously a specific operationalization, that generates 'sufficiently well' the data under consideration. The term 'sufficiently well' refers to the adjustment between precision, tolerance or error in the specification of the initial experimental conditions and the precision, tolerance or error in the implied results. The determination of what is 'sufficiently well' lies within the particular domain of research and the particular community of researchers involved.

The independence but coherent parallelism between a model for a phenomenon and the analysis of data on the phenomenon are rendered explicit with this definition of a model. A model can imply a certain type of organization of observable data. A coherent data analysis (an analysis whose internal mechanisms do not conflict with those hypothesized by the mechanism of the model) should result in an organization of the data that is 'sufficiently well' adjusted to that implied by the model. Inversely, the resultant organization of observed data by a form of data analysis can suggest certain, often several, compatible models that could engender the given data.

The above terms of 'sufficiently well adjusted' and 'suggest certain compatible . . . ' reveal the approximate nature of the reciprocal implication between analysis and model. This approximate nature is very likely the source of the problems concerning the rejection of a model by (the analysis of) a certain experiment. Inversely, to say that a particular model is the only model possible for a phenomenon is to say that there is a necessary or logical implication between the model and all possibly compatible forms of analysis, and that all these forms of analysis suggest one and only one compatible model. This has never proven to be the case, for very long, in any field of science.

This coherent parallelism implies not only that models can be the basis for and inspire new analyses, but that analysis can be the basis for and inspire new models, without either a model or an analysis proving the other to be incompatible or 'wrong'. Indeed, this mutual inspiration between models and analysis evolving under the persistent insistence upon coherence, compatibility, and being 'sufficiently well adjusted', is very likely the source of most scientific knowledge and development.

Ascending and descending methodologies

Recent studies of 'hidden subpopulations' using traditional sociological research methods have revealed a distinction between ascending methodologies adapted to the study of small or local populations and descending methodologies adapted to general populations. Data intensive sampling and hierarchically ascending classification analysis, and its more advanced form of cross-classification analysis, together form a coherent and rigorous ascending methodology for studying hidden or specific subpopulations. Their problems with the calculation of general population characteristics and the explanation of variance have been the subject of recent research. Through the complementary combination of ascending and descending methodologies, this recent work has largely resolved these problems and provided both a formal and an operational tie between these two methodologies.

Implicit in the minds of most social and behavioral science researchers is an association, on the one hand, between the problem of studying social groups or types of social behavior that are not accessible by established means of sociological research ('hidden populations'), and, on the other hand, the use of research methodologies based on intensive, detailed, data collection strategies ('snowball sampling', 'experience sampling', 'life histories') and their associated methods of analysis ('qualitative research designs'). Explicitly, this identifies 'established means of sociological research' with large-scale representative surveys ('quantitative research') and opposes them to 'qualitative' counterparts. Though the problem of studying hidden populations is real, as is the adequacy of intensive data collection strategies for studying hidden populations, the opposition 'qualitative' – 'quantitative' is far more a social product of institutional conflict than a formalized mathematical reality (Combessie, 1985; Wilson, 1986). Indeed, most social researchers have abandoned this opposition while acknowledging and adapting the complementary nature of these different methodologies (Combessie, 1986).

But the difficulty of studying hidden populations does reveal an opposition between extensive survey methodologies and intensive data collection methodologies. This opposition distinguishes between what we have called DESCENDING METHODOLOGY and ASCENDING METHODOLOGY (van Meter, 1985; DSP, 1986; Kaplan et al., 1987). This opposition can be found both in data collection and in methods of statistical analysis. Descending methodology involves strategies elaborated and executed at the level of general populations. They therefore necessitate highly standardized questionnaires and rigorous population samples, and, for historic and economic reasons more than methodological considerations, usually involve traditional statistical analysis. This methodology has been typically used by national governments in order to make statistical inferences and decide future social policy. The strict scientific rigor of this methodology, even in its most exemplary use, can be easily criticized (Guttman, 1984), but this does not reduce the usefulness of its results. However, there are problems and hidden populations are probably the most important there are for descending methodologies.

Ascending methodologies involve research strategies elaborated at a community or local level and specifically adapted to the study of selected social groups; for example, a hidden population. In order to be efficient, the means of data collection are usually selective and intensive. Snowball sampling, experience sampling, life histories and ethnographic monographs are typical forms of data collection in ascending methodology. Methods of analysis in this type of methodology must also be adapted to the specific form of data furnished and also to the specific objectives of the research. Typical forms of ascending data analysis are social network analysis and classification analysis, often called 'cluster' analysis.

But the specific adaptation of ascending methodology is not obtained without the loss of easy generalizability. In exchange, descending methodology cannot reach hidden populations without specific adaptations. Indeed, that is exactly what the President's Commission on Organized Crime (PCOC, 1986, p. 340) was proposing when it recommended 'oversampling' high school dropouts and people without residence in the National Institute on Drug Abuse (NIDA) annual High School Senior Survey and biannual Household Survey of drug use. Similarly, ascending methodology, such as network analysis, can be employed in the study of large populations, though at great material cost and with rigorous standardization; the best example is Joel H. Levine's *Atlas of Corporate Interlocks* that covers the entire world population of corporations (Levine, 1988).

Polythetic and monothetic classes

It is astonishing that in spite of the high quality intellectual effort invested in this field, experts have managed to touch upon the question of classification analysis without clearly developing further research in this field. It is often assumed that the difficulties of clarifying 'cut-off points' and delimiting syndromes must be worked out in the practice of classifying. In clear language, the problems of operationalization could (will) be worked out in the process of classification. This ignores an abundant scientific literature on the question in the domain of classification analysis.

From this literature, we take the concept of a monothetic class A which is defined as a subset of entities x such that each entity, member of A, written $x \in A$, has a specific characteristic V, written $V(x)$ or x satisfies V. Moreover, if x does not satisfy V, written $-V(x)$, then x is not of member of A, $x \notin A$. Also if $V(x)$, then $x \in A$. Thus $x \in A \longleftrightarrow V(x)$; x is a member of A if and only if x satisfies V. For example, the subset A of male respondents in a survey is a monothetic class. If $x \in A$, then x is male, and if x does not belong to A, then x is female.

A polythetic class B is a subset of entities y such that $y \in B$ implies that y satisfies an important but unspecified number n of characteristics, $VB=(V1, V2, \ldots, Vn, Vn+1, \ldots Vb)$, associated specifically with class B. This does not mean that if $z \in B$, then automatically z will satisfy any specifically chosen $V \in VB$. It also means that if z satisfies all $V \in VB$, z is not necessarily a member of B.

It is clear that this formal definition of a polythetic class is the generalization of that given below for a Weberian ideal type and also that given above for a syndrome.

Those methods of classification analysis that are hierarchically ascending, formally construct polythetic classes. Hierarchically ascending means that resemblance between entities is used to form classes of those entities which resemble each other the most. Therefore, the first classes formed are composed of those entities which resemble each other the most. The later the class is formed, that is to say the higher in the hierarchy, the less its member entities will resemble each other. See the hierarchy or tree of classifications in Fig. 6.1. This also means that for hierarchically ascending methods, each level in a tree of classifications corresponds to a particular and distinct classification of the entire population under investigation and with successively fewer but larger classes of entities. The final classification or level, of course, is composed of one unique class including the entire population.

A specific type of hierarchically ascending classification analysis, called automatic classification (Lerman, 1981), allows the application of minimal criteria which permit a formal systematic means of reducing or summarizing the often considerable list of variables or dimensions involved in classification analysis. In automatic classification analysis, proximity between entities or subjects analyzed is measured by a similarity indice calculated over all variables taken into consideration (Prod'homme et al., 1983). It allows us to construct classes based on the 'maximum likelihood of association' ('vraisemblance de lien' in French) between two subjects that emphasizes the resemblance between two classes more than the distance that separates each of them from nearby large classes of subjects (SAS, 1985).

The classifications based on inter-subject resemblance are then arranged in an ordered hierarchy or tree by this method which also establishes, for each level of the hierarchy, the statistical probability or likelihood of the occurrence of that particular classification, given the original null hypothesis that all characteristics are normally distributed. The evolution of this local statistic, associated with each level of the hierarchy of classifications or classification tree, permits the identification of local minima where improbable and therefore significant classifications are situated. By this means, one can identify within the successive classifications the more significant groups of subjects or nodes which, by their construction, form polythetic classes. Moreover, this same process reveals the development and evolution of such significant groups throughout the hierarchical tree of classifications, starting with the first and most detailed classification (each subject constitutes his or her own individual

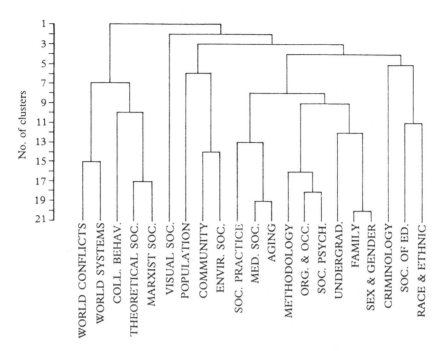

Fig. 6.1. An example of ascending hierarchical clustering.

class) and extending all the way to the final and roughest classification (everyone in one single class).

Cross-classification analysis is the Cartesian crossing of two automatic classification analyses of the same data. It reorganizes a two-dimensional data set (subjects by variables) by projecting on to the set the results of an automatic classification analysis of the individuals (or rows of figures) and of the descriptive variables (or columns of figures) as can be seen in Fig. 6.2.

In this manner, all initial data can be directly presented along with the organization due to the cross-classification analysis, thus permitting comparative or critical analysis of the same data. This method was employed in order to find the significant nodes or polythetic classes mentioned in the preceding paragraph, and also in order to extend in an unlimited fashion the application of classification analysis to any finite population, no matter how large (Faugeron & van Meter, 1987).

This latter result is of a certain significance due to the fact that classification analysis of large data sets has been inhibited up until now by its heavy requirements in computer time and memory capacity. Furthermore, the groups or units of individuals/variables found by cross-classification analysis met the same criteria as the blocks obtained by block modeling methods in social

ITEMS

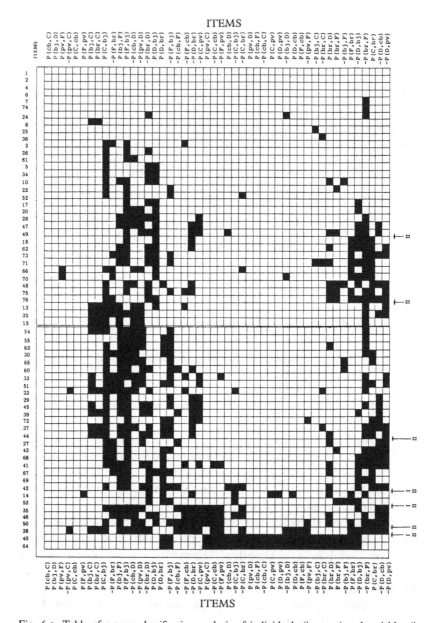

ITEMS

Fig. 6.2. Table of a cross-classification analysis of individuals (in rows) and variables (in columns). This data set includes all experimental data from a genetic psychology experiment with children between the ages of three and six years. Roman numerals I and II indicate the levels of the significance classes and, respectively, second most significant levels of the classification analysis of the individuals. Note the formation of blocks of individuals/variables which are either mostly black, mostly white, or an aleatory mixture of white and black.

network analysis (van Meter, 1986) and is the methodological basis for an ongoing sociological survey of cocaine use (Kaplan et al., 1985).

These groups of individuals/variables are of course polythetic classes and are rather stable units of analysis. This stability allows the construction of classification grids that characterize the subset of variables for each group. This stability also permits the use of these groups in further cross-classification analyses where the initial results concerning a 'state' of behavior (the initial blocks of individuals/variables) are then submitted to a cross-classification analysis over a certain period in time. Thus, one can construct a polythetic class corresponding to a 'syndrome' which would be a stable block generated by the cross-classification analysis of individual 'states' crossed with chronological time. In turn, the individual 'states' will have resulted from an initial cross-classification analysis of individuals crossed with descriptive variables. This particular adaptation of cross-classification analysis forms the methodological basis of current research that employs the Experience Sampling technique of gathering repeated measurements of behavior and mental state at randomly selected moments in the daily life of an individual. ES studies of anxiety and drug abuse will be used here to illustrate the polythetic cross-classification technique.

The experience sampling of anxiety disorders and drug craving: some working hypotheses

In the biological and behavioral sciences, supplementary methods have been developed that have provided a deeper understanding of the fundamental features of mental disorders. To a large extent, these advances have relied on the creative use of technology, producing methods ranging from CAT and NMR scans in neuropsychiatry to new electronic ambulatory signaling devices, currently used in the behavioral sciences for the study of subjects in their natural settings, such as for ESM.

The ESM techniques have not yet been tested to determine what they have to offer in terms of reclassifying mental disorders. They have been experimental. The challenge to these new techniques that provide repeated measures of a mental state within the real time and context of a subject's daily experience, is to integrate and test classical diagnostic approaches. There is already evidence accumulating to suggest that this will be a fruitful undertaking (deVries, 1985, 1987; Delespaul & deVries, 1987; Dijkman & deVries, 1987; deVries et al., 1986, 1987; Csikszentmihalyi & Larson, 1984).

The diagnostic dilemmas surrounding anxiety, agoraphobic and panic disorders provide a good test case. Complex variables at the behavioral, mental state, temporal and situational levels play a crucial role in this diagnostic controversy.

In spite of the epidemiological significance of anxiety disorder (Pitts, 1971;

APA, 1980; Robins et al., 1984) and the search for metabolic or biological factors (Klein & Rabkin, 1981; Crowe et al., 1980; Sheehan et al., 1981; Pitts & McClure, 1967; Appleby et al., 1981; Marks & Herst, 1970; van den Hout & Griez, 1984a, b) there is still no convincing mechanism underlying anxiety that accounts for all cases. Moreover, exact behavioral and phenomenological descriptions of anxiety phenomena are lacking. Therefore, a desirable strategy for research would be precise descriptions of the symptomatology and the variability of anxiety over time, that could be linked to biological data.

Recent advances in the field support this suggestion: Hibbert (1984), Ley (1985) and Borkovec (1985) offered behavioral, dynamic, affective and ideational descriptions of anxiety and panic. Ambulatory monitoring of physiological measures have further demonstrated that anxiety periods in normals as well as spontaneous or situational panic attacks in patients are phenomenologically similar (Margraf et al., 1987) and subject to diurnal and situational influences (Taylor et al., 1986; Freedman et al., 1985).

The ESM may be added to these methods, since it is ideally suited to assess rapid within-day fluctuations, as well as variability across real life situations. It provides a quantified description of patterns in the build-up and decay of situations (Dijkman & deVries, 1987). Moreover, the detection of time-patterns, situational and state effects in onset, maintenance and diminution of anxiety could perhaps help resolve the current debate on the relationship between general anxiety disorders, panic disorders and agoraphobia (Emmelkamp, 1982; Griez & van den Hout, 1983a, b; Sheehan, 1982; Zitrin et al., 1978; Arrindell, 1980; Spitzer & Williams, 1984).

The ESM questionnaires are filled out ten times a day for six days, at preselected random moments, when a beep (wrist-watch device) signals the subject to do so. Each subject provides about 50–60 descriptions of his momentary state, context, etc. Subjects are further described by cross-sectional psychometric measures, such as demographic and anamnestic information, DSM-III diagnosis, self-reports: e.g., STAI (Spielberger et al., 1970; state and trait anxiety), Fear Questionnaire (Marks & Matthews, 1979; avoidance), Zung & Durhan (depression scale, 1965), a biological index of reactivity to CO_2 inhalation (SUDS) (Griez & van den Hout, 1983a, b), and a behavioral measure of avoidance (time alone on the street during an exposure task).

In ESM, time-sampled variables take the following form:

(1) Frequency counts and means: thoughts, mood, activities, social context, etc.

(2) Variability of anxiety/panic symptoms over time (items based on a 'repeat diagnostic' factor of DSM-III criteria): individualized complaints and other psychological variables, such as mood, etc.

88

(3) Relationship between the presence of symptoms of anxiety/panic and psychological variables: thoughts, mood, etc.

(4) Relationship between the presence of anxiety/panic symptoms and the physical and social context: anxiety in agoraphobic situations, relationship with presence of intimate persons, etc.

The predictive power of ESM variables in discriminating anxiety disorders is applied to the following questions:

(1) Can we identify contextual variables or dimensions that differentiate anxiety disorders?

(2) Does the classification of anxiety patients based on relevant contextual dimensions correspond to the diagnostic criteria of DSM-III, or can we supplement or further differentiate the existing system with a more functional and ecologically valid classification scheme?

(3) Can we replicate these findings using a discriminant analysis to predict the 'diagnosis' from contextual variables?

Before this can be accomplished, some methodological and practical problems remain: how should a cross-classification be performed on these data; how should we deal with the specific characteristics of ESM data (i.e., repeated measures, combinations of nominal and ordinal scales and Likert items); what form will the results take?

Some of these questions have easy answers and others require more work. For example, items with reasonable distribution scores should be selected and scales with extremely skewed answers should be discarded. The data should be analyzed using every time beep as a unit of analysis. Further, analysis could proceed using one individual at a time as well as with individuals grouped in diagnostic classes. After this step, we plan to determine whether the cross-classification of ESM data could reveal types that can be compared to results of other methods; i.e., diagnosis, cross-sectional tests. From this analysis, two categories could emerge:

(1) A type characterized by differences in behavior over time: STATES,

(2) A type of individual characterized in terms of these states: SYNDROMES.

For the first type (STATES), all measurements (60 time beeps) should be used as separate cases. For the second type (SYNDROMES), individuals will be cases and the states, the variables, or the types of states could be classified for one individual. In Fig. 6.3, a scenario for such a two-step analysis is presented.

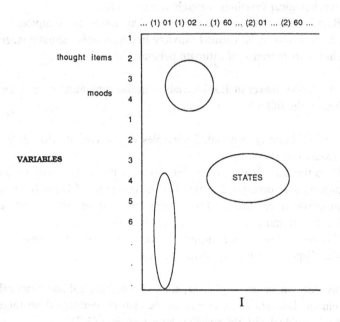

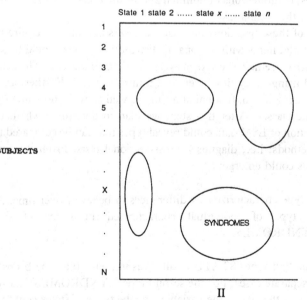

Fig. 6.3. I, Cross-classification I: beeps × variables. II. Cross-classification 2: states × subjects.

In this way, the relevance of temporal, contextual and psychological variables gathered using the ESM technique will be used in reclassifying anxiety disorders. It should provide a more comprehensive description of clinical anxiety syndromes that would be of significant help in guiding therapeutic interventions.

In drug abuse research (Kaplan et al., 1987), the ESM cross-classification methodology would serve two functions:

(1) The recognition of patterns of use.
(2) The relationship of these patterns to probabilities of consequences.

An approach would be to consider each of these patterns of use to compose a polythetic class. Elements in each use pattern or polythetic class have certain characteristics in common, but do not have other characteristics. A critical value could be established to ascertain the 'grade of membership' (Woodbury et al., 1978) in each class; i.e., how may of which common core characteristics an individual drug user has to show in order to belong clearly to the class. Once the individual drug users could be distributed between the emerging classes, these patterns could be compared with similarly constructed classes of consequences.

A cross-classification would reveal the relative weights of subsequent use patterns and consequences in the general population. Given the existence of this methodology, it now becomes possible to discover patterns of use based on very simple observational studies of the experience of drug users. As suggested by the WHO (1981), subjective reports of craving are much more sensitive than psychological or behavioral measures. Craving thus provides a clue to the class of variables that would be most effective in describing use patterns.

A study currently being conducted by Kaplan et al. (1987) employs the technique described above for anxiety: ESM studies with the goal of obtaining data on the experience of craving. Craving is hypothesized to be the fundamental mechanism underlying the patterns of problematic drug use.

The literature on craving is long and characterized by stormy controversies that focus on the measurement of the subjectivity of the concept. This problem can in part be overcome by a method such as ESM that relies on randomly elicited self-reports of subjective experience. The reliability of self-reports can be determined and controlled. Moreover, the craving literature has already isolated two components of craving:

(1) A *negative component* related to the attempt to nullify the discomforts of not having the drug (the withdrawal symptom) in an attempt to feel normal, usually in the midst of a situation where the possibility of loss of control is present.

(2) *A positive component* related to a desire to feel different and oriented toward fantasies of use of large amounts of the drug.

The study operationalizes these two components in a 'craving module' of self-reported questions imbedded in a larger instrument described above. The module consists of seven-point Likert scales that index subjective characteristics that represent the two components. The module elicits at the moment of the beep the following questions on the seven-point scale:

(1) Are you thinking about using?
(2) Do you feel stoned?
(3) Do you have yourself under control?
(4) Do you feel restless?
(5) Do you need dope in a hurry?
(6) Do you need money desperately?
(7) Are you sick?

The goal of the cross-classification analysis would be to do a within-subject analysis with each beep representing a 'patient-time' (Woodbury et al., 1978), cross-classified with the Likert items and the pen coded items. A comparison of between-subject analyses could determine whether the patterns are subject-specific or more dependent on temporal or contextual factors measured by the self-report.

Hypotheses to be tested by this type of analysis would be of the following kinds: the 'goodness of fit' between the ascending hierarchical classifications and the use patterns; the positive component of the craving module is more useful as a means of classification than the negative component. Applications of the results of this analysis should be useful in revising the standard diagnostic categories used in clinical evaluation (e.g., the DSM-III) and the standardization of a case index for epidemiological research and forecasting.

Concluding remarks: toward Weberian ideal types

Adequate classification presents a universal problem that is manifest across many scientific disciplines. We hope to have shown in this chapter that progress in cross-classification analysis and time-sampling methods in social and behavioral science resolve many of the problems in the operationalization of classification research as well as in interdisciplinary comparison and communication.

One of the most useful conceptual categories for this task is that of Max Weber's ideal types. Weber presents three stages in the use of ideal types in social science research. The first stage is the comparison of individual elements or cases before attempting to construct types from these elements. The second is the development of systematic criteria that permit the selection of those elements that constitute a type that will be submitted to the three tests described in the next paragraph that determine if the type is an 'ideal type'. The third is the confrontation between the ideal type and each element to determine the latter's degree of association or deviation from the ideal type (Weber, 1947a).

Indeed, a 'type' can only be an 'ideal type', according to Weber, if it successfully passes three tests. Firstly, the test of coherence which requires that no information or data on the subject matter openly contradict the hypothesis incorporated into the ideal type. Secondly, the test of simplicity which requires the inclusion in the ideal type of only those elements found to be indispensable; that is to say, if an element is omitted, the description or results do not remain the same. Thirdly, the test of experimental validity which requires the correct anticipation of the processes characterized by the ideal type (Weber, 1947b).

It is obvious from this extended definition that current social and behavioral science use of the concept of an ideal type is a probabilistic generalization of the concept defined by Weber. No one requires a test of simplicity for the data considered to constitute an ideal type and individual exceptions are widely admitted in ideal types as they are currently employed. What is essential is that almost all of the information is not openly contradictory with the hypothesis involved and that all the elements retained can be explicitly characterized in a probabilistic manner.

It is clear from the formal definitions given above that a polythetic class is the generalization of an ideal type as defined by Weber and also of a syndrome as defined by the WHO (1981). Together, through the ESM and cross-classification analysis, we can coherently operationalize these concepts in behavioral science research. This methodology also furnishes the researcher with a formally established and concise subset of variables associated with each syndrome. In their simplest form, these subsets of variables are classification grids, the establishment of which clearly furnishes the necessary results for the construction of a model of the phenomenon under investigation. The use of this methodology ensures the compatibility of any such model. The construction of different models from this common basis can permit fruitful comparisons which, in turn, will raise new questions and problems of analysis and reclassification in social and behavioral science research.

PART III

Experience Sampling studies with clinical samples

*Psychotic Disorders: Chapters 7, 8 and 9
*Anxiety, Mood, Multiple Personality, and Eating Disorders: Chapters 10, 11, 12, 13 and 14
*Substance Abuse: Chapters 15 and 16
*Stress and Psychophysiologic Studies: Chapters 17, 18 and 19

7

Variability of schizophrenia symptoms[1]

MARTEN W. deVRIES
and PHILIPPE A. E. G. DELESPAUL

The issue of mental state variability is central to the understanding of psychiatric pathology in general and schizophrenia in particular. Historically, psychiatry has been interested in these phenomena. Kahlbaum (1863), Kraepelin (1896) and Bleuler (1911) about a century ago, richly described the symptoms and course of schizophrenia. Since then, theorizing and studies of schizophrenia have been varied and many, but currently researchers tend to avoid phenomenological descriptions. Only a small group has investigated the actual course, changes, stages and fluctuations in schizophrenia (Strauss et al., 1985). Even less is known about fluctuations of symptoms, mood, thought and behavior in real-life situations, although these issues are the bread and butter concerns of clinical psychiatry.

Currently biological formulations receive much attention in schizophrenia research. Most studies emerging from prominent institutes use new diagnostic techniques such as MRI, PET scans, and CBF that promise to bring to fruition the search for functional and anatomical abnormalities in schizophrenia. Epidemiological researchers ponder issues such as cross-national prevalence differences and unequally distributed birth rate frequencies over the months of the year, of persons developing schizophrenia later in life. Psychological scholars focus on intellectual and cognitive factors such as loss of abstracting ability, perception and attention difficulties, and problems with faulty associations and thinking, all of which are tied to slow learning and adaptive liability (Rabin et al., 1979). These studies have enhanced our knowledge of schizophrenic symptomatology. Unfortunately, the interactive, social and behavioral aspects of the disorder that have been illuminated over the last 30 years were not researched as intensively. Therefore, new studies in all fields of schizophrenia research need to be augmented as far as possible by phenomenological and behavioral descriptions of schizophrenic symptoms over time.

The schizophrenia syndrome is today generally considered a disorder marked by a vulnerability to time-limited, acute illness episodes that occur throughout the lifespan. Studies have shown that specific factors leading to

[1]Appeared in part in *Schizophrenia Bulletin* (1989), **15**, 2, 223–44.

exacerbations of the illness do not differ from precipitating factors in other illnesses, but that persons with schizophrenia seem to react to these influences more severely and maladaptively. Although the meaning of the concept is not well worked out, a general agreement has evolved that patients with schizophrenia are environmentally vulnerable. Patients with schizophrenia are postulated to be less able than normal individuals to maintain homeostatic control in the face of environmental disruptions. This has lead to successful treatment strategies that have stressed the management of environmental changes, particularly in the family (Leff & Vaughn, 1985).

Most of the studies on changes in mental state of subjects with schizophrenia have focused on the issue of expected outcome over time. Particularly the long-term follow-up studies of Bleuler (1978) and Ciompi & Müller (1976) are instructive. Their work can be summarized as follows: 15–25% of subjects developing schizophrenia at some point in their life willl be 'cured' some years later and remain symptom-free for the rest of their lives; 30–40% will follow an episodic course leading to repeated rehospitalization but also potentially long symptom-free periods during which they have no residual handicaps; 10% will stay chronically incapacitated for the rest of their lives. Unfortunately, we do not know how we can change these patterns of outcome. Most factors associated with poorer outcomes are demographic, such as never having been married, month of birth, place of birth, etc. and it is clear they are not easily changed. Pathological aspects such as acute vs. chronic onset and subtyping are also related to outcome. Finally, Cloninger et al. (1985) have suggested that maximum predictability of poor outcome can be reached using an index composed of symptoms such as delusions of persecution and control, specific mood-incongruent delusions and auditory hallucinations. These outcome-related characteristics all deserve much attention but fall short in their usefulness for designing therapeutic interventions.

Until now, studies of the course of schizophrenia have been less common. Except for the staging of the onset of psychosis (Chapman & Chapman, 1980; Docherty et al., 1978) we have not learned much. Bleuler (1978) differentiated a linear course from an episodic one. Strauss et al. (1985) describe eight specific principles of longitudinal course during the first year following a psychotic episode. Strauss stresses key components such as the nonlinearity of course, identifiable phases such as 'moratoria', 'changing points', 'ceiling effects' and 'getting a foothold', the time-decay of vulnerability and phases of environmental responsiveness to the patient. This description of course over an entire year is a step forward in clinical understanding but more is needed, for it is still not enough to describe the individual's relationship to contextual and temporal factors, while not understanding their subjective illness experience.

Can we indeed find an increased vulnerability, evidenced by cognitive and mood disturbance in certain settings, that differentiate patients with schizophrenia from non-psychiatric populations? Setting effects have not been well-studied, despite the strong therapeutic claims made by the family and expressed emotion researchers (Leff & Vaughn, 1985). Supportive evidence for setting effects have come from behavioral observation. Reynolds (1965), while seeking periodicity in schizophrenic symptoms with behavioral observation techniques, noted instead considerable contextual influences on maladaptive behavior. Setting-dependent symptom reactivity has also been reported in observational studies of schizophrenia (McGuire & Fairbanks, 1977; McGuire & Polsky, 1979). These authors suggest that persons with schizophrenia are less able to stabilize their behavior after a stimulus change and therefore demonstrate greater thought disorder in the presence of increased affect and interpersonal stimulation. This often results in a rigid and withdrawn defense strategy that is the hallmark characteristic of the illness. In all these studies, variations between patients in reaction patterns and sensitivity were also noted. Similarly, deVries (1983) observed in a pilot study of paranoid and undifferentiated subjects with schizophrenia that the undifferentiated group was more sensitive to social stimuli.

Subjective self-reports of symptom fluctuations as they occur in relation to environmental influences can be illuminated by the repeated non-retrospective self-reports of experience that we employ. Since settings have been shown in retrospective, cross-sectional studies to differ in their pathogenicity, we would expect to find this too in prospective studies. So we expect, as Leff & Vaughn (1985) did, that some settings increase pathological responsiveness, while others do not.

The experience sampling method

ESM is a data-collecting method using random time-sampling procedures to gather repeatedly and non-retrospectively self-reports of experience (deVries, 1987; Csikszentmihalyi & Larson, 1987). It borrows from a variety of time-sampling approaches that date at least from the ethnographies of Malinowski (1935) to the large time-budget studies of today (Robinson, 1977; Szalai et al., 1972). Further contributions have been made by the more systematic application of time observation techniques in naturalistic field studies (Barker, 1968, 1978; Chapple, 1970; Monroe & Monroe, 1971a, b), by ethological research strategies applied in psychiatry (McGuire & Polsky, 1979; Reynolds, 1965), by 'spot observations' in ethnographic fieldwork (Whiting, 1977) and by the behavioral monitoring techniques (Nelson, 1977). These approaches have described the behaviors of subjects and patients in great detail, but not the subjective experience of individuals. ESM on the other hand is intended to catch the experiential dimension of mental state variability.

The ESM is an assessment technique designed to obtain repeated self-reports, using an electronic beeper that signals subjects to fill in small questionnaires at preselected but randomized time points each day over a number of days. The subjects carry a beeper and a booklet containing the report forms into the places and during the activities of their normal day and make the required assessments within this context. For method, application, validity and reliability, see the appropriate chapters in this volume.

Study

Purpose of the study

In this chapter we will present a study demonstrating that it is possible and interesting to set up research on repeated non-retrospective self-reports of experience, even with severely disordered mental patient populations. The core isssue is the description of variability and context relatedness of symptoms over time.

The different subtopics studied were: (1) the mental state description of the subjects; (2) the use of time and context; and (3) the effects of context on mental state.

Subjects

All psychiatric patients were being treated actively in health care facilities when participating in the study. Cross-sectional measures were gathered before the repeated-measurement period.

The study was conducted on a group of nine severely disordered persons. All were diagnosed as having schizophrenia by DSM III criteria and had a 7 'plus' score on the Strauss & Carpenter (1981) 12 symptom list, a cross-cultural research criterion used in the International Pilot Study of Schizophrenia. The patients were drawn from extremely ill ambulatory and hospital populations who had illness careers exceeding 10 years; all were under 40 years old and on medication. In addition, seven non-psychiatric subjects (academic-level professionals in this pilot study) were sampled.

Method: an ESM application

ESM application In the ESM application used in the study reported here, subjects were signaled 10 times a day (once in each 90-min timeblock between 7.30 a.m. and 10.30 p.m.) for six consecutive days. Randomizing the occurrence of beeps throughout the day minimizes subject reactivity, assures contextual and concurrent validity and presents a clear picture of situational and diurnal variations in experience.

Subjects were seen by the researchers for a briefing session in which the diagnostic assessments were done and the sampling procedure as well as technical details concerning the beeper, were explained. This face-to-face contact is crucial in order to develop a good research alliance.

After the sixth sampling day we meet again with the subject for a debriefing session. Then we checked the missing data with him as well as the answers that were expected to lead to coding difficulties.

ESF: questions, variables and coding   The repeated self-report questionnaire is based on the mental state examination in psychiatry and called an Experience Sampling Form (ESF). The ESF is constructed using closed Likert-type scales and open questions.

(a) Closed Likert-type scales: The Likert-type scales are set up using a modular format, with subsets requesting responses on scales referring to 'thoughts', 'mood' and 'physical concerns' (Table 7.1). Data of individual scales belonging to a 'module' are summarized to a 'module score' by taking the mean of these Likert scales in such a way that a high score is always a positive emotion or affect. Factor analytical studies confirm the internal consistence of these different modules. The thought assessments follow dimensions described by Hurlburt (1980), while mood can be traced back to the classic studies by Izard (1972).

Table 7.1. *ESF 7-point Likert scales[1] within pre-defined subsets (modules)*

'thoughts'	pleasant; clear; excited; normal
'mood'	cheerful; secure; social; relaxed; calm; friendly
'physical concerns'	hungry; tired; not feeling well

[1] 1 = not at all; 7 = totally true.

A specific deviance and psychopathology-module was developed for the assessment of schizophrenic symptomatology and is displayed in Table 7.2.

Table 7.2. *Likert scales[1] related to schizophrenic symptomatology*

I hear voices
I'm suspicious
I cannot express my thoughts
My thoughts are influenced (by others)
I can't get rid of my thoughts
I feel unreal

[1] 1 = not at all; 7 = totally true.

Table 7.3. *Open-ended questions with coding information*

Where are you?	home; relatives; network; health care facilities; public places; . . .
What are you doing?	nothing; self-care; household; work; leisure; travel; . . .
Who are you with?	alone; with family; friends; colleagues; strangers; . . .
What are you thinking?	— congruency of thought and activity ('online') — pathology ('goofs'): focused thinking; daydreaming; worrying; preoccupation; circular thoughts; psychotic/derealized; . . .

(b) Open questions: The open-ended questions are coded by the research team and assess the social and physical context in which the above-mentioned aspects of mental state take place. The coding categories are briefly described in Table 7.3. The assessment of 'thoughts' ('What are you thinking?' question) is difficult to operationalize. Two additional variables are derived. The *first* one assesses the congruency between the thought and the activity, e.g. when a subject is washing dishes and thinking about a quarrel on the previous day it is assessed as 'off-line'. On the contrary, a subject washing dishes and asking herself where she left the towel is clearly 'on-line'. The *second* variable assesses the pathologic aspects in the thought process. It forms an ordinal scale from no pathology to severe illness. This variable, as well as the previous one, refers primarily to the thought content. Some examples can elucidate this 'thought-pathology' variable. The woman washing dishes can think of the towel and will be assessed as 'focused'; she can think of the children at school and then will be assessed as 'daydreaming'; when expressing some disturbance referring to the children who are late from school she is 'worrying'. When she thinks without cause of what could happen to the children at school she is 'preoccupied' and when this is described as happening frequently, it is a 'rumination'; if she cannot stop them, it is assessed as 'circular thoughts'. Considering a situation where she describes her hands dissolving in the water she is clearly hallucinating and will be scored 'derealized'. Coding this variable accurately usually requires additional information on the life habits of the subjects and often further questioning in a debriefing interview (see Delespaul & deVries, 1987).

Results

Mental state   The problem operationalized in this part is: Do severely disturbed psychiatric patients describe themselves differently, in comparison to the normal controls, on selected experiential dimensions? Table 7.4 summarizes our results.

Based on the Likert scale self-assessments, only the module assessing soma-

Table 7.4. *Between group statistics*

Item group	Schizophrenia (N = 9)	Normals (N = 7)	t-statistic
Thoughts			
Likert Module	4.73 (0.65) (N = 8)	5.35 (0.68) (N = 6)	t(12) = −1.73 n.s.
'on line' (0 = off/1 = on)	0.52 (0.18) (N = 9)	0.74 (0.15) (N = 7)	t(14) = −2.62 P<0.02
'goofs' (1 = normal/5 = mad)	1.75 (0.83) (N = 8)	1.13 (0.15) (N = 6)	t(12) = −1.82 n.s.
Mood			
Likert Module	4.66 (0.37) (N = 7)	5.12 (0.67) (N = 6)	t(11) = −1.57 n.s.
Somatic aspects			
Likert Module	3.43 (1.72) (N = 6)	5.96 (0.91) (N = 6)	t(10) = −3.18 P<0.05
(Hunger − not feeling well)	5.53 (0.75) (N = 6)	5.96 (0.91) (N = 6)	t(10) = −0.90 n.s.

tically related experiential aspects separated the groups significantly. The other variables were in the expected direction but failed to reach significance, probably because of the small sample size. Interpretation of the only significant module is difficult because of the broad range of aspects covered by the scales (hunger – tiredness – not feeling well). After removal of the 'tiredness' variable the difference is no longer significant. A separated treatment of the Likert-scales would be more appropriate in the future.

As could be expected, the schizophrenic subjects were rated less 'on-line', indicating less congruency between their thoughts and activities. Normals showed less psychopathologic thought content on an assessment of thought quality, the 'goofs' – variable. Only the 'on-line' variable significantly differentiated the two groups (see Table 7.4).

The use of time and context   The information gathered concerning the social environment at the moment of the beep was coded and collapsed into the categories 'alone'/'not alone'. As expected, patients with schizophrenia spent more time alone (41%), as compared with 31% for normals. This last figure matches the 'alone' time in other studies of normal populations (Csikszentmihalyi & Larson, 1984). Differences between in- and outpatients should be noted. The clinical population, although small, is almost never

Table 7.5. *Time spent alone*

Schizophrenia (N=9)		Normals (N=7)	t-statistic
41%(±35)		31%(±27)	t(14)=0.65 n.s.
ambulatory (N=7)	clinical (N=2)		
51%(±34)	10%(±14)		t(7)=1.60 n.s.

alone, while the ambulatory, treated patients with schizophrenia were even more often alone than their normal counterparts. This low 'alone' frequency for clinically treated schizophrenics is a consequence of the living situation on the crowded hospital wards where being alone and consequently to enjoy some privacy is almost impossible. Contrary to their clinical colleagues, ambulatory treated schizophrenics are alone very often, even more than normals. The meaning of this difference in frequency of alone time should be evaluated further in relation to the mental states reports in this situation to determine its clinical significance.

Setting effects and experience The influence of setting on mental state was assessed using the 'number of persons present at the beep' variable and a global mental state measure composed of the combined thought and mood scales. We hereby hoped to determine 'the context of disability' (see Fig. 7.1). Both schizophrenics and normals had relatively 'depressed' mental states when alone, reaching an optimal level in a 1–3 persons company range. The groups differ when more people are present. Then we see a clear drop in mental state self-evaluation for subjects with schizophrenia but not for normals.

Many interpretations are possible, but the data are primarily of interest because it seems that a crowded setting is extremely troublesome for these schizophrenic patients. Crowdedness is an aspect of the setting where we most often treat them, the acute hospital unit. Ambulatory treatment without alternatives for social contacts may also create troublesome situations because the frequency of 'being alone' is extremely high in this group and this is associated with relatively depressed mental states. This information, if replicatable in a larger standardized sample, could provide us with important data for optimizing living environments for subjects with schizophrenia. We plan to study specific social activities and contexts to clarify this relationship further.

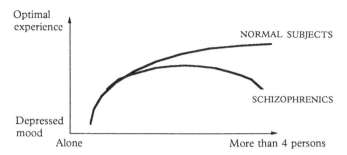

Fig. 7.1. Thought/mood combined score related to the number of persons present.

Case presentations

Other contextual aspects were explored on a casuistic basis to demonstrate more complex situational relationships with mood and thoughts. They warn us of the pitfalls of interpretations based on group-level aggregated data.

Case 1

A woman in her mid-forties, formally educated as a bacteriologist, who had a ten year history of paranoid schizophrenia, was sampled over three consecutive days with a mean beep frequency of six per day. She showed a repetitive late afternoon increase in problematic thoughts. The morning periods, during which she felt better, were spent carrying out domestic tasks. In the late afternoon, she was generally alone without specific tasks and in this situation she became preoccupied with herself physically. Her delusions had a professional component such as 'bacteria crawling on her skin'. Revealing is the pattern of the third day where beep signals capture a delusional period followed by the patient subsequently studying an anatomy text. On debriefing it was confirmed that her studying functioned as an intellectual coping strategy, which served as an attempt to organize disturbing delusions.

To substantiate and confirm adaptive patterns of this sort, a longer sampling period with a higher beep frequency is required. In this way we could collect more observations in the situation of interest and enhance the power of the test of the 'environment/mental state' – covariation hypothesis.

Case 2

The complexity of the relationship between context and fluctuations in experienced mental state is also illustrated in the following case.

A 53-year-old married woman was seen in ambulatory care for an endo-

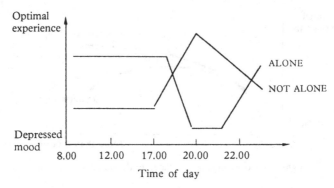

Fig. 7.2. Case presentation of within-day pattern of thought assessment in 'alone' vs. 'not alone' situations.

genous depression with psychotic features. The graph (Fig. 7.2) presents her thought scores (mood data were similar: $r=0.56$) for the 'alone'/'not alone' conditions in a within-day format computed by collapsing the six sampling days to a 'mean' day. The within-day data can be divided into three time-blocks. During the first phase, until 5.00 p.m. the most positive thoughts and feelings occur when alone. In the second phase (5.00 p.m. to 8.00 p.m.) social contact clearly enhances feelings, although the alone condition also shows a slight positive trend. After 8.00 p.m. a drop in experienced mental state in the 'not alone' situation can be observed. Clearly the simple contextual association with the number of people, as found in the first study, cannot account for the complex interactions we observe in this idiographic analysis when 'time of the day' is introduced as an additional variable.

Case 3

ESM data may simply be presented by graphing a person's coded activities and plotting the frequency of severity of symptoms over the time period assessed. These plots or troublesome thoughts and mood in relation to social activities and context in turn become a powerful clinical tool for the therapist and the patient alike. For the therapist, it actualizes the patient's life and generally produces empathy; for the patient, it enhances positive transference, the feeling of being cared for and often provides useful information. An example suggests how these data may function clinically.

Alfred is a 28-year-old man, first diagnosed at the age of 22 with undifferentiated schizophrenia. His other DSM-III diagnoses were passive dependent personality disorder and hypertensive illness. He had been employed as a dishwasher and store clerk, and had lived alone or with his parents in a relatively unstressful environment over the last eight years. Since he was diagnosed the patient was treated steadily on 20 to 30 mg of Stelazine which allowed him to function socially at a marginal level. The patient was referred for two reasons: the exacerbation of his schizophrenia as well as a hypertensive crisis which had required intensive medical intervention. On ESM assessment it was found that, rather than being present throughout the day, the patient experienced anxiety and increased blood pressure primarily at 11.00 a.m. each day while at work. At this time, as a dishwasher, he had to sort silverware – spoons from forks – on an automated conveyor belt system during the pre-lunch rush. In this anxious state his blood pressure increased markedly often to 180/120. In the clinical setting, the agitated patient with rampant high blood pressure appeared puzzling. The time assessment, however, linked the problem to a specific environment that the patient experienced as socially and cognitively distressful and pointed to a clinical intervention. The circumstances were explained to his employer with the suggestion to change the patient's work tasks. The employer cooperated and over the next three weeks the patient's blood pressure returned to near normal, a quite remarkable change since his extremely high blood pressure over the previous two months had lead to intensive treatment with Aldomet, Propranodol and Valium in addition to the Stelazine. After three weeks, the patient was again assessed with the ESM and an increase in the patient's agitation between 10.00–11.00 a.m. was again noted. At this time, the lunch-work shift, made up primarily of female workers, came to prepare the noon meal. This brought up a host of fearful, sexual and aggressive feelings in the patient which he experienced as psychological disorganizing. This situation uncovered new psychotherapeutically useful information about the nature of the patient's relationship with women and particularly his mother, relationships which he was previously unable to discuss. A focused psychotherapy approach was thus possible and resulted in a relatively symptom-free year. While this information could have been derived from careful clinical interviewing, other medical workers missed the importance of the environmental influence. The ESM assessment method brought it to the fore. In this case, it proved doubly powerful since it provided a capacity for both a medical and a social intervention as well as guiding a psychotherapeutic approach. It is important to remember that the patient during interview had been unable to communicate the linkage of these events.

We think the case of Alfred is a striking example of the clinical usefulness of ESM.

Discussion

In this study we have demonstrated the promising usefulness of repeated self-report-methodology in natural environments, for the elucidation of questions related to the experience or mental state of patients with chronic schizophrenia in the context of changing social aspects in their daily life.

As a group, our patients felt best in a small social environment, characterized by the presence of one to three persons. Being in the company of more people, as well as 'being alone', was more troublesome.

These results, if replicated in larger studies, have direct implications for the organization of care-taking facilities for the chronically mentally ill. As far as these data are considered, the crowded hospital ward is not the optimal choice for a treatment environment, while ambulatory treatment can lead to a dramatic rise of 'alone' time, which is equally disturbing. Optimalized care-taking facilities should be organized to avoid these 'contexts of disability' and create opportunities to let the patients live and be treated in small-scale environments.

These results are not unexpected. Nevertheless, the cases presented show us that optimal environments are more differentiated and complex at the level of individual patients. Furthermore, even the global conclusions at the group level may be inaccurate due to the nature itself of the ESM sampling technique. Events such as being 'alone' or 'not alone' do not occur in a randomized way in the daily life of patients, but may be an active choice, even a coping strategy, reacting upon existing mental state changes. In this way the depressed mood in the alone situation can be a result of the active withdrawal of the patients when they are bothered more by delusions and hallucinations. The same hypothesis can be made concerning the more depressed mental state in the large social environment, where withdrawal can be reached in the anonymity of the crowd.

The discussion goes on concerning the actual application of the ESM: the relevant items to ask, the way to present them, the coding of the open-ended questions and the pooling of the items within the a priori modules. Nevertheless, the protocol used to collect data appears satisfactory. The assessment method is time-consuming, but this does not lead to excessive dropouts. Problematic, however, is a heavy reliance on debriefing information to clarify self-reports.

We are well on our way to develop an ESM file of psychopathological subpopulations. Standardization in the thought and mood modules, as well as in the environmental context scales and the flexible module for specific research questions ('psychopathology-module'), provide a workable combination. Lastly, our preliminary investigations in environmental (co)variability with mood/thought fluctuations are promising. Development in the exploration of time-dynamic properties of the data are also expected.

In order to clarify these possibilities of phenomenological elucidation, we plan to carry out further idiographic and nomothetic explorations within increasingly well-defined pathologic populations at both the biological and psychological levels, to experiment with various formats (increased sampling frequency, etc.), to investigate further the therapeutic relevance of ESM and to examine its capacity to illuminate contextual relationships as well as to clarify temporal or diurnal patterns.

8

The daily life of ambulatory chronic mental patients[1]

PHILIPPE A. E. G. DELESPAUL
and MARTEN W. deVRIES

Time-sampling research using self-report instruments has described the daily life patterns of people in different nations (Szalai, 1972; Robinson, 1977) and communities (Barker, 1968, 1978) and subjects of different ages (Csikszentmihalyi & Larson, 1984). These studies present a rich body of significant findings that differentiate behavior and activities within subjects over time and between categories of subjects. In spite of the accruing evidence for the variability of human reactivity and behavior, recent static pathological typologies for use in neuropsychiatric research (Crow, 1980, 1982; Andreasen, 1982; Pao, 1979) and bureaucratic third-party reimbursement schemes (Mason et al., 1985; Sinclair & Alexson, 1985; Widem et al., 1984; Rupp et al., 1984) stress the general view that chronic mental disorders are invariable over long periods of time. Nevertheless, there are studies to the contrary suggesting that subtypes of schizophrenia evolve in relation to context and life stages (Kendler et al., 1985) and that have traced the increased morbidity of illness throughout the life cycle (Bleuler, 1978; Ciompi & Müller, 1976). Recent work in schizophrenia research has taken a more detailed look at the onset of the disorder (Donlon & Blaker, 1973, 1975; Docherty et al., 1978; Chapman & Chapman, 1980), its relapse (Heinrichs & Carpenter, 1985) and recovery from acute episodes (Szymanski et al., 1983). These inquiries suggest that it would be wise to take a closer look at chronic illness and take variations in social environment (Zubin et al., 1985) and changes in the vulnerability of the subject over time more fully into account (Strauss et al., 1981, 1985).

Although prognosis for the schizophrenic person is likely to remain relatively poor, a better understanding of the coping strategies of mental patients in daily life is extremely relevant for providing more appropriate clinical interventions that may enhance the quality of their lives. Accordingly, in this paper we will present and discuss a more detailed analysis of data gathered over a sequence of days in the lives of chronic mental patients than is typically offered. Continuous observation of the mental state of chronic mental

[1] This work appeared in *Journal of Nervous and Mental Disease*, 1987, **175**, 9, 537–44.

patients, however, is not entirely new, although it has recently become an increasingly active area of research. The variability in positive symptoms has been described in thought disorders (Harrow & Marengo, 1986; Marengo & Harrow, 1987), in the fixity and intensity of delusions (Garety, 1985), and in hallucinatory experiences (Junginger & Frame, 1985; Mott et al., 1965). Fluctuations of negative symptoms have also been observed in two longitudinal studies carried out on hospital wards by Reynolds (1965, 1976). The effects of environmental changes on behavior and pathology have been studied by McGuire and his associates on acute wards (McGuire & Fairbanks, 1977; Whitehead et al., 1984), and the influence of the family environment has recently been fruitfully explored by Expressed Emotion researchers (see Leff & Vaughn, 1985, for summary).

We use self-reports in our study of the daily life of chronic mental patients, a technique recommended by leading researchers in this field (Bannister, 1977; Wynne et al., 1978; Bellak, 1979; McGuire & Fairbanks, 1977) as a means of understanding the moment-to-moment experience of patients in their natural settings. We use the ESM, a randomized time-sampling procedure for self-reports (see Csikszentmihalyi & Larson, 1987; deVries, 1987), to overcome the shortcomings of retrospective recall in psychiatry research (Lamiell, 1981).

The potential treatment applications of this research are complementary to but different from approaches that seek to change the family environment as a treatment goal (Bernheim & Lehman, 1985; Falloon, 1985; Falloon et al., 1984; Anderson, 1983). Our focus is on the individual and his or her self-reported experience, with the therapeutic goal of providing context-related specific information to the patient and his or her therapist about optimal and deviant functioning that may be used to improve the individual coping style.

Our aim in the present study was to focus attention on descriptions of daily life, mental state fluctuations, and the relationship between them. Three general questions were examined:

(1) Are there differences between patients and normal groups in organization and time allocation in daily life? (Here we expect more restricted social networks and activity spectra in the chronic population.)

(2) Are there differences in self-reported mental states? (Here we expect lower global ratings of mood, thought, and motivation in the patient group.)

(3) Is there an interaction of social environment with mental state? (Here we anticipate, based on current theories and data about other disorders, that these patients will be more vulnerable to external stimuli and report a stronger cognitive and emotional reactivity to environmental influences.)

Methods

Subjects

The sample consisted of 11 Dutch ambulatory chronic mental patients who were representative for this country on demographic (age, sex, social status, and employment) and diagnostic variables (see Romme et al., 1985). Due to the unique emphasis in the Netherlands on early detection and prevention, as well as a tendency to avoid the 'schizophrenic' diagnosis (Romme, 1978) only 22% of our patients had been given that label. The DSM-III diagnoses (American Psychiatric Association, 1980) for the 11 subjects were as follows: organic (one); schizophrenic (two); other psychotic (two); affective (two); somatiform (two); and adjustment disorders (two). Anxiety disorders were excluded and are described elsewhere (Dijkman & deVries, 1987). These subjects were less severely ill than the hospitalized sample we studied earlier (deVries et al., 1984, 1986). We are aware that a research design that defined pathological subpopulations more specifically would have been preferable, but this refinement awaits a larger sample.

All subjects were referred to the research groups by their therapists for additional diagnostic information. The average duration of illness was 15 years, with 2.5 hospitalizations per subject, and scores on a functional checklist showed marginal functioning. The group mean on the Brief Psychiatric Rating Scale (Hedlund & Vieweg, 1980) was 27.4, well within the range of the pathologic samples described by Overall (1974).

Compliance with the experience sampling procedure was good. All 14 subjects whom we approached agreed to participate, but data from three subjects (21%) were discarded, primarily due to reporting problems caused by inadequacy in the introductory procedures when the project was begun. This low rate of refusal, along with high compliance in filling in the booklets, is found for almost all subjects in spite of the effort it takes, especially in the few first days, to respond to 10 signals a day. In the more severely ill hospitalized sample we previously described (deVries et al., 1984), however, we found that pathology could interfere with compliance, resulting in a dropout rate of 25%. For example, one subject, a 35-year-old man, refused to carry a pager, explicitly declaring that he did not want to be associated with the pager-carrying hospital staff. Another subject feared radiotransmitted control of his thoughts by the pager. In the present study the data from the mental patients were compared with data on a normal control group of 11 adult men randomly selected from a census list (three of these additional control subjects refused to participate). The control subjects were sampled during the same period and had the same mean age, but a greater percentage were employed and married.

Research procedure

Subjects were referred by their therapists, who also provided demographic and medical history information. Introductory 'briefing' interviews were carried out in the subjects' homes. The purpose of the research was explained, informed consent was obtained, and the person's chief psychological and somatic complaints were determined for later study in the repeated diagnostic modules. The use of the Experience Sampling Forms (ESF) was explained, and a practice session was conducted in which the subject filled out an ESF under supervision. Any problems encountered were discussed, the signaling device explained, and the subject was given the telephone number of the interviewer, whom he could phone if a problem arose. Subjects were then sampled over six days, after which a 'debriefing' interview took place in which the reason for missing information was ascertained and additional information was gathered to limit potential coding problems with the open-ended questions.

Sampling method

The six consecutive days included a weekend, so that subjects' total scores slightly underestimated working-day information. A SEIKO RC-1000 watch was used to signal subjects to fill out the ESF 10 times a day in a random schedule between 7.30 a.m. and 10.30 p.m. More than 80% of the forms were filled out adequately by both subject groups within 10 min of receiving the signal. Of the first signals of each day, 40% were lost, primarily because subjects were asleep. A small response decay of 10% on the fourth day occurred in both samples, but compliance returned to normal on days 5 and 6.

ESM booklets

Subjects received a set of six ESM booklets, one for each day; these contained ESFs, a sleep assessment form to be filled out in the morning, and a retrospective day report to be used in the evening to record information about unusual events, as well as eating times and other regular events. The booklets were identical for both samples with the exception of a module assessing psychopathology, which was given only to the patients (Table 8.1).

The ESF asked classic mental status information (e.g., Ryback et al., 1981), using 26 Likert-type scales scored from 1 to 7 that allowed the recording of within-day variability of mental state. The scales are grouped in four subsets or modules defined by factor analysis, assessing: thought (Hurlburt et al., 1984); mood (Izard, 1972); activity-motivation (Klinger et al., 1980) (see Table 8.2); and, for patients only, psychopathology (see Table 8.1). Open-ended questions are also asked (see Table 8.3), allowing the coding of thought/activity congruence, thought content, and the presence of psychopathology.

Table 8.1. *7-point Likert scales related to psychopathology*

I hear voices
I'm suspicious
I cannot express my thoughts
I can't get rid of my thoughts
I feel unreal

1 = not at all; 7 = totally true.

Table 8.2. *ESF 7-point Likert scales, within previously defined subsets of thoughts, mood, motivation and physical concerns*

About the *thoughts:*	About activity *motivation:*
pleasant	like to do this
clear	active
excited	in control
normal	can concentrate on this
About *mood:*	About *physical concerns:*
cheerful	hungry
secure	tired
social	not feeling well
relaxed	
calm	
friendly	

1 = not at all; 7 = totally true.

Table 8.3. *EFS open-ended questions with coding information (codebook available)*

About *context* (with coding categories)	Additional *thought* variables
Where are you (home versus family – network – health care – work – public spaces)	Congruence of thought and activity
	Thought pathology (focused thinking – daydreaming – worrying – preoccupation – circular thoughts – psychotic/derealized)
What are you doing (nothing – self care – household – work – leisure – travel	
Who are you with (alone vs. being with family – friends – colleagues – strangers)	Thought content (nothing – leisure – travel – selfcare – friends – sex – aggression – money – religion – work – past – environment – ESM – future – abstract thoughts – miscellaneous)

Additional open-ended questions describe the daily life of subjects on four dimensions: what activities are carried out, when, where, and with whom. These categories are coded using procedures introduced by the larger time-budget studies (Szalai, 1982; Robinson, 1977; Wicker, 1984). The interrater reliability on the coded categories using Cohen's unweighted Kappa was found to be between 0.73 and 1.00. Two forced choice questions, finally, assessed physical posture and the ingestion of psychoactive substances such as medication, alcohol, coffee, and drugs.

Filling out the ESF takes two to five minutes. Nine percent of the responses by patients were invalid or left missing compared to only 2% by control subjects.

Methods of analysis

Because each subject's repeated self-reports over the six-day period cannot be regarded as strictly independent measures, we have taken a conservative approach, calculating a single mean value per subject for each Likert-scale item in the ESF for use in further analysis.

For all subjects, the Likert-scale items were then collapsed over the four modules of *thoughts*, *mood*, *activity motivation*, and *physical concerns* by calculating the mean of the relevant item scores (see Table 8.2). For patients, an additional score was calculated for items on the psychopathology module.

Results

The data presented are an attempt to map the daily lives of chronic ambulatory mental patients, describe their self-reported mental states, and depict changes in mental state in relation to characteristics of the social environment. Data were compared with those from normal control subjects. All analyses were performed for 11 subjects in each group (patient data are always presented first, followed by data from control subjects).

Psychological environment

Daily life activity subcategories, 'where', 'with whom', and 'what' a person was doing, were coded with good interrater reliability (Kappa=0.94, 69, and 0.85, respectively). Normal and disturbed groups were represented in all the coded contextual subcategories for place, activities, and persons (see Table 8.3), suggesting an unexpected similarity in social environments between normal subjects and chronic patients. However, the six *Where* categories, the six *What* categories, and the five *With Whom* categories showed significantly different distributions between patients and non-patients: Where ($\chi^2[5]=24.63$, $P <0.001$); with whom ($\chi^2[5]=89.9$, $P <0.001$); and what ($\chi^2[4]=32.99$, $P <0.001$). Thus, the differences in daily life reports are clearly a matter of degree rather than kind, with the patients showing more restricted patterns on all three variables. For instance, patients were more frequently at home (71% of the moments sampled vs. 55%), alone (37% vs. 30%), and spent more time 'idling' 'doing nothing in particular' (9% vs. 2%) than controls. Patients also did not use their spare time for purposeful activities as often as normal subjects. This was especially true when patients were at home, where 'idling' rose to 13% but did not change for normal subjects. Furthermore, in the evening, when time spent in organized leisure activity almost tripled for normal subjects, it remained unchanged for patients. The demographic differences between the groups, such as in employment rates and sex of the subjects, may have contributed to variations in time allocation over the course of the day. These factors will be examined further in a larger study.

Assessment of mental state

A number of dimensions of thought were coded: thought content using 16 coded categories (Kappa=0.72); a 'thought' self-assessment measure representing the subject's mean score on four Likert scale items (see Table 8.2); a measure of congruence between thought and activity (Kappa=0.71); and a measure of thought pathology coded on an ordinal scale from normal to severe psychopathology (Kappa=0.75).

Thought content frequency distributions were significantly different ($\chi^2[16]=31.00$, $P <0.005$). Diffuse thoughts dominated in the patient group (abstract thoughts, day dreaming, or specific worries about health, the past, and relatives; total $= 40\%$), while thoughts of normal subjects had primarily concrete content such as work, leisure, and self care (total $= 48\%$). The patient's average thought self-assessments were significantly less positively scored (see Table 8.4), although this rating was still fairly positive (overall $\bar{x} = 4.51$). The thoughts and activities of the chronic patients were significantly less congruent than those of control subjects (28% vs. 56%), indicating that the patients tended to report that their thoughts had drifted from 'here and now' activities and concerns more often. On the other hand, the thoughts of normal subjects were most often prosaically targeted; they seemed merely to paraphrase their current activities. The ordinal coding of 'thought pathology' (see Table 8.3) demonstrated significantly different frequency distributions for both groups ($\chi^2=24.6$, $P <0.001$). Using 'daydreaming' as the normal/abnormal cutoff, however, we see that thoughts of mental patients, like those of control subjects, were mostly codable as 'normal' (72% vs. 100%).

The self-assessed mood measure representing the subject's mean mood scores on the six Likert-scale items (see Table 8.2) also differentiated the groups (see Table 8.4), with normal subjects reporting more positive overall moods. Further, patients scored both thoughts and mood equally high ($t[9]=-0.81$, n.s.), whereas normal subjects reported higher mood scores than thought evaluations ($t[10]=-3.71$, $P <0.01$). Whether the similarity of mood

Table 8.4. *Overall group comparisons on mental state*

Variable Description	Chronics			Controls			Test
	$\bar{x}$	SD	n	$\bar{x}$	SD	n	
Thoughts	4.329	0.849	9	5.412	0.697	11	$t(18) = -3.1$ $P<0.01$
Mood	4.468	0.955	9	6.266	0.372	11	$t(18) = -5.76$ $P<0.001$
Psychopathology	5.196	0.816	9	—	—	—	—
Activity–motivation	4.029	0.378	9	5.538	0.626	11	$t(18) = -6.33$ $P<0.001$
Psychological complaint	4.040	1.618	9	6.423	0.822	11	$t(18) = -4.28$ $P<0.001$
Somatic complaint	4.070	1.251	10	6.230	0.892	10	$t(18) = -4.44$ $P<0.001$
Hunger	6.026	0.637	9	5.923	0.529	11	$t(18) = -0.53$ n.s.
Tired	4.461	1.939	10	6.167	0.784	11	$t(19) = -2.691$ $P<0.01$
Not feeling well	4.915	1.289	9	6.394	0.777	11	$t(18) = -3.176$ $P<0.005$

and thoughts for this patient group is due to a decreased capacity to differentiate the items of the two modules or whether these mental state aspects influence one another more in patients than in normal subjects, who seem to assess mood and thought independently, is a question for future and more detailed research. However, a different result has already been obtained from a more severely ill group of chronic patients. In these, markedly incongruent thought and mood was characteristic of the population (deVries et al., 1984, 1986).

The specific symptom variables were composed of personally identified psychological and somatic complaints. These were established during the briefing interview and were subsequently reported on a seven-point Likert scale at each signal. Patients rated both assessments less positively than normals did (see Table 8.4). Although not a significant finding, psychological complaints were the most troublesome for patients whereas normal subjects were bothered most by their self-defined somatic problems.

The above trends (Table 8.4) reappeared on the activity motivation and somatic ratings. The patient sample scored lower on the motivation for activity cluster (see Table 8.2) and reported feeling significantly less well and more tired. The subjective experience of hunger did not differentiate the two groups.

From these data we can conclude that on almost all variables the patient group scored differently from the normal group. This confirms a number of theoretical expectations and indicates methodological validity.

Interaction of mental states and the social environment

The mental states of patients and normal subjects in different daily life situations were compared by selecting two dichotomized variables ('alone' vs. 'being with others' and 'being at home' vs. 'out in the community') to explore illustratively the effects of the social environment. These global categories had previously differentiated reactivity patterns within a group of anxiety patients (Dijkman & deVries, 1987) and acutely psychotic individuals (deVries et al., 1986) and were used there to determine whether the impact of these categories on mental state also differentiated the normal subjects from the chronic patients.

For the categories coded by the researchers, thought/activity congruence and pathological thought, significant differences were found on the two dichotomized social dimensions. Chronic patients differed from normal subjects in showing less thought and activity congruence when at home $(\chi^2[2]\chi16.10$, $P <0.001$, vs. $\chi^2[2]=0.5$, n.s.) and when they were alone $(\chi^2[2]=5.68$, $P <0.05$ vs., $\chi^2[2]=0.02$, n.s.). Patients also registered slightly more pathological thought content when they were alone $(\chi^2[5]=29.92$, $P <0.001$, vs. $\chi^2[5]=1.35$, n.s.) or at home $(\chi^2[5]=14.41$, $P <0.02$, vs. $\chi^2[5]=0.005$, n.s.). A closer look at these data indicates that daydreaming increased markedly when the chronic patients were at home or alone and shifted to more focused thinking when they were with others or out of the house.

We next asked if the self-assessment categories of mental state could discriminate between the groups when subjects were alone or not alone. We were interested in determining only the impact of the social environment on each group, regardless of its direction. To do this we normalized the data by subject and computed new subject means for variables in the alone/not alone situation. The absolute value of the difference in the alone vs. not alone condition was taken to signify environment reactivity. On this measure, the chronic patient showed greater reactivity in thought, mood, and activity motivation measures than did normal subjects. In Table 8.5, t-test results for all mental state variables are shown.

Exploring the normalized variables measured at each point in time in order to determine the direction of the reactivity for the chronic subjects, we found mood to be significantly elevated in social situations $(t[503]=-2.74, P <0.01)$, suggesting a moderate trend toward positive experiences for the patients as a

Table 8.5. *Group differences in reactivity to the social environment (absolute differences between alone/not alone)*

Variable Description	Chronics			Controls			Test
	x	SD	n	x	SD	n	
Thoughts	0.456	0.134	9	0.301	0.237	11	$t(18) = 1.744$ $P<0.05$
Mood	0.530	0.442	9	0.085	0.069	11	$t(18) = 3.313$ $P<0.005$
Psychopathology	0.366	0.337	9	0.153	0.265	9	$t(16) = 1.489$ n.s.
Activity–motivation	0.535	0.386	9	0.231	0.162	11	$t(18) = 2.302$ $P<0.025$
Psychological complaint	0.458	0.464	9	0.240	0.240	11	$t(18) = 1.189$ n.s.
Somatic complaint	0.516	0.433	10	0.291	0.291	8	$t(16) = 1.353$ n.s.
Hunger	0.689	0.661	8	0.368	0.321	11	$t(17) = 1.411$ n.s.
Tired	0.746	0.782	10	0.474	0.320	11	$t(19) = 1.061$ n.s.
Not feeling well	0.345	0.461	9	0.415	0.535	8	$t(15) = -0.288$ n.s.

group. When the data were analyzed at the subject level, however, the distinctions between normal subjects and patients disappeared, indicating the importance of individual differences within each group.

Mood variability during the reporting period did differentiate the groups. Mood stability over time was assessed by computing median lag correlations between 90-min periods. Patients in this study reported more stable mood over a longer period than normals (r at lag 1: 0.49 vs. 0.32; r at lag 2: 0.30 vs. 0.10), in contrast to the more severely ill subjects studied earlier who reported instability for all mental state dimensions (deVries et al., 1984, 1986).

Discussion

In this chapter we have presented a quantitative description of fluctuations in mental states in some key aspects of daily lives of chronic mental patients and non-psychiatric controls using the ESM. Although the patient group was diagnostically heterogeneous, it was representative of an ambulatory chronic population in many social life and illness course variables. Comparing this group with normals on time allocation patterns and mental state reports and also with the effects of the social environment on mental state, we found differences between the groups on all three categories. In time allocation, differences were found in the daily organization of activities and places frequented as well as in time spent alone and socially. Mental state reports also differed for thought content, thought self-assessment, mood level, mood-thought congruency, and mood stability. Finally, environmental effects on mental states were illustrated by increased psychopathology, increased abstract thought, and a propensity to daydream more frequently when alone or at home. Although these group differences indicate both the construct and predictive validities of the approach, they should not obscure the large individual differences in responsiveness to the environment that exist.

In spite of their chronic deficits and handicaps, the patients demonstrated only relatively minor differences from control subjects and from subjects studied in the general population in their daily time-budgets (Szalai, 1972). Their chronically ill condition, then, did not dramatically affect the activities they performed or the content of the thoughts they had. Differences between the groups were primarily variations in relative frequencies of activities, places, and social situations, that is, differences of degree rather than of kind. This suggests that, at least on the global measures used in this study, ambulatory chronic patients can lead relatively 'normal lives' in the community and make use of socially available places and activities essentially similar to those of their non-ill counterparts. Studied in greater detail, however, patients in our study tended to lead less varied lives when compared with normal subjects. They also used time in a less organized fashion and reported 'doing nothing' more often than did normal subjects. Although they did spend more time alone, the data contradict the view that chronic ambulatory patients are socially isolated and withdrawn. Patients generally reported feeling as well or better when away from home in the company of others than normal subjects did.

In their reported mental states, however, the patients differed significantly from control subjects on almost every measure. Although mental states in both patient and control groups were not static but fluctuated in relation to context and time, the patients demonstrated greater reactivity to environmental influences. Again, patients rated their mental states as relatively positive, and diagnosable psychopathology occurred infrequently, in only 28% of all reports. However, they reported fewer congruent thought and activity scores, more abstract thoughts, fewer positive moods, and less pleasant cognitive self-assessment; they also felt less well physically and were tired more often than normal subjects.

The stability of mental state from one point in time to the next was greater for the patient group than for normal subjects. This finding contradicts the pilot data (deVries et al., 1984) gathered from actively psychotic individuals (all diagnosed as schizophrenic), who demonstrated great instability of thought and mood. Our ambulatory patients who were in remission, thus reported not only a more stable mood than the acutely psychotic subjects did but also, although to a lesser extent, than the normal subjects did. It is possible that this difference is related to the diagnostic heterogeneity of the current group because the inclusion of subjects with affective disorder may have contributed to the group's overall mood stability. Alternatively, the more severely ill hospitalized schizophrenics may have been more sensitive to environmental stresses. In any event, the differences found between the two patient groups suggested that severity of illness is a major determinant of stability in daily routine and mental state.

The 'environmental vulnerability' of individuals with chronic mental disorders predicted by expressed emotion research (e.g., Leff & Vaughn, 1985), also modestly characterized our chronic patients, who have seemingly reorganized their daily lives after the acute phase of their illness in order to minimize further stress. Their mental state reports show the degree of stabilization and reorganization that can take place in such a population, and that, while leading far from static lives or having static mental state, they seem to have succeeded at their restabilization. As they adapted their daily routines to the level of their own vulnerability, the ambulatory patients' mental states were more stable than those of anxiety subjects (Dijkman & deVries, 1987) or of the previously studied chronic and acutely psychotic patients who showed a greater instability and departure from normal daily routine.

Although more detailed categories of events than those we have reported here are available for analysis at the individual level and for clinical applications, the small sample size did not allow coding of more specific environmental factors. The environmental categories used, alone/not alone and home/not home, although sufficient for the purpose of the present study, are still too broad to achieve our goal of describing generalizable and meaningful environmental contexts of experience, which may account for our failure to find a significant impact of the social environment on mental state after the sample is normalized at the subject level. More detail may be introduced as the sample size increases both by the analysis of low-frequency events (Stone & Nicolson, 1987) and by combining factors such as place, person, and activity to characterize situations more adequately.

The individual differences among chronic patients in response to the social environments are one of the key findings of this study. ESM can be useful clinically in providing detailed descriptions of psychopathology, stress, or vulnerability at the individual level, and thus offers a personalized treatment approach with a greater potential for success than one derived from group data. In therapy, for example, we can use ESM data to capture healthy moments and problematic situations. Contexts that promote well-being may then be identified and their conscious selection encouraged, while overly problematic ones may be avoided. Moreover, situations important for a patient's wellbeing may be uncovered for use in behavioral didactic or supportive therapeutic approaches. Individual rehabilitation thus becomes feasible using ESM (Massimini et al., 1987).

ESM has thus proved to be an effective method for gathering information with satisfactory descriptive power about the daily lives of chronic mental patients and to provide valid assessments of different aspects of mental state that may be further applied in treatment. However, the data presented here are correlational and preliminary and should be read with some caution, particularly because they may have been influenced by Dutch cultural and health care factors, small sample size, and subject heterogeneity. These are issues that we expect to clarify in a larger study.

9

'Goofed-up' images: thought sampling with a schizophrenic woman[1]

RUSSELL T. HURLBURT
and SUSAN MELANCON

There are, in the psychiatric and popular literature, both true and fictional accounts of the experience of being schizophrenic (e.g., Beers, 1908; Green, 1970; Sechehaye, 1951). Such narrative descriptions are powerful human documents, and have profoundly influenced the practice of psychiatry (Kaplan, 1964, p. 146).

With few exceptions (e.g., Custance, 1952), such descriptions are written retrospectively, during remission or years after the episodes described, and are thus vulnerable to the distortion of selective memory, forgetting, condensation of events, details within events, etc. The time-sampling methods described in this book were explicitly developed to minimize the distortions due to retrospective reporting. While those time-sampling studies are quantitative analyses, a variant of the 'beeper' method can be used to create narrative descriptions that are not retrospective (or only slightly so), and thus also minimize distortion.

This method generates narrative descriptions of the moment-by-moment inner experiences of subjects, descriptions that are impossible to generate by any other method. The authors are preparing[2] a collection of such experience descriptions of normal and disturbed subjects to exemplify the range of human experience. We provide here an excerpt from the description of a young schizophrenic woman to demonstrate how this descriptive time-sampling method can augment the understanding of schizophrenia provided both by retrospective narrative descriptions and by quantitative time-sampling methods.

This example may prove useful if readers pause before reading further to ask themselves what is generally understood by psychiatric professionals about how schizophrenics experience their inner world. Our own impression is that such a general understanding is likely to be vague and indefinite, perhaps

---

[1] This work appeared in the *Journal of Nervous and Mental Disease*, 1987, **175**, 9, 575–8. © 1987 Williams & Wilkins.

[2] Now published as Hurlburt, R. T. (1990). *Sampling Normal and Schizophrenic Inner Experience*. New York: Plenum Press.

including such phrases as distractible, feeling the pressure of thoughts, and lack of involvement or centeredness in experience. Although these phrases may or may not be accurate descriptors of the momentary experiences of schizophrenics in general (we need to collect more samples to answer that question properly), they do not characterize adequately the experiences of the young woman we will call Jennifer, whose inner experience was, as we will see, primarily visual, brightly detailed, but distorted.

Our goal here is not to claim that Jennifer is typical of schizophrenics in general. Instead, our aim is to demonstrate that it is possible to generate descriptions of inner experience and that such descriptions may significantly enhance our understanding of the inner world of schizophrenia.

Case description

Jennifer Knoll (not her own name) was a 23-year-old female resident of a relatively structured and restrictive psychiatric halfway house. She had been diagnosed as paranoid schizophrenic four years earlier, based primarily on her reports that she heard annoying voices, which frequently triggered sadness and crying. She had spent much of the last four years in inpatient psychiatric facilities or halfway houses and had volunteered to participate in the sampling study. At the time of sampling, she was performing quite well in her residential activities, and the residential treatment staff decided near the end of the sampling period to 'graduate' her to a less restrictive cooperative apartment administered by the same mental health care provider group. She received haloperidol (10 mg/day) throughout the sampling period and attributed to it a reduction in the presence of the annoying voices. Although these voices were occasionally dimly present during the two-week period in which the sampling took place, the beep used in our experiment (details below) never occurred during one of those episodes.

In this descriptive variant of the time-sampling method, Jennifer was beeped through a small earphone at random times. Her task at each beep was to 'freeze' the ongoing inner experience that was occurring at the moment of the beep and immediately to write down in a notebook a description of that inner experience. The beeps occurred randomly with an average interval between them of 30 min. Each day, she sampled until about 10 beeped experiences had been described, and then met with the authors (either the same day or the next day) to discuss each sampled experience in detail. Each sample was discussed until Jennifer and the authors agreed that everyone understood what Jennifer's inner experience was like at the moment of the beep. It was possible to discuss between five and 10 samples in a session that lasted between 60 and 90 min. The beep-freeze-write-discuss procedure continued daily for about two weeks, after which the authors prepared a written description of Jennifer's sampled experiences. This description was then reviewed by and discussed with her, and her suggestions for very slight alterations were incorporated.

In general, Jennifer's inner experience can be characterized by the frequent presence of vivid inner visualizations. Most of her experiences included visualizations of some kind, ranging from simple inner 'copies' of portions of her present environment to highly abstract, colorful visual presentations that had no apparent meaning. Visualizations were experienced to the front and back of her visual field, to the right and left, straight on or from an angle, tilted or vertical, with or without sounds and movement, and veridical or 'goofed up' with extraneous lines and blurs. Words were also present in her inner experience, both spoken subvocally in her own voice and visualized as handprinted, frequently colorful, and frequently 'scrunched-up' displays. Color was important not only as an aspect of inner experience, but also as a frequent focus of attention in both her internal and external world, as in noticing the electric blue of a Royal Crown Cola can. Accompanying these cognitive characteristics were clear bodily feelings, quite distinctly localized in some particular part of her body, most frequently her heart. The present description, however, will focus on only one aspect of her inner experience, namely, distortions in visual images.

Many of Jennifer's images (19 of 71 samples) were distorted or goofed-up in some way that was neither meaningful to her nor obviously related to the image. These distortions occurred on a continuum of severity. At times, for example, the images were just slightly tilted or details in the visualizations were slightly incorrect, such as seeing a yellow glass when in fact the glass was blue. On the other hand, at other times portions of images were entirely obliterated or blurred or altered in a fairly dramatic way.

The most common distorting characteristic was Jennifer's perception that either an entire image or certain details within an image were 'kind of crooked', that is, were tilted in some way rather than vertical. For example, she was sitting at a house meeting, listening to one of the other residents (Bill) talk. At the moment of the beep, Jennifer was looking down at the floor but picturing an image of Bill sitting on the couch across the room. The image was an accurate copy of Bill that day, and was in front of her and to the right, where Bill was in fact sitting. Details within the visualization were all the correct size and distance away as if Jennifer was not in real life looking at Bill sitting on the real couch. In other words, this was a realistic image, distinguishable from reality primarily by the fact that Jennifer was not in real life looking at Bill at that moment. However, the entire image, and everything within it, was tilted, with the right side up at about a 45-degree angle. Underneath the part of the image that was tilted up seemed to be a black, empty space that was not visible on the other sides of the visualization. While in the above sample the entire visual image was rotated, Jennifer also had images in which the image itself was straight, but some details within the image were crooked. For example, when beeped while gathering up her makeup in preparation for leaving for the weekend, Jennifer saw an image of her makeup case, viewed from the back, as if she were looking at the reflection of the actual case in her mirror. In this image, the mirror and reflections of a hot-water pot and some jars of tea that were sitting on her countertop were vertical. However, the makeup case and the items within it (such as the nail polish and lipsticks) were slightly tilted.

In other samples, Jennifer's images were altered in ways that resembled graffiti. For example, she was reading the newspaper index page and had just finished reading the word 'television'. At the moment of the beep, Jennifer had just raised her eyes from the paper to look out at the room, but she was paying attention, not to the room she was seeing, but to an image of a tilted color television set. On the television screen in the image was a dark-haired man standing behind a round, chest-high, white podium or altar-like structure. The top of the podium, however, was obliterated by a rather messy black rim or ring that Jennifer could see was not a part of the actual podium structure. This black rim seemed fuzzy, like a flat splotch of scratched-out lines across the place that the podium was on the screen. Jennifer did not know of any significance underlying either the appearance of the altar-like podium or of the graffiti-like obliteration. She was definite, however, that the black pattern was not a part of the podium, but was in front of it, blocking out the top of the podium from her view. This entire image was tilted about 45 degrees, and the man and the podium were also tilted.

Jennifer frequently (10 of 71 samples) saw hand-lettered representations of words in her images, and such visualizations could be goofed up also. For example, she saw the red word 'sugar', floating above a transparent glass, and the word was nearly obliterated by red lines crossing through its letters. She also frequently (16 of 71 samples) had visual images that were concrete representations of the real existing situation Jennifer was in at that moment. Some of these re-creations of the physical world contained particular details that were slightly modified from the external reality she could have been viewing if she had turned her attention to it. For example, Jennifer was sitting at a living room table, smoking a cigarette. At the moment of the beep, she was gazing idly at the blue wall across from her and behind the table, but paying attention to an image of Ben, one of the other residents in her halfway house, who was sitting on the opposite side of the table. This image also simultaneously included a picture of her tall blue glass of ice tea. Jennifer's image of Ben was viewed slightly up and to her front right, in the same place that he was actually sitting. This image accurately portrayed the physical Ben sitting across from her, except that the real Ben was holding a yellow glass, not a blue one. The image of Jennifer's own big blue glass of tea was positioned lower at her left side, which was where her glass was physically placed at the time. In this image, her glass had a lid on it but no straw. In reality, however, Jennifer's drink did have a straw in it, but no lid. Thus, the imaginal picture she was viewing was basically true to external reality, but some minor details were slightly modified.

Discussion

This case shows quite clearly that one schizophrenic patient's everyday experiences were predominantly visual and that many of those everyday inner visual experiences were goofed up in some more or less important way. There are a number of features of this case that are significant.

The diagnostic descriptions of distortions in schizophrenic experience are bizarre delusions and hallucinations. This example shows that a schizophrenic's distortions may also occur on a much smaller everyday scale.

Most descriptions of schizophrenic distortions are of reality-based perceptions or of the intrusion of distortions into perception. This case demonstrates that the distortions occur also in what are readily recognized by the patient as inner images.

Jennifer described these goofed-up images in a matter-of-fact way, recognizing that they were in fact goofed-up, but not registering surprise or curiosity about it. We interpret this to indicate that such distortions were common for Jennifer. Thus we conclude that Jennifer's adjustment must be to an inner world in which representations cannot be relied upon to reflect reality. The treatment staff noted that Jennifer frequently spilled things, and before sampling they had interpreted this behavior as possibly aggressive or manipulative. The description of tilting in images suggested to them the alternative interpretation of Jennifer's inability to recognize departures from the vertical at any given moment. This interpretation is, of course, speculative, but it does exemplify the restructuring that can take place by observers following sampling and the difficulties such distortions may present for a patient's experience and behavior.

The case highlights the range of flexibility of the time-sampling procedures. Whereas most sampling studies are highly quantitative, qualitative reports are also possible. It is further our impression that our understanding of subjects is more complete in the present descriptive study, than in any of our previous quantitative studies (Hurlburt & Melancon, 1987).

The present case can serve as an example of the way in which descriptive time-sampling studies can influence quantitative studies. For example, before Jennifer's study was prepared, we would not have predicted, based on her diagnosis or clinical observations, that distortions in images have not been considered in any quantitative sampling studies, including those reported earlier in this issue. Detailed explorations of this kind could thus discover new variables that may be added to the variable set used in future quantitative studies.

We should note the need for descriptive detail in these narratives. As we continue to sample schizophrenics, it may be that it is not distortions in images that emerge as the most important characteristic, but some other aspect, which was only mentioned in passing in Jennifer's account. The accounts must be descriptively rich enough so that characteristics, important tomorrow but less vivid today, can gradually emerge.

We note that the descriptive method seems to exert a therapeutic effect on our subjects. We found this in an earlier case study (Hurlburt & Sipprelle, 1978) using a somewhat less detailed method. Now our preliminary observations are that the focusing of attention on the subject's actual perceptions seems to facilitate growth in both normal and disturbed subjects.

Last, we should note that this procedure, in our experience, exerts a powerful effect on all participants, not unlike transference and countertransference. Individuals considering attempting such studies are advised to be prepared for such eventualities.

10

The social ecology of anxiety: theoretical and quantitative perspectives[1]

CHANTAL I. M. DIJKMAN-CAES
and MARTEN W. deVRIES

Anxiety disorders and agoraphobic symptoms have had a long history: For more than a century they have been the subject of clinical and theoretical interest in psychiatry (Da Costa, 1871; Freud, 1924). Today, through the application of rigorous diagnostic procedures, anxiety has been recognized as an epidemiologically significant disorder, especially in women (Pitts, 1971; American Psychiatric Association, 1980; Robins et al., 1984).

In recent years most research has focused on the possible underlying mechanisms of anxiety. Genetic and endocrinological explanations, particularly the finding that sodium lactate and carbon dioxide precipitate panic attacks, stimulated the rapidly advancing search for metabolic or biological factors (Pitts & McClure, 1967; Marks & Herst, 1970; Crowe et al., 1980; Appleby et al., 1981; Sheehan et al., 1981; van den Hout & Griez, 1984a, b). Nevertheless, a mechanism underlying anxiety that accounts for all cases is still debated, and exact behavioral and phenomenological descriptions of anxiety phenomena are generally lacking. A precise description of the symptomatology and the variability of anxiety over time and place that could further be linked to the growing biological data base is necessary.

Recent advances in the field support this suggestion: Hibbert (1984), Borkovec (1985), and Ley (1985) have offered behavioral, dynamic, affective, and ideational descriptions of anxiety and panic. Ambulatory monitoring of physiological measures has demonstrated that periods of anxiety in normal subjects are phenomenologically similar to spontaneous and situational panic attacks in patients (Margraf et al., 1987) and both are subject to diurnal and situational influences (Freedman et al., 1985; Taylor et al., 1986).

The Experience Sampling Method (ESM) may be added to other approaches because it is ideally suited for assessing rapid within-day fluctuations as well as variability across real-life situations. It can provide a clear quantitative description of predictable patterns in the build-up and decay of anxiety and of its relationship to mood, setting and situations. Moreover, the

[1] This work appeared in *Journal of Nervous and Mental Disease*, 1987, **175**, 9, 550–7.

detection of time patterns, and situational and state effects in the onset, maintenance, and diminution of anxiety may help to elucidate the behavioral relationship between general anxiety disorder, panic disorder, and agoraphobia that is the subject of much debate (Zitrin et al., 1978; Arrindell, 1980; Emmelkamp, 1982; Sheehan, 1982, 1982; Spitzer & Williams, 1984).

ESM provides information at the levels of both the person and the group. At the person level, knowledge about the use of time and the circumstances in which anxiety occurs supplies relevant and clinically useful information about the coping strategies of an individual patient. At the group level, existing psychological, sociological, and anthropological theories about anxiety and avoidance behavior can be re-examined in the light of ESM data and incorporated into a new frame of reference for classifying and understanding anxiety disorders. In this paper a socioecological frame of reference will be discussed to clarify innovative theories of anxiety as they apply to quantitative data on anxiety gathered with the ESM.

Theories of 'place' and agoraphobia

The circumstances and predictability of anxiety are most clear in agoraphobic subjects. By definition, we expect anxiety to increase when these subjects are out of the house or alone at home (e.g., Chambless & Goldstein, 1982). A thought-provoking theoretical formulation about the mechanism by which situations and contexts affect agoraphobic behavior is offered by the Dutch sociologist van Zuuren (1982), who isolates 'behavioral freedom' and 'acknowledgement' as the crucial characteristics of situations. She then hypothesizes that behavioral freedom in the absence of socially organized normative rules, as well as a lack of acknowledgement by relevant others, results in a loss of identity.

Van Zuuren's typology characterizes various social situations, such as going into crowded places or to parties, being with an intimate person or being alone, in terms of their degree of acknowledgement and behavioral freedom. Both normative and situational aspects of identity in agoraphobia can be related to this typology. Agoraphobics experience difficulty both when normative directions are lacking and when they cannot identify themselves with a fixed role. In situations in which behavioral prohibitions exist, but for which agoraphobics feel that expectations or rules about how one should behave are absent, deficiencies in their sense of 'identity' come forward. They feel 'at a loss' if they cannot act in conformity with a specific role and if they are not continuously acknowledged by relevant others. According to van Zuuren, it is primarily because of the lack of acknowledgement that agoraphobics experience discomfort in public – especially in anonymous – places as well as in solitary situations.

Moreover, agoraphobia and perhaps other anxiety disorders are largely influenced by culture. Each culture ascribes a different meaning to behavior and the experience of stress. Accordingly, different manifestations of anxiety exist across cultures (Good & Kleinman, 1984). In Western European countries, for example, the prevalence of agoraphobia in the nineteenth century has been attributed to social and cultural developments by de Swaan (1981). His argument is based on historical accounts of the 'disappearance' of women from the streets in the nineteenth century. He notes that with industrialization our cities grew enormously and became crowded by individuals from the lower class; beggars and jobhunters were described as filling the streets. For the 'petit bourgeois' middle class, it became increasingly difficult to maintain distance from these individuals. Men could not avoid them, because they had to leave home to go about their daily business, but the behavior of women of the time could be controlled by men. Limitations were thus imposed on their out-of-the-home behavior in order to protect them from dangerous, rough, insulting or – even worse – seductive contacts with the mob. Interestingly, however, as women acquired more freedom at the end of the nineteenth century and could even appear unaccompanied on the streets, the prevalence of agoraphobia rose. From a quite different perspective, then, de Swaan (1981) joins Freud (1924), in describing agoraphobia as the learned fear of the street or market place. It can be argued, moreover, that the cultural historical view of the street as a threatening place with potentially dangerous erotic and seductive encounters for women still holds.

From a more functional viewpoint, de Swaan relates agoraphobia to the dependency of nineteenth century women on their protective father or 'chaperone': 'The nineteenth century child-woman disappeared but the agoraphobic woman continues to compel others to protect her as a child, and in so doing she imposes her dependence upon others who find themselves forced to act in the family drama according to her directions' (de Swaan, 1981, p. 367). In this, like system theorists, de Swaan explores the functional aspects of agoraphobia from a historical perspective and points out that it is the collusion between partners that prevents them from a feared separation, inherent in the symbol of the street and open space; 'and thus the ideal nineteenth century bourgeois family is compulsively reproduced by contemporary phobic couples' (p. 367).

Rules of avoidance and their consequences are not just a Western phenomenon. Across cultures, prescribed avoidance behaviors that are often based on the fear and avoidance of sexual contact have been described in detail in the ethnographic literature (e.g., Malinowski, 1927; Wilson, 1951). For example, precise and rigid behavioral rules exist for the avoidance of intimate contact between members of the same family or kin group as well as with other defined categories of persons. The strain involved in abiding by these rules may involve significant social stress, and the reality of breaching them may have profound psychological consequences that account for a certain percentage of mental health admissions in both Western and developing countries (Tseng & McDermott, 1981).

The symbolic, emotional, and economic significance of social settings has also been examined in different cultures. Bohannan (1963) offers a useful and psychologically significant account of social situations and the rules that guide social and economic interactions within them. He describes three economic domains related to specific places, each of which is governed by a different degree of economic reciprocity. They may be visualized as concentric circles, of which the center is the home, the place of positive reciprocity or of 'giving without expected return'. The next consists of the village, extended kin group, or neighborhood in which the theme of 'balanced reciprocity' prevails, based on the assumption that you will 'get back what you give'. The outer ring is the marketplace or city, in which negative reciprocity, 'a get what you can' approach, guides economic as well as social interactions. Simply put, the marketplace or town is a relatively dangerous place, an area in which one has to engage, negotiate, and protect oneself. This is precisely the place onto which many phobic anxieties are projected.

Carrying this idea further, we suggest that the sequential mastering of the different areas of reciprocity is a development task. First, the child is usually exclusively at home with the mother, then with mother and father, and later moving about in the neighborhood at large (Fortes, 1958). An individual's opportunity to practise interactions in the balanced reciprocity domains of the neighborhood and village may be a crucial developmental step toward the establishment of a later capacity to function in the marketplace. Practice may be offered differentially less to women than to men, perhaps accounting for the predominance of women with phobic or avoidance problems.

Guidano & Liotti (1983) further suggest that agoraphobic patients may have had childhood experiences that comprise serious obstacles both to their autonomous exploration of the extradomestic environment and to the active separation from protective persons. If they are overprotective, moreover, parents are apt to discourage their children from leaving home even for a short while, citing reasons such as the child's supposed weakness and the potential difficulties or dangers in the outside environment. Agoraphobics thus may miss opportunities to practise in the balanced reciprocity domain, leading to later problems in adapting and coping, especially in a negative reciprocity domain. Through the use of the ESM, it is now possible to determine empirically whether agoraphobic patients demonstrate avoidance not just in the negative reciprocity area as expected, but also in a paucity of interactions registered in the neighborhood or balanced reciprocity domain.

The historical, cultural, and ontological perspectives on agoraphobia noted above introduce the ideas of 'place' and social activities into traditional psychological formulations of anxiety. These perspectives can be examined more carefully by using quantified data gathered from the time sampling of representative moments in the daily life of anxious people.

The Experience Sampling Method

The first objective of the ESM is to obtain self-reports about a representative sample of mental reactions to moments in a person's life. The subjects carry a 'wrist terminal watch' that signals them on a programmed random schedule, with 10 beeps a day between 7:30 a.m. and 11:00 p.m. The mean interval between two signals is 90 min; the minimum interval is 15 min. Because the set of signals is to be representative and unpredictable, randomization is essential, to prevent the person receiving the signals from anticipating them. When signaled, the person completes a self-report form that includes a range of questions about his or her objective and subjective states. Reports also include information about where they are, what they are doing, and who they are with, as well as their thoughts, moods, activities and (individualized) somatic and psychological complaints. A pathology module based primarily on the DSM-III criteria for panic attacks was included specifically and exclusively for the use of anxiety patients and their controls in reporting anxiety and panic symptoms. The repeated administration of this module may be regarded as a form of repeated diagnosis.

Subjects who met DSM-III criteria for panic disorder, general anxiety disorder, or agoraphobia (with and without panic) were recruited from three mental health care settings: a behaviorally oriented phobia treatment ward, a psychotherapeutic unit, and several ambulatory mental health care teams in Maastricht (the Netherlands). They were usually referred to the ESM research group by the mental health clinicians.

In the 'briefing' phase, the method was introduced using standardized instructions to the patient. Two individualized complaints (a psychological and a physical one) to be assessed during the research period were selected. In addition, subjects completed the State-Trait Anxiety Inventory (STAI; Spielberger et al., 1970), as well as the Fear Questionnaire (Marks & Matthews, 1979) and were instructed to fill out the checklist every time a beep was heard on the random-signal watch. The ESM data were then collected during the next six days. After the sixth day another meeting with the subject was arranged. In this 'debriefing' phase, information about possible missing data and the impact of the beeper on the patient's daily life was gathered. In a separate interview, the therapist provided information about the patient's life history.

ESM data at the aggregated level

Data from a pilot study of 10 anxiety subjects are reported here. The research group consisted of four agoraphobic subjects with panic attacks (two women and two men) and three male patients with panic disorders (without

Table 10.1. *Results of cross-sectional anxiety inventories for different groups compared to those reported by Spielberger (1979) and Marks & Matthews (1979) for comparable groups*

Questionnaire	Panic with avoidance		Panic without avoidance		Other disorders		Range scale (min–max)	Anxiety patients (Spielberger)	
	Mean	SD	Mean	SD	Mean	SD		Mean	SD
STAI state anxiety	55	5.50	50	7.55	61	10.38	20–80	58	12.3
STAI trait anxiety	60	5.92	60	6.68	66	4.51	20–80	54	11.5
								Phobic patients (Marks & Matthews)	
Fear questionnaire									
Total phobia	59	4.77	27	10.03	72	7.87	0–120	47	19.3
agoraphobia	32	5.94	9	4.12	28	5.45	0–40	17	10.0
blood-injury	15	8.70	5	3.42	22	4.51	0–40	15	10.7
social phobia	12	7.53	13	9.90	22	2.16	0–40	15	8.5

avoidance). We feel that, except for questions of validity, the use of normal control subjects is insufficient when specific variations in symptoms are the focus of research. For this reason, a group of three women with other DSM-III disorders (somatoform disorder, histrionic personality disorder) and concomitant anxiety complaints was studied, in addition to five male and five female normal control subjects. Anxiety phenomena in persons with and without diagnosed anxiety disorders could thus be compared.

Table 10.1 shows the mean scores of our subjects on the anxiety inventories given at the start of the study, as well as the scores for other, comparable groups (Spielberger et al., 1970; Marks & Matthews, 1979). These data are not available for the normal control group, but other studies (Spielberger, 1979) suggest a mean state score of 35 and a mean trait score of 36 could be expected for normal subjects.

As can be seen, the anxiety groups scored high on both the Trait and the State Inventories. Curiously, the control group with 'other disorders' scored even higher. On the Fear Questionnaire, agoraphobics with panic scored higher on the agoraphobia subscale and reported more avoidance behaviors overall than did the non-avoidant panic disorder group. In the panic disorder group, only one subject scored above 20 on the social phobia scale. Here again, however, the group with other disorders scored high on all subscales, indicating a high amount of avoidance behavior in various situations that was not recognized by the clinicians who diagnosed them.

The small size of the sample shows the preliminary character of these data. However, the findings of this pilot study not only demonstrate the possibilities offered by ESM research when it is aggregated at the level of the diagnostic group but also offer intriguing directions for future research.

To illustrate the theoretical propositions outlined earlier, we will focus here on the descriptions of various social situations as they interact with the different groups. Avoidance behaviors may be deduced from subjects' descriptions of their behavior in different contexts, such as being at home for most of the time or going out only with intimate persons; these data are coded from answers to the questions: 'Where are you now?' and 'Who are you with?' (Delespaul & deVries, 1987). These coded answers are displayed as frequency counts in Figs. 10.1, 10.2. Significant differences emerged between groups on the question 'Where are you now?' ($\chi^2(9)=79.4$; $P <0.001$). Avoidance – defined here as staying at home most of the time – characterized all the patient groups (in more than 80% of all sampled cases), but not the normal control group (Fig. 10.1).

On the other hand, differences in social contexts (With whom?) were also significant ($\chi^2(12)=141.2$; $P <0.001$). Agoraphobics, but also patients with other disorders, had very few social contacts outside their families: they reported being with their family in more than two thirds of all cases. In

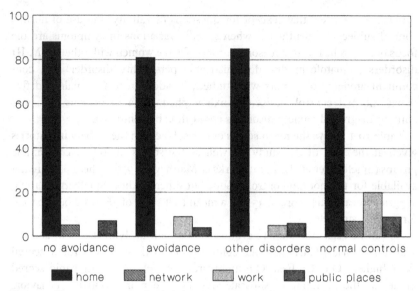

Fig. 10.1. Frequency counts of coded answers on the question 'where are you?' for different groups.

contrast, subjects in the panic disorder group were more often alone and spent almost as much time with their friends as with their family (Fig. 10.2). Frequency counts of contexts thus show clear differences between the groups under investigation, indicating restricted mobility patterns for agoraphobics and the subjects with other disorders, who avoid leaving home or being alone.

Because of the small sample size and the low frequency of some events, relatively few descriptions of 'avoiding' subjects away from home are recorded. Still, the findings do raise a set of interesting questions that should be explored further. Because both the avoidance and non-avoidance groups were defined on the basis of DSM-III diagnoses and descriptive cross-sectional techniques such as the Fear Questionnaire (Marks & Matthews, 1979), it is striking that in the random sampling of their experience they do not differ and report remaining at home for approximately the same amount of time.

This discrepancy between moment-to-moment reports and retrospective recall may prove understandable after more detailed examination of these phenomena. ESM research may clarify these findings by classifying the nature of activities in large samples. The type of activities engaged in, the social domains in which they take place, and the chosen companionship outside the home can then be compared for avoiders and non-avoiders in order to eluci-date discrepancies between avoidance behaviors that are retrospectively reported and those actually displayed.

Using a larger sample, an 'individualized fear questionnaire' recording both 'safe' and 'threatening' situations for individual patients will be administered.

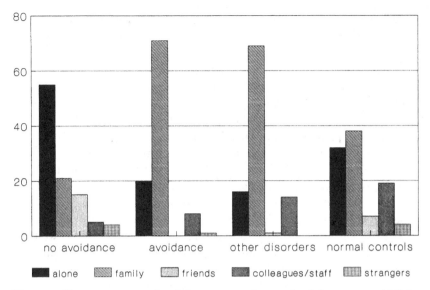

Fig. 10.2. Frequency counts of coded answers on the question 'who are you with?' for different groups.

These data will then be compared with avoidance and anxiety reported when subjects are actually in these situations. Ongoing mood states also need to be taken into account. It may be that agoraphobic patients go out only when they feel good and therefore do not experience anxiety. An analysis of sequences of experiences, using techniques such as cross-lag analysis in larger samples, can control for mood and state occurring prior to activities outside the house.

At the case level, however, clear relationships between anxiety and context may be ascertained. The theoretical and practical implications of the ESM results are illustrated in the following case.

The case of Mrs A

Mrs A is a 38-year-old part-time store clerk who has been married for 19 years to a partially disabled craftsman. They have two boys, aged 13 and 17. Mrs A was the last-born in a family of eight children, that may be characterized as a 'classic workers family', in which the father rose early to go to work and returned late and exhausted at the end of the day.

The mother was the predominant socializing figure in the household and is remembered by Mrs A as a strong disciplinarian. Mrs A was well protected by her older siblings and had a strong identification with her mother. Twelve years ago her mother died of cancer and since that time Mrs A has remained preoccupied with thoughts and dreams about her. Moreover, she saw herself as partially responsible for her mother's death, because she left home 'early' to marry and go to work. Her present problem began five years ago, when she experienced a panic attack on a flight to Africa at the start of her first major vacation with her husband, the first time that she had taken a trip outside of the region in which she grew up without her children or siblings. Since this episode she had increasingly frequent panic attacks, developed a fear of leaving home and began to avoid public places. She was also bothered by a suspicious preoccupation with her husband's extramarital sexual behavior, which both she and her husband describe as unrealistic.

At the time of the study, she had been treated for about half a year with psychodynamically oriented therapy that focused on mourning the loss of her mother as well as on the acceptance of her femininity and sexual independence. This treatment had been successful to the extent that she was less confused, had fewer panic attacks, was able to work occasionally, and was less bothered by sexual suspicions. Accompanied by members of her family, she was also able to take the bus to the shopping center of a nearby city and to shop for short periods of time. However, fear of the street, shops, and buses, still kept her home most of the time.

During the study she filled out the ESFs in a very dutiful manner. Her chief complaints of panic and feeling faint, formulated in the briefing phase, did not occur during the research period. Although the panic attacks had become rare, the item 'feeling anxious' could be related to where and with whom she was, as well as to her activities, thus illustrating contextual influences on her mental state.

Mrs A's high anxiety can be expected in two settings: when she is alone in the house with nothing to do and when she is out. Looking at the ESM findings, it is first of all remarkable that she is at home most of the time (in 84% of all cases). When her husband or sons are out, she is almost always alone at home (in 35% of all cases). Thus she has very little social contact in general and none in the neighborhood in which she has lived for some time. In addition, when alone she is predominantly occupied with cleaning the house, almost literally cleaning away her discomfort.

This pattern corresponds quite well with the hypothesis proposed by van Zuuren (1982) for agoraphobics: Mrs A experiences anxiety most in public places and when she is alone with nothing to do, but if she is engaged in housekeeping activities such as cleaning the house, she experiences less discomfort. When she is cleaning – although there is no direct acknowledgement by others – her identity is maintained by a strong identification with her mother, a perfect housekeeper, who was also usually at home with her eight children. Just like her mother, she conforms to the role of a 'good house-keeper', a role that structures her behavior and mental state.

These data may also be understood in the historical perspective offered by de Swaan (1981) and its theoretical emphasis on the socially prescribed behaviors and avoidance patterns described in the cultural literature. In this view, Mrs A was a simple country girl who imposed on herself the difficult task of behaving like a modern, independent, self-confident woman in a large city. In the small village where she lived, however, she remained very dependent, first on her parents and siblings and later on her siblings and husband. She did not acquire the social skills and the assertiveness required to manifest her independence, nor did she gain experience with the role requirements for the kind of woman she imagined herself wanting to be. She literally jumped from her mother's lap into the city streets. On the few occasions that she was able to go to the city alone, her experience was marked by panic, fear of separation from her husband, and her own sexual confusion, perhaps experienced in terms of physical sensations of fainting and ruminating thoughts about her husband's supposed infidelity.

The possible therapeutic use of these explanations should be considered. In actuality, the idea of the psychological impact of 'domains of reciprocity' on human interaction and individual experience does lend itself to practical therapeutic interventions, and combined with the ESM data, supplemented the understanding gained in psychotherapy and resulted in a simple behavioral strategy that could be added to the treatment. The approach was based on Mrs A's paucity of interactions in the neighborhood, the 'balanced reciprocity domain'. On the hypothesis that her current lack of social interactions in the neighborhood mirrored her experience in her 'overprotected' childhood, a treatment strategy was then implemented in which she was instructed to practice specific social interactions in the familiar surroundings of her neighborhood, such as with a neighbor or a storekeeper.

Although this technique is not different from generally accepted behaviorally oriented therapy, it does go a step further. ESM quantitatively located not just periods and sources of high anxiety, panic, or social avoidance – as behavioral monitoring would – but also brought to light Mrs A's limited interactions in the neighborhood and village. This 'insufficiency' in daily experience that had marked much of her life might have gone unnoticed if only the periods of illness, and not her range of experiences, had been the focus of research. Thus, by providing information about this individual's daily life, ESM allowed the application of a remedial development and behavioral strategy that permitted the patient to develop the coping skills that could support her identity across a larger number of social settings while she was building on the intrapsychic gains established in psychodynamic psychotherapy.

Discussion

In this chapter we have demonstrated that ESM is a useful device for providing a quantitative phenomenological description of anxiety. This in turn allows us more fully to understand and integrate theoretical propositions about anxiety, panic, and avoidance and to develop more focused therapeutic strategies. Psychological, historical, cultural, and developmental perspectives on anxiety and avoidance behavior have been presented in a socioecological frame of reference that helps to clarify the interaction between anxiety symptoms and the environment in which they occur. We then presented quantitative data gathered with ESM to illustrate these theoretical applications.

Although based on a limited number of subjects, our group findings allow us to formulate some tentative conclusions that offer guidelines for further exploration of the basic interaction between anxiety and context.

Interestingly, patterns of restricted mobility and avoidance were demonstrated in all of our groups of patients, indicating that avoidance may be a general coping strategy in psychiatric illness. Further, situational and contextual factors play an important role not only in situational panic but also in 'unpredictable' anxiety. So it is not unrealistic to suggest that when temporal and contextual patterns can be described in greater detail, there will be no need to use concepts such as unpredictable anxiety. Detection of hitherto hidden but predictable patterns of anxiety could lift the curtain off these now obscure disorders.

While our discussion of the implications of the aggregate findings in the anxiety subjects must stand up to the scrutiny of future research, our case description illustrates the importance of situational and contextual aspects in anxiety. It also demonstrates how ESM data can be helpful in establishing therapeutic approaches that are optimally suited for an individual patient.

II

Consequences of depression for the experience of anxiety in daily life[1]

MARTEN W. deVRIES, PHILIPPE A. E. G. DELESPAUL and CHANTAL I. M. DIJKMAN-CAES

What clinicians have long noted, recent systematic studies have demonstrated, that anxiety and depression commonly coexist (Roth & Mountjoy, 1982; Hamilton et al., 1984; Dobson, 1985). Many patients with anxiety present with concurrent depressive symptoms and many depressive patients present with concurrent symptoms of anxiety. The past or concurrent incidence of major depression in a sample of agoraphobic panic patients for example may be as high as a 70% (Breier, Charney & Henninger, 1986). Moreover, those individuals with mixed disorders seem to suffer from greater morbidity and poorer psychosocial outcomes (Stavrakaki & Vargo, 1986; Van Valkenburg et al., 1984; Klerman, 1986; Paykel et al., 1973).

In spite of this clinical significance, understanding of the phenomenon and treatment possibilities are incomplete. Experts still disagree about the interaction of depression and anxiety and suggest that this interaction is an artifact of measurement. Previous studies have relied on lifetime prevalence rates or cross-sectional assessments of anxiety and depression without the advantage of clear exclusion criteria that enhance the reliability of diagnosis. Cross-sectional studies about the comorbidity of anxiety and depression have often not been helpful (Mullaney, 1987; Stavrakaki & Vargo, 1986), partly because we have little information about the experience of comorbidity or knowledge about the co-occurrence of symptoms. This paper explores an alternative assessment approach, the Experience Sampling Method (ESM), to highlight daily experiences of subjects with anxiety and depression. ESM supplements traditional cross-sectional assessment methods by providing daily life descriptions and self-reports of mental states gathered within the context in which they occur.

The point of departure for the ESM research is that diagnostic categories provide inadequate descriptions for planning treatment and understanding

[1] Parts of this Chapter have appeared in *Anxious Depression. Assessment and Treatment*, eds. G. Racagni and E. Smeraldi, 1987. New York: Raven Press.

mental disorder; 'diagnosis is insufficient for treatment' (Klerman, 1984). In-depth investigations into the personal experience of psychopathology may be more useful, particularly when complex or chronic disorders are the focus of concern. In this Chapter we describe how temporal and contextual factors interact in anxiety patients with significant depression and discuss the clinical relevance of these findings.

Specifically, variations in time allocation, self reports of mental states across the day and recovery rates from anxious moments are explored to determine whether they differentiate anxiety subjects varying in the degree of comorbid depression.

Methods

ESM measurement of mood and anxiety

In spite of agreement about the importance of environmental factors in anxiety, panic, and depression, we know little about the diurnal and temporal aspects of mood and anxiety, and their interaction in daily life. The ambulatory monitoring of patients is ideally suited to clarify these issues. Recent studies employing such methods have compared the shape of circadian rhythms of depressed and normal persons and demonstrated that variations in affective symptoms are common in both (Monk et al., 1990). The ESM technique, which employs random, repeated self-report measures, was developed in the late seventies and early eighties (Csikszentmihalyi & Larson, 1984; deVries et al., 1986, 1987). ESM uses a 'beeper' to signal subjects randomly, within 90-min periods, to fill out self-reports 10 times per day for one week in the context of a person's natural environment. The ESM has proven capable of capturing mood and anxiety fluctuations sensitively in clinical populations over time and in different contexts. Previous studies have shown mood disturbances to co-occur in daily life with a variety of disorders such as bulimia and anorexia (deVries, 1985; Johnson & Larson, 1982), multiple personality disorder (Loewenstein et al., 1987), panic, anxiety (Dijkman & deVries, 1987) and schizophrenia (Delespaul & deVries, 1987; deVries, 1985, 1987; deVries et al., 1984, 1985, 1986). In these studies the ESM assessment of mood correlated significantly with social behavior and activities as well as aspects of psychopathology, motivation, and thought, while retaining its independent factor structure. The implication for the study reported here is that mood and anxiety may be defined independently by means of a number of the ESM variables. The interplay of mood and anxiety in daily life may therefore be successfully explored.

Subjects

This report is based on a sequential sample of admissions of patients with a primary complaint of anxiety to two ambulatory settings that specialize in the treatment of anxiety. The sample is equally derived from a hospital outpatient and community clinic during the spring and summer of 1986. Diagnostically, the group demonstrated significant depression and anxiety which co-occurred with panic attacks and agoraphobia. The group is similar to the patients defined by Van Valkenburg et al. (1984) and the anxious depression group (Overall, 1974; Paykel et al., 1973).

Our goal in this project was to describe anxiety patients with low and high levels of cross-sectionally measured depression using the criterium of less than 1.00 SD below or more than 1.00 SD above the population mean on the Zung scale for depression (Zung & Durhan, 1965). Eleven of the first 15 subjects sampled had high scores on the Spielberger Trait Inventory for Anxiety (STAI) (Spielberger et al., 1970). The criterion used was 1.00 SD above the population mean. This was expected in the caseload of an anxiety clinic. Of these 11 subjects, none scored 1.00 SD below the population mean for depression, five scored 1.00 SD above the mean and the remaining six scored in the intermediate group. The remaining four of the original 15 subjects were spread over the remaining cells too sparsely to be analyzed in this study. Although there was some overlap in the STAI and Zung measures, which might contribute to the co-occurrence (Dobson, 1985), the clustering of all individuals near the high anxiety, high depression range was an interesting finding supporting the prevalence of the comorbid phenomenon. We restricted our research to two groups with similar sex distribution, a high anxiety/moderate depression group ($N=6$) and a high anxiety/high depression group ($N=5$). The study thus compared two high anxiety groups that differed by 1SD on reports of mood disturbances measured on the Zung.

Findings

The two groups were compared using three types of data. First, we present variations in ecological descriptions and time allocation; second, we present differences in the self-rating of mental state; and third, we describe temporal characteristics of depression and anxiety.

Table 11.1 shows differences in frequency distributions of the ESM variables between the two groups. For all coded ESM categories (except congruence of thought and activity), strong differences were found. The groups differed on thought content, expressed psychopathology, where they were, what they were doing, and whom they were with.

A more detailed breakdown of these differences in global categories is instructive. For example, thought-content differentiated the groups. In this

Table 11.1. *Differences in frequency distributions of nominal variables between groups with high anxiety/medium depression and high anxiety/high depression*

	χ^2 of frequency distributions	Significance
Thought/activity congruence	$\chi^2(2) = 4.11$	n.s.
Thought content	$\chi^2(16) = 57.88$	$P<0.001$
Psychopathology	$\chi^2(5) = 31.48$	$P<0.001$
Where	$\chi^2(6) = 13.06$	$P<0.05$
What	$\chi^2(6) = 31.84$	$P<0.001$
Who	$\chi^2(6) = 54.43$	$P<0.001$

cluster, thoughts about leisure were found 10% of the time in the medium-depressed group and 21% in the highly-depressed anxiety subjects; 'thinking about nothing' was found in 1% of the medium group and 8% of the high group, and thoughts about work were found in 11% of the medium group and 25% of the high group. For the category psychopathology, in this case excessive worrying and rumination, it occurred 2% of the time in the medium group and 11% in the high group. In terms of activities, the medium group was found to be involved in self-care 7% of the time and the high group 14% of the time, and inversely the medium group was caring for others 18% of the time, but the high group did so only 7% of the time.

The social variable 'whom they were with' also differentiated the groups. Although both groups were alone a relatively equal amount of time, 21% and 26%, the medium-depressed group interestingly spent 47% of their time with family and the highly depressed only 33%. For friends and colleagues this relationship switched, and the medium depressed group was with friends 13% of the time and the high group 23% of the time. The actual time and places frequented, provide an indicator of the social time-space utilization of these subjects. The medium-depressed group reported significantly more time out of the home. When medium-depressed subjects were at home during the day they were likely to stay there for an average of 4.3 h. In the highly-depressed anxiety subjects this period was seven hours. When they went out of the home, medium-depressed anxiety subjects spent average periods of five hours at work and 50 min in the homes of relatives or friends, while the highly-depressed subjects spent only 3.5 h at work and 3 h with relatives and friends. Social support seems very important for the highly-depressed subjects. In one out of four observations those subjects went to the home of a relative or friend before going to work. This was never the case in medium-depressed anxiety subjects. In short, the medium group demonstrated a more diverse and dynamic network as shown in the pattern of time use, including long travels and public places, as well as reporting more transitions from place to place. The highly-depressed anxiety subjects were primarily sampled in a familiar environment.

In summary, the highly-depressive group had more idle thoughts, ruminated more and experienced less-focused thoughts. They allocated the most time to self-care and reported less care and involvement with others. Socially, the high-depression group worked and used transport less, was at home more and with the family less both in and out of the home. They also tended to report more diffuse and vague somatic and psychological complaints than the moderately-depressed group. These findings are in accordance with the clinical characteristics of this group of having a higher degree of morbidity than individuals with only anxiety or depression alone.

Self-ratings of mental state

While frequency distributions clearly differentiated the two groups on ecological and time-allocation variables, the psychological reactions to similar situations, such as being alone or being at home, did not differentiate the groups significantly. A difference was found for the entire group, however, on the item that rates whether thoughts are focused on ongoing activities. This measure differentiated both groups from other ESM samples of mental disorders. For example, in contrast with schizophrenics, who are markedly more incongruent when they are alone (Hurlburt et al., 1984; deVries & Delespaul, 1984), both anxiety groups were less congruent when they were away from home. The anxiety group then, interestingly, reports more disorganization when they are with people. In summary, self-ratings of mental state, daily mean measures of affect, motivation, and reactions to situations did not differentiate the medium- and highly-depressed groups.

Diurnal patterns and recovery rates

Diurnal patterns in anxiety and depression scores in the highly- and medium-depressed groups were explored applying a linear regression technique to the entire sequence of beeps per subject and collapsing over subjects per group. For the moderately-depressed group, no daily pattern was found for anxiety or depression symptoms, but for the highly-depressed group, a within-day significant fluctuation was found for depression ($t=2.06$, $P < 0.04$). This significant effect was produced by one subject who demonstrated a strong late-in-the-day mood upswing ($t=-3.93$, $P < 0.001$). This finding was supported by a trend in the other four subjects. Interday differences per subject were also detected, but at the group level this effect disappeared.

We next asked whether we could separate the two groups on other temporal dimensions such as the recovery rate from high-anxiety states. To demonstrate this, we tracked the flow of the symptom within the day from a point minimally one SD below that individual's mean mental state on anxiety. The

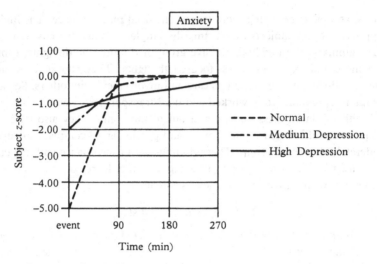

Fig. 11.1. Recovery to baseline from anxious events. Differences between normals, medium- and highly-depressed anxiety subjects.

'symptom event' was followed over subsequent signals that day to manufacture a recovery or decay curve of intense anxious episodes for each group. Figure 11.1 shows these recovery curves in the course of the day in relation to the mean for each group, medium- as well as highly-depressed anxiety subjects, while data on 10 normal control subjects are included for comparative purposes. On this graph, we see that the high-depression group recovers to baseline from anxiety more slowly.

For the normal group, rather than a gradual decrease of anxiety, we observe a precipitous return to normality, the absence of anxiety. This suggests that the recovery from anxiety states occurs at different rates across groups varying in the type and severity of psychopathology.

Discussion

Although the difference between the two groups defined on the Zung and STAI scales were subtle and often not readily discernible clinically, marked differences characterized the daily activities and experience of the anxiety subjects on ESM measures. This was particularly true for behavioral and activity data but also diurnally in terms of each group's differential capacity to recover and rebound from high anxiety episodes.

ESM self-report scores differed significantly for thought content, psycho-pathology, and the time allocation of activities. Mean self-report scores of the repeated measurement of mental state did not separate the groups significantly nor did the sensitivity to situations. Anxious depression therefore appears relatively context-independent. Further, social behavior and changes in daily life activities provide a good indicator of changes in mental state, better perhaps than the self-perception of state.

From the slow decay of anxiety in the high-depression group, we may tentatively conclude that depression in a day-to-day sense alters the individual's sensitivity to anxiety and that depression plays a major role in the phenomenology of anxiety. Since recovery rate is related to the duration a subject spent in a symptomatic condition, these data begin to suggest that depression may be a crucial factor influencing or altering an individual's capacity to experience or cope with anxiety. The findings presented, when pursued further and in larger samples, could lead us to a more comprehensive description of the co-occurrence of mood and anxiety that may help solve diagnostic controversies, and provide new avenues for treatment.

12

Dysphoric moods in depressed and non-depressed adolescents

WILLIAM A. MERRICK

'The psyches of all persons with psychiatric illnesses are guided by normal psychological processes.' (Freud 1901)

The blurring of the boundary between sanity and insanity has led to a view of normal men as creatures subject to psychopathological processes rather than leading to the exploration of the similarities and differences between groups of individuals and their experience. This paper takes this perspective by investigating in what way the experience of dysphoric mood in a group of depressed adolescents is similar to or different from that experienced by non-depressed adolescents?

The essential symptom of a 'clinical depression' is the presence of a relatively persistent dysphoric mood or anhedonia, the loss of interest or pleasure in most of one's usual activities. However, because normal people experience dysphoric moods from time to time, psychiatric diagnostic systems like the DSM-III-R (A.P.A., 1987) must distinguish between pathological variants of a depressed mood, characteristic of only a few people at particular times in their lives, and the normal emotional experience of a depressed mood, characteristic of many people from time to time. Accordingly, the use of the term 'depression' is often inexact. The distinction between depression as a syndrome and depression as a mood must be clarified. It can refer to a normal emotional experience, a state of dysphoria, or a clinical psychiatric syndrome.

There has been little research investigating the nature of the relation between the experience of dysphoria in clinically depressed and non-depressed samples (Hamilton, 1982). Studies which have attempted to address these issues have been limited by two major impediments – the use of data which introduce a retrospective bias, and the assessment of depression in clinical settings.

This is of particular importance for understanding depression in childhood and adolescence. Although many investigators have reported that children as young as six years old meet adult criteria for a depressive syndrome

(Puig-Antich et al., 1978), the validity of the diagnosis of depression in these age groups may be questioned, since we lack knowledge about the phenomenology of mood states and do not have direct measures of precipitants, persistence and reactivity of dysphoric states in children. Are children who are diagnosed as depressed a true mirror of adult depressions? What is the comparability of the illness in different age groups? The difference between syndrome and subsyndromal levels is of exaggerated importance here because children's sense of time is so different from that of adults and therefore, a retrospective bias is all the more relevant. Children's moods are also more variable across situations than are those of adults; the assessments of mood states in the settings in which they naturally occur are all the more critical in the study of childhood depression. A means to assess directly dysphoric moods in the settings in which they occur naturally and to assess these with some degree of ecological and temporal validity is now available to psychiatric researchers in the form of the Experience Sampling Method (ESM). The present study used this technique to measure the 'topography of everyday experience' (Csikszentmihalyi & Larson, 1984) including everyday moods and situations of three samples of adolescents.

Methods

Procedure

The ESM used with ambulatory subjects in the present study was similar to that used in many previous studies (Csikszentmihalyi & Larson, 1987; deVries, 1987). Data were collected from an intake interview that was used to orient subjects to the beeper method and to gather data about the person. In this 'initial interview', the 17-item Children's Depression Rating Scale – Revised (Poznanski, Freeman & Mokros, 1983) (CDRS-R, an observer-rating scale of depressive symptoms in prepubertal and adolescent samples), the 27-item Children's Depression Inventory (Kovacs, 1985) (CDI, a self-report measure of depression severity based on the attribution theory of depression), the Diagnostic Interview Scale for Children (Costello, Edelbrock & Costello, 1985) (DISC, a highly structured diagnostic interview schedule which provides up to 27 diagnostic groupings based on DSM-III nomenclature), and a questionnaire to assess demographic characteristics were used.

Subjects were asked to complete one ESM form every time they were beeped, randomly eight times per day. Subjects were asked to answer questions specific to depressive symptoms relevant to the study, such as items having to do with the experience of negative, causal self-attributions for the occurrence of good and bad events.

Subjects

The 28 subjects involved in the present study included 14 boys and 14 girls, adolescents, ranging in age from 11 to 18 with a mean age of 15 years, who were divided into three groups on basis of present and past psychiatric status. The first group, the Currently Depressed (CD) group consisted of seven adolescents who met DSM-III criteria for in-childhood depression and who at the time of the assessment were still clinically depressed. They suffered from Major Depression, Bipolar Disorder, or Dysthymic Disorder. The second depressed group, the Previously Depressed (PD), consisted of seven adolescents who were clinically depressed prepubescently, but who were not clinically depressed at the time of this assessment in their adolescence. The third group consisted of 14 adolescents who had taken part in a larger study of adolescent experience (Csikszentmihalyi & Larson, 1984). These 14 normal controls (N.C.) were similar in age, sex, and socio-demographic characteristics.

Assessing dysphoric mood

Dysphoric mood was defined by six variables assessed at each beep by means of Likert scales: sadness, loneliness, grouchiness, anger, boredom, and anhedonia. These variables were used to analyze the severity of dysphoria along three different axes; frequency, intensity, and duration. The first assessed frequency of dysphoric moods in order to answer the question: 'Do depressed kids experience dysphoria more frequently than do non-depressed kids?' The second assessed intensity of dysphoric moods in order to answer the question: 'Do depressed kids experience dysphoria more intensely than do non-depressed kids?' The third assessed persistence of dysphoric moods in order to answer the questions: 'When depressed kids experience dysphoria, does it persist longer than do the dysphoric periods of non-depressed kids and does it last for the length of time specified by the DSM-III-R'.

Results and discussion

Frequency of dysphoric moods

The first assumption regarding group differences in severity of dysphoric moods is that depressives should be more frequently dysphoric than non-depressives. Table 12.1 presents the results of a comparison of the frequency of six dysphoric moods. These support the assumption for four of the six items. The Table lists the frequency with which the subjects responded that, at the time of the beep, they were experiencing that mood in a euphoric range (e.g., at least some happy), in a dysphoric range (e.g., at least some sad), or in a middle range that was in a range that was neither euphoric nor dysphoric. As

Table 12.1. *Frequency (%) of beeps in euphoric, middle, and dysphoric range*

Variable	Group	Euphoric range N	%	'Neither' range N	%	Dysphoric range N	%	χ^2 value	P
Sad	NC	523	(60.3)	265	(30.6)	79	(9.1)		
	PD	128	(67.4)	46	(34.2)	16	(8.4)	11.46	0.003
	CD	131	(54.8)	59	(24.7)	49	(20.5)		
Lonely	NC	488	(56.7)	267	(31.0)	105	(12.2)		
	PD	118	(63.1)	58	(31.0)	11	(5.9)	31.17	0.001
	CD	104	(43.9)	67	(28.3)	66	(27.8)		
Grouchy	NC	471	(54.3)	233	(26.9)	163	(18.8)		
	PD	108	(57.4)	59	(31.4)	21	(11.2)	4.38	N.S.
	CD	123	(51.7)	64	(26.9)	51	(21.4)		
Angry	NC	536	(62.2)	232	(26.9)	94	(10.9)		
	PD	105	(55.9)	60	(31.9)	23	(12.2)	4.89	N.S.
	CD	130	(54.6)	63	(26.5)	45	(18.9)		
Bored	NC	347	(40.1)	242	(28.0)	276	(31.9)		
	PD	115	(61.5)	43	(23.0)	29	(15.5)	53.42	0.001
	CD	72	(30.6)	46	(19.6)	117	(49.8)		
Pleasure*	NC	—	—	—	—	—	—		
	PD	51	(32.1)	38	(20.0)	91	(47.9)	26.66	0.001
	CD	159	(24.9)	42	(17.7)	136	(57.4)		

*Item not assessed in NC sample.

is apparent from the Table, sadness, loneliness, boredom, and anhedonia are experienced more frequently in clinically depressed samples than in the non-depressed sample, whereas grouchiness and anger are *not* experienced more frequently in one sample or the other.

Intensity of dysphoric moods

The second assumption regarding group differences in severity of dysphoric moods is that depressives should feel dysphoria more intensely than do non-depressives. Tables 12.2 and 12.3 present the results of a comparison of the intensity of six dysphoric moods and the results support this assumption for all of the items. Listed are the mean intensity levels reported by the samples when they were signaled. For each of these, the CD sample reported feeling most dysphoric while the PD sample reported feeling least dysphoric.

Table 12.3 compares the groups on a measure of mood intensity which examines only those instances in which a dysphoric mood was present to some

Table 12.2. *Average* (SD) *levels of mood intensity for various dysphoric moods*

	Normal control	Previously depressed	Currently depressed	F value	P
Absolute values:					
sad	3.09 (1.23)	2.89 (1.35)	3.55 (1.57)	15.09	0.001
lonely	3.11 (1.26)	2.82 (1.29)	3.85 (1.85)	32.92	0.001
grouchy	3.35 (1.42)	3.12 (1.42)	3.58 (1.49)	5.42	0.005
angry	3.09 (1.36)	3.05 (1.48)	3.50 (1.57)	8.17	0.003
bored	3.85 (1.51)	2.93 (1.68)	4.31 (1.94)	37.29	0.001
pleasure*	— —	5.09 (2.83)	3.20 (2.89)	44.44	0.001

*Item not assessed in NC sample.

Table 12.3. *Dysphoric episode severity index (counting only those in dysphoric range)*

	Normal control	Previously depressed	Currently depressed	F value	P
Absolute values:					
sad	4.32 (0.67)	4.47 (0.87)	4.93 (1.15)	21.262	0.001
lonely	4.33 (0.64)	4.28 (0.69)	5.16 (1.27)	46.628	0.001
grouchy	4.62 (0.88)	4.51 (0.93)	4.81 (1.06)	2.666	N.S.
angry	4.49 (0.88)	4.51 (0.92)	4.86 (1.16)	5.884	0.003
bored	4.83 (0.99)	4.84 (1.13)	5.41 (1.13)	18.756	0.001
pleasure*	— —	6.66 (1.76)	6.12 (1.67)	0.495	N.S.

*Item not assessed in NC sample.

degree. These findings support those of the analysis above, except that the significance of the difference for 'grouchiness' drops out. In other words, looking only at those times in which there was some degree of dysphoria present, there was a significant difference between the groups regarding how intensely they felt dysphoric, and the CD group experienced each of these moods more intensely than the other two groups.

Duration of dysphoric moods

The third assumption regarding group differences in severity of dysphoric moods is that when they feel dysphoric, depressed patients will feel depressed for a longer period of time than non-depressed individuals. The criteria state

Table 12.4. *Persistence of dysphoric moods: average number of consecutive beeps in dysphoric range (rating of 4 or more)*

	Normal control	Previously depressed	Currently depressed	F
Sad	2.31	1.72	2.81	1.189
Lonely	1.81	2.10	3.38	4.257*
Grouchy	2.53	2.28	2.72	0.185
Angry	2.13	2.35	2.90	0.808
Bored	3.33	2.36	3.75	0.996
Pleasure	N/A†	2.36	2.74	0.224

*$P<0.05$.
†Item not assessed in N.C. sample

that they should feel depressed for 'most of the day, nearly every day . . .' as specified by the DSM-III-R (A.P.A., 1987, p. 218).

Table 12.4 presents the results of a comparison of the persistence of dysphoric moods. The results of these group comparisons provide only limited support for the first of the two descriptions. With only one exception, depressives were not any more likely to have their dysphoric moods last longer than the other groups. Further, in only one case did these moods last for most of the day.

From these Tables, then, it would seem that at least two of the three assumptions commonly made about clinically depresssed and non-depressed people's moods are valid, but that the third may not be. These ESM data suggest that the CD group experiences dysphoria more frequently and more intensely than do the PD or NC groups, but that the persistence of dysphoric moods does not differentiate the groups as expected. All groups, however, demonstrated fluctuation in mood.

Mood and situations

What are the circumstances under which a depressed person experiences more dysphoria and are these circumstances different from those under which non-depressed persons are more dysphoric? The situational specificity and temporal lability of mood states in relation to descriptions of where subjects were, what they were doing, and with whom they were, yield interesting data.

Locations

A breakdown of the locations in which the three samples reported spending their time can be expressed in relative frequencies. The CD group, spent more time at home (51.9% vs. 33% PD and 23% NC) whereas the percent of time spent in public places was very low (12.5% vs. 18% PD and 13% NC) when compared to the other two groups.

The location within the home where the CD group reported being most frequently, was the living room; for 50% of the time that the subjects spent at home, a location generally removed from their peers, these depressed youngsters surprisingly chose the most public room in the house, the living room. This represents nearly a three-fold increase over the amount of time either of the other groups spent in *their* living rooms (30% PD and 18% NC). For both the PD and NC groups, the bedroom was the most frequented location (CD 18% vs. PD 33%, NC 33%).

Activities

The CD group spent significantly less time (27.2%) carrying out 'productive' activities such as schoolwork or job while PD spent 36% and NC 40%. All groups devoted the same amount of time to leisure activities (approximately 44%). Looking at the leisure activities more closely, we see that CD youngsters report more television watching than socializing with others. One-third of the CD group's leisure time was spent passively, watching TV, and another quarter spent in reading and thinking. Socializing accounted for only about a quarter of their leisure time activity. This pattern stands in sharp contrast to that found in the non-depressed groups. These groups spent five to six times as much time socializing as they did watching television, reading, or thinking.

Social context

The CD group spent more time alone (42.1%) in comparison to either the PD (23.0%) or the NC (27.9%) groups. Of the time spent with friends, the CD group spent only 4% with more than one member of the opposite sex which accounted for about half of their beeps when with their friends. More surprisingly, of all 239 beeps reported by the CD group, there was not a single report of being in the company of only one member of the opposite sex. A striking lack of heterosexual contact at this critical developmental time for the CD group.

The analyses presented thus far have been cross-sectional comparisons between the groups, but how do affects vary in different settings and over time? Are friendship patterns, peer pressures, and social interactions *as* crucial to adolescent development as they are to the onset and maintenance of depressive symptoms in adolescents?

Figure 12.1 presents the mean intensity levels of sad moods in social settings, alone, with family, friends and class. This figure demonstrates that while the CD group feels more dysphoric, and shows greater sensitivity and vulnerability to different settings, their moods have the same pattern across social

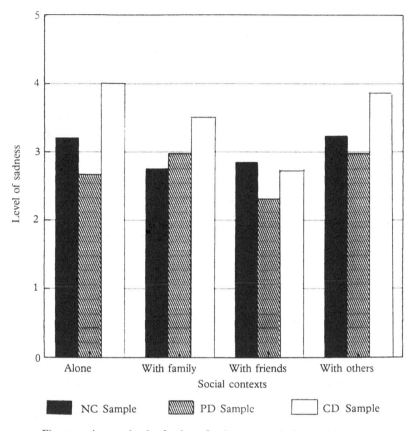

Fig. 12.1. Average levels of sadness for three groups in four social contexts.

settings as the other two groups. All three groups were *least dysphoric when they are with friends* and most dysphoric when they were alone. This pattern holds for all the six variables studied, sadness and loneliness, grouchiness and anger, and boredom and anhedonia.

The mood fluctuations of the depressed adolescents suggest that the depressed group may be more sensitive to the social context of situations. For all six items, the CD group demonstrates the widest swings. Both elements of contextual sensitivity and emotional lability are present as is demonstrated by the great standard deviation in all six of the variables assessed (refer to Table 12.2).

Diurnal variation in mood

There was no evidence for a diurnal mood pattern in these adolescent patients. The persistence of any given mood state seems quite short and did not differentiate between depressed and non-depressed groups. The mood level, also, did not change drastically over the course of a day. Fluctuations were not patterned and were linked to social aspects of situations.

Discussion

Although the sample was small and the data were analyzed exclusively at the beep level (see Harson & Delespaul, this volume), the results of this study suggest that there are both similarities and differences between adolescents with and adolescents without psychiatric illness. More importantly, though, these results suggest that, for temporal patterns, the processes governing the experience of dysphoria are very similar between the two groups.

Even in normal teenagers, adolescence is a time of wildly erratic moods and very great contextual sensitivity. They always have their 'feelers' out. Depression seems to exaggerate these normal developmental characteristics and processes. Yet, significant group differences in time-budgets, the social choices made, mental state reports, situational sensitivity and mood lability were found. These quantitative experimental differences in experience present support for the concept of adolescent depression as a valid psychiatric syndrome, particularly if these findings are replicated in studies investigating the experience of depressions in adults. Most importantly, however, the daily life data presented here provide clinically useful insights into the world of depressed adolescents such as the limited nature of their heterosexual contact, their increased time at home in isolated, passive leisure activities, as opposed to the more productive and social activities of their non-depressed peers. These findings on their marked contextual sensitivity are of direct therapeutic importance.

13

Capturing alternate personalities: the use of Experience Sampling in multiple personality disorder[1]

RICHARD J. LOEWENSTEIN,
JEAN HAMILTON, SHERYLE ALAGNA,
NANCY REID and MARTEN W. deVRIES

Despite the classic single case studies of multiple personality disorder by Ludwig et al. (1972) and Larmore et al. (1977) and more recent descriptive and psychophysiological studies of larger series of multiple personality (Bliss, 1980; Horevitz & Brown, 1984; Kluft, 1984a, b, 1985; Putnam, 1984; Putnam et al., 1983), much of the literature on the disorder consists of parital, single clinical case reports from which sweeping conclusions are drawn.

We describe the application of ESM, a new behavioral time-sampling method, to the assessment of rapid mood, self-perceptual, and clinical state changes in a woman with multiple personality disorder. The purpose of the study was to examine the utility of experiential sampling in the study of a clinical syndrome characterized by frequent, rapid state changes (switching of multiple personality alternates) that were readily apparent to the treating psychiatric staff but were of uncertain periodicity in non-clinical, everyday situations. We also wished to make a contribution to the systematic study of the phenomenology of multiple personality disorder.

ESM permits comparison of a naturalistically derived sample of the patient's own experience with clinical observations, standardized single-time-of-day rating instruments, and psychophysiological and other laboratory measures. Subjects collect data about their own experience at different times during the day. ESM can help characterize clinically significant, within-day variations in mood, behavior, and experience such as the immediate precipitants of switch processes or mood changes. It helps to minimize the biases that may occur with single-time-of-day reports based on retrospective, global recall of symptoms or precipitants of symptoms. ESM has been used in the study of normal subjects (Larson & Csikszentmihalyi, 1983), schizophrenic patients

[1] Appeared in: *American Journal of Psychiatry*, 1987, **144**, 1, January issue. © 1987, the American Psychiatric Association. Reprinted by permission.

(deVries & Delespaul, 1989), and patients with eating disorders (Larson & Johnson, 1981; Johnson & Larson, 1982), but the range of its applications to clinical psychiatric research has not been fully explored (Hamilton et al., 1984).

In this report we will use the relatively neutral terms 'alter' and 'alternate' whenever possible instead of 'personality'. We know of no well-accepted rigorous definition of the term 'personality' in the literature. We feel that it is more important to characterize the variety of discrete behavioral states seen in multiple personality disorder without implying prematurely that they conform to a particular form of superordinate psychological organization.

Method

The patient

Ms A, a white woman in her thirties, had a childhood history of severe physical, sexual, and emotional abuse and met all three DSM-III criteria for multiple personality disorder. Her initial clinical presentation has been described in detail in a prior communication (Putnam et al., 1984). She was admitted to the National Institute of Mental Health (NIMH) in-patient service on an emergency basis because of suicidal ideas and mood swings. Initially she received a diagnosis of rapid-cycling or mixed-state bipolar illness and was treated with lithium and fluphenazine, with little response. Subsequently, the treating psychiatrist (R.J.L.) identified five separate alters with different names and stated ages, mannerisms, styles of dress, postures, dominant moods and/or activity states, and vocal and cognitive styles. It became clear that the apparent rapid-cycling observed on admission had been a manifestation of rapid switching of alternates. Over the next six months, 16 additional alters were described. Characteristics of and pseudonyms for the main alternates described in this study are presented in Table 13.1. The patient gave oral and written consent for research participation and publication of her history. All names and demographic data pertaining to the patient have been altered to preserve anonymity.

Procedure

The patient was studied in two three-day periods during the first and third weeks of the final month of her three-month NIMH in-patient stay. During the study the patient was free to enter and leave the hospital on her own schedule and had visitors. Between 8:00 a.m. and 11:00 p.m. during each period, an electronic beeper was used to signal the subject to fill out self-reports according to a preselected, randomized time schedule generated by a random-number table. Each rating form asked for the following information: (1) time of day;

Table 13.1. *Characteristics of the main alternates of a woman with multiple personality disorder studied with the ESM*

Name	Current age	Sex	Reported basic affects, purpose, and characteristics	Reported additional characteristics	Reported age when fully in existence	Stated precipitant of creation[1]	Identification or shaping factors	Amnesia score[2]
Jennifer Sue	Early 30s	Female	'Host personality' (8); fearful, depressed, amnesic	Sexuality, motherhood	There since the beginning		Attempted to follow manifest conventions of family of origin	4+
Jennifer	Early 30s	Female	An organizer; rational, orderly, cognitively oriented, little overt affect	College degree in social science	7 years	Verbal and physical abuse by mother, responded by not showing feelings	Intellectual interests	1+--2+
Taylor	Adult (20s)	Neuter to female	A protector; independent, aggressive, joking, pacing	Interested in cars, athletics; has mechanical aptitudes not shared by others	9 years[3]	'Unfair' discipline by a teacher in school, punched the teacher	Identification with grandfather; 'maybe what they really want is a boy'	2+
Regulator	Adult	Neuter to male	'Memory trace personality' (8) (i.e., denies amnesia); 'control of others' access to time'; little physical ability	The internalized 'voice of the father'; seen as very punitive; demands suicide by the others or punishes them for indiscretions	About 5–6 years	Being beaten by father, terrified of attacks at home	Identification with/introjection of aggressor; 'if we took the father inside, we thought maybe we could control him . . . , but it didn't work'	0

[1] Often alternates are described as 'existing' before fully coming into being.
[2] 4 = severe, 0 = none.
[3] May have existed at a younger age but with similar characteristics.

(2) 'who was "out",' referring to the alternate 'in control of the body' before the beep; (3) whether a switch had occurred or whether time had been 'lost' (psychogenic amnesia experienced) since the last signal; (4) contextual information such as where she was, whom she was with, and what she was doing; (5) motivational information such as why she was doing what she was doing and her wish to be doing something else, measured on a 10-point scale; (6) responses to 13 dichotomized mood adjectives on a seven-point scale; (7) global reports of physical symptoms; and (8) the main global mood or feeling state as she was beeped. The reliability and validity of the method have been detailed elsewhere (Larson & Csikszentmihalyi, 1983).

During each study period a number of data were collected. The treating physician and a second rater (N.R.) made separate blind predictions of the percentage of time each alter would be out during an average day and the proportion of time – from high to low – that an alter would tend to be out. In addition, blind predictions were made about the different alternates' responses to the mood and motivational scales. The raters also developed brief global descriptions of each alter. Data were also collected about the switch process itself. All reports of switches were mapped according to the time of day and who was out before and after. Switches were examined to see if any kinds of situations and mood or feeling states were related to the frequency of switching or to the emergence of specific alters.

We gathered qualitative data by examining the handwriting style and other idiosyncratic features that characterized the self-report forms completed by the different alternates. ESM data were also compared with clinical observations from individual and group psychotherapy and from the hospital milieu.

Results

There were 21 responses in the first study period and 10 responses to 16 signals in the second. Although 21 alternates had been identified clinically, only seven ever responded to the beeper signal, alone or in combination. The latter was subjectively experienced as either a transitional state in which one alter was departing while another took over or as several alternates out together. Only four alternates – Jennifer Sue, Jennifer, Taylor, and the Regulator – responded more than once (Table 13.1). In the first study period Jennifer Sue responded 33.3% of the time; Taylor, 25%; the Regulator, 16.7%; and Jennifer, 12.5%. This frequency was significantly correlated with that predicted by the therapist ($r=0.82$, d.f.$=4$, $P <0.05$), and there was a similar trend in the ratings of the second observer ($r=0.78$, d.f.$=4$, $P <0.10$). In the second study period only three alternates responded: Jennifer Sue answered 80% of the beeps, and Jennifer and Taylor responded to the others. On the basis of reports of who was out before and after a signal, we concluded that the beeper itself did not usually provoke a switch. On the basis of reports of amnesia and switching between the signals, we extrapolated that Jennifer Sue not only responded most often but was also out the longest total time of all alternates during both study periods.

Because multiple personality disorder is characterized by complex psychogenic amnesia, there may be 'amnesia for amnesia' and alters may underreport switching (Kluft, 1984a, b). We attempted to cross-check for this by discussing with several alters on each study day whether additional amnesia had occurred but had not been reported. Although we cannot exclude this possibility, all alters vehemently insisted that the ratings were completed accurately.

In general, the alternates were cooperative in filling out the study materials. The exception was the Regulator, who was viewed by both raters as the least likely to cooperate with the study. This prediction was confirmed: the Regulator did not complete any of the ratings aside from self-identification.

During the first study period there were 11 switches reported between 24 beeper signals (range=3–5 per day). There were only three switches reported for the second condition (range=0–2 per day). Forty-three percent of all switching occurred in the morning, and 47% occurred in the afternoon and evening. Switches were reported between night-time sleep and waking beeps, although no changes were reported after an afternoon nap. On three occasions during the first study period (Fig. 13.1, day 2, open circles) additional ratings were completed, apparently owing to malfunction of the beeper. Data collected at these points were completely consistent with those generated at other times during the study. Figure 13.1 shows a graphic representation of the alternates' responses to the beeper signals, as well as their responses to several of the self-report items.

Examination of the actual rating forms revealed striking differences in how the forms were used by the different alternates. Some showed little variability in marking scale items, whereas others consistently rated themselves at the extremes. For example, Jennifer Sue mainly used the 0 or 5 rating on the 7-point scale but left other items blank. Jennifer used the 3, 0, and 6, while Taylor preferred the 3 and 4 but used the entire range of the scale, leaving a different set of items blank. One alternate usually circled the items, while another characteristically marked through them. These characteristics remained quite constant among the responding alternates.

Mood states were examined on the basis of the rating scale data for the three alternates who responded completely and often enough for analysis. Analysis of variance showed a significant difference on 'weak–strong' mood ratings among alternates, with Jennifer feeling the strongest (mean ±SD score=6.0 ± 0), Taylor the weakest (score=1.5 ± 1.7), and Jennifer Sue in between (score=4.6 ± 2.3) (F=3.62, d.f.=2.17, P <0.05). There was also a non-significant trend among the alternates in the 'hard to concentrate' and

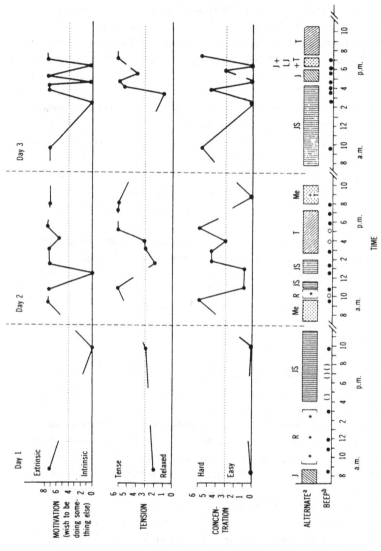

[a]J=Jennifer; JS=Jennifer Sue; T=Taylor; R=Regulator; LJ=Little Jenny, a child alternate; and Me=possibly Jennifer, possibly another alternate.

[b]●=Answered beep, ( )=unanswered beep, O=additional rating completed.

Fig. 13.1. Self-ratings of alternates of a woman with multiple personality disorder in response to randomly timed electronic beeps.

alert-drowsy' ratings, with Taylor being the most different from the other two. Her respective scores were 5.5 ± 1.9 and 3.0 ± 0, compared with Jennifer Sue's scores of 3.9 ± 3.1 and 4.9 ± 1.4 and Jennifer's scores of 1.0 ± 1.7 and 6.0 ± 0.

Prior research on ESM has documented a within-person correlation between mood and motivational variables, which differ between people (Larson & Csikszentmihalyi, 1983). This researcher has also shown that the 10-point wish-to-be-doing-something-else scale is a robust measure of the extrinsic/intrinsic dimension of motivation, with high scores indicating a lack of intrinsically motivating rewards for what one is doing (Csikszentmihalyi & Graef, 1980). When we examined the correlations between the wish-to-be-doing-something-else scale and several mood adjectives for the alternates, we found that Taylor was again the most different from Jennifer Sue and Jennifer. Although the individual correlations were not necessarily significant, owing to small degrees of freedom, the differences among alternates were clearly apparent from the pattern of positive as opposed to negative values. That is, when Taylor wished to do what she was doing, she felt sad vs. happy ($r=0.58$), and sociable vs. lonely ($r=-0.50$). In contrast, when Jennifer so wished, she felt happy ($r=-1.0$), tense ($r=0.87$), and lonely ($r=0.97$). In comparison, Jennifer Sue felt sad ($r=0.58$), relaxed ($r=-0.11$), and sociable ($r=-0.17$). These differences between alters are as different as those reported to occur between different persons previously studied with ESM (Larson & Csikszentmihalyi, 1983).

We compared the raters' global descriptions of the alternates to the self-report data. Some of the raters' descriptions were discrepant with each other and with the self-report data. For example, the therapist described Jennifer Sue as anxious, angry, depressed to the point of meeting DSM-III criteria for major affective disorder, and extremely troubled by chronic amnesia, headaches, fugues, and dissociative experiences. On the other hand, the second observer saw Jennifer Sue as relatively competent, energetic, and unimpaired. On the ESM mood scales, however, Jennifer Sue's scores were not significantly different from those of the other alternates. She actually scored between Jennifer and Taylor on those self-ratings which always showed differences between the alters.

The greatest discrepancy between raters' predictions and the ESM data occurred between Jennifer and Taylor. Clinically, Taylor seemed the most energetic, resourceful, assertive, humorous, and optimistic. She was a self-described 'protector' who usually gave the appearance of hypomania, cracking jokes and pacing through the room. Yet on self-reports, Taylor reported feeling the weakest, least alert, and least able to concentrate. Jennifer, who described herself as decorous and 'rational' and who appeared clinically to be relatively emotionless, emerged on the ESM data as the most alert, strongest, and most able to concentrate. In fact, the rank order of mood ratings for these two alters was the reverse of that predicted. When the alternates' main mood when signaled was assigned to global positive or negative categories and analyzed, Jennifer showed positive moods 66% of the time, compared to 20% of the time for both Jennifer Sue and Taylor.

Discussion

The ESM data suggest that switching of multiple personality alternates can be documented in a naturalistic study outside the usual clinical contexts. Although we encountered 21 alters in therapy, only seven ever answered the ESM signal and only three were frequent responders. Indeed, the data operationalize Braun's definition of 'host' personality (Jennifer Sue) as the one who has 'executive control of the body the largest percentage of the time at a given time' (cited in Kluft, 1984a, b). We also documented the phenomenon of consciousness (several alternates out together) that has been described in the clinical literature on multiple personality disorder (Bliss, 1980; Kluft, 1984a, b).

Our data complement the clinical observation that relatively few multiple personality alters have frequent or habitual access to full control of the body at times of reasonably good day-to-day functioning, although others may manifest themselves intrapsychically or coconsciously or only come out for particular activities, in response to specific situational triggers, or at times of stress (Putnam et al., 1984). Stress may lead to more frequent switching in patients with multiple personality disorder. This in turn may lead to a vicious cycle in which the switching itself becomes an additional stressor, leading to more symptoms and dysfunctional behavior. Misdiagnosis may be quite likely at these times, as occurred with Ms A (Putnam et al., 1983, 1984).

The multiple personality alters displayed some characteristics that were as different as those which occur between separate individuals who have been studied over time with ESM (Larson & Csikszentmihalyi, 1983). These ranged from highly idiosyncratic styles of marking forms and using rating scales to quantitative differences on the mood and motivational scales by the alternates.

The most puzzling aspect of the study was the discrepancy between the predicted mood states for Jennifer, Jennifer Sue, and Taylor and the actual results. This may have been a transient circumstance related to Jennifer's and Taylor's insistence at that time in therapy that they had decided to fuse and exchange characteristics. If so, it is remarkable that ESM captured the change. Another explanation is that the actual internal experience of multiple personality disorder alternates may be far more complex than the seemingly rational, internally consistent, and plausible manifest explanations for their behavior – especially as presented quite early in treatment (R.P. Kluft, personal communication).

These discrepancies may be related to the defensive function of the alter personality system – both in the everyday and intrapsychic senses of the term. Current research strongly indicates that multiple personality disorder develops as a childhood defense against overwhelming trauma – usually ongoing, severe child abuse (Putnam et al., 1983; Kluft, 1984, 1985). The giddy, apparently hypomanic protector alter may not only have functioned to handle vulnerability to new external dangers, as she proclaimed, but may also have represented an intrapsychic attempt to protect against a chronic internal experience of despair and helplessness. Except for conversion disorders – with which they are historically linked – the dissociative disorders may be the only DSM-III conditions in which phenomenology can be directly correlated with readily inferred intrapsychic events. Ironically, we generate the data for this hypothesis with ESM, a behavioral method.

Because of the intrapsychic functions of the alter personality system, multiple personality disorder should not be conceptualized as a static entity. The alter personality system may be consistent and repetitive in many respects but fluid and dynamic in others. The relation between enduring and abiding characteristics of multiple personality disorder alternates and those activated by dynamic and situational factors is an important area for future research. This view may also help to reframe the longstanding debate over iatrogenesis in multiple personality disorder by leading to a clearer articulation of the specific dynamic, defensive, and representational aspects of the multiple personality disorder alters as they appear during psychotherapy.

The discrepancies between predicted mood states and actual self-reports illustrate concretely how easily these patients may mistakenly be given other DSM-III diagnosis instead of or in addition to multiple personality disorder. We had continued to consider the presence of true affective illness in this patient owing to the apparent depressive symptoms in Jennifer Sue and hypomanic symptoms in Taylor. The ESM data suggest, however, that dissociative and dynamic factors led to apparent phenocopies of other psychiatric syndromes, as has been suggested in larger series of patients with multiple personality disorder (Putnam et al., 1983; Kluft, 1984; Bliss, 1984). The implications are that clinicians should be cautious and that extensive, longitudinal, and in-depth clinical material should be gathered before symptoms of multiple personality disorder are ascribed to or 'explained' by the presence of other DSM-III diagnoses such as borderline personality disorder or primary affective disorder, as has happened in several single case reports (Buck, 1983; Benner & Joscelyne, 1984; Coryell, 1983). With respect to axis II diagnoses, reports of larger series of patients with multiple personality configurations, not just borderline personality disorder, may accompany multiple personality disorder (Horevitz & Braun, 1984).

Finally, this study illustrates the potential utility of ESM for examining aspects of the treatment of multiple personality disorder and possibly of other conditions. The literature describes patients with mixtures of well-developed adaptational characteristics along with significant regressive potential who can become highly symptomatic in a relatively instructed in-patient hospitalization. Regression may be countered by setting clear treatment goals and firm limits, which may include an enforced discharge date from the hospital (Wishnie, 1975; Gunderson, 1984). During her NIMH in-patient stay, Ms A became difficult to manage as dysfunctional, highly symptomatic alters became very prominent. It was finally decided to give the patient a firm 30-day limit for her remaining hospitalization, with either discharge or transfer to another facility mandated at the end of that time. The ESM study occurred during the final hospital month. Although an ESM baseline was not obtained before the study, in this instance the ESM data fit well with the clinical data. During the last month in the hospital, the symptomatic and dysfunctional alters primarily retreated into the background. Behavior across the whole alternate personality system of the patient was relatively adaptive and symptom free.

In summary, we have shown that ESM is a useful, relatively simple method for studying aspects of the phenomenology of multiple personality disorder that can easily interface with other research methods such as psychophysiological measures and single-time-of-day rating instruments. In addition, ESM may show promise in the study of the phenomenology and treatment of other psychiatric disorders, especially those with frequent state changes or symptoms apparently generated by behavioral triggers.

14

Bulimia in daily life: a context-bound
syndrome

REED LARSON and LINDA ASMUSSEN

Introduction

The sudden widespread appearance of bulimia nervosa in the last 15 years has
given psychiatry the opportunity, usually reserved for pathologists, to test its
skills at identifying, describing, and developing a treatment for a new disorder. Given this challenge, controversy quickly emerged between those who
sought to assimilate it into existing nosology and those invested in defining
bulimia as a new disease entity. One viewpoint has seen the cycle of binge
eating and purging that characterizes bulimics as merely a new symptomatic
expression of existing disorders, particularly affective disorders. Another has
sought to characterize it as the manifestation of a novel condition with a unique
internal organization.

In this paper we demonstrate that information on the day-to-day patterns of
patients' lives can be useful in clarifying the structure of pathology associated
with a condition such as bulimia. In particular, we show bulimia to be associated with a disturbed experience of daily solitude. Since the controversy about
bulimia is most acute for the substantial subclass of bulimic patients who have
never met the criteria of anorexia nervosa, we will focus on this group. We also
demonstrate that information on daily life, which describes the disease as
patients experience it and localizes its manifestation, is particularly useful if
our goal is to engage patients as allies in a process of treatment.

Bulimia and depression

The controversy about bulimia turns on a question of figure versus ground, on
whether one stresses an overall pattern of cognition and affect or whether one
emphasizes the unique focal symptoms that revolve around patients' peculiar
relationship with food. Global personality assessments of normal-weight
bulimic patients reveal characteristics associated with affective disturbance.
These patients report dysphoric moods, poor self-esteem, high levels of guilt,
external locus of control, helplessness, and suicidal ideation (Johnson &
Conners, 1987), defining features of depression. A majority report that these
symptoms of depression occurred prior to the onset of bulimia (Walsh et al.,

1984), and family studies show a high incidence of depression and alcoholism among first-degree family members (Herzog, 1984; Johnson & Conners, 1987). Finally, bulimics have been shown to have neuroendocrine abnormalities similar to those found among patients with major depression (Gwirtsman, Roy-Byrne, Yager & Gerner, 1983; Hudson, Pope, Jonas, Laffer, Hudson & Melby, 1983), and double-blind studies indicate a positive response by bulimics to antidepressant drug treatment (Hughes, Wells, Cunningham & Illstrup, 1985; Pope, Hudson, Jonas & Yurgelun-Todd, 1983; Walsh, Stewart, Roose, Gladis & Glassman, 1984).

Many normal-weight bulimic patients, however, do not meet the full set of criteria for depression. Cooper & Fairburn (1986) compared a sample of bulimics with a sample of patients diagnosed with major depressive disorder and found less sadness, less suicidal ideation, and less sleep disturbance, but more inner tension and pessimism among bulimics. Laessle, Kittl, Fichter, Wittchen & Pirke (1987) found that nearly half of their clinical sample did not present enough symptoms to meet DSM-III criteria for major affective disorder. In a study of 108 bulimic women, Hatsukami, Eckert, Mitchell & Pyle (1984) found that only 43.5% of their sample met DSM-III criteria for affective disorder either at the time of assessment or in the past, and less than half of their sample scored moderate to high on the Beck Depression Inventory. In a review of literature, Hinz & Williamson (1987) conclude that there are not enough data to warrant classification of bulimia as an affective disorder and cite several studies that challenge some of the bases for the initial argument. Stern and colleagues (1984) failed to find significantly higher incidence of affective disorder in first-degree relatives of bulimics than in the control group. Halmi (1985) reviewed findings related to neuroendocrinological differences between those with bulimia and affective disorders and argues that they preclude the classification of bulimia as an affective disorder. Laessle et al. (1987) also suggest the possibility that the depressive symptoms associated with bulimia may be a result rather than a cause of the abnormal eating behavior of bulimics, in other words that the disturbing pattern of behavior leads to negative affect.

Perhaps the biggest challenge to the assertion that bulimia is an affective disorder is evidence, much of it from clinical impressions, that bulimics appear outwardly to be well-adjusted. Their depressed affect is not readily visible to others, and they do not appear to suffer from the debilitating amotivation and poor concentration associated with depression but rather often seem to be functioning quite competently. Boskind-Lodahl (1976) described a sample of 15 bulimic women participating in group therapy as '. . . high achievers academically and above average in intellect' (p. 348). Similarly, others have characterized bulimic patients using adjectives such as 'bright', 'articulate', 'intellectually gifted' and 'perfectionistic' (Herzog, 982; Dym,

1985; Rizzuto, 1985; Saunders, 1985; Browning, 1985). Rizzuto (1985) noted that bulimics are '. . . usually employed, work steadily, are reliable and responsible, and stay in the same job for a long time' (p. 197). Reports of personal characteristics and social competencies further evidence the appearance of normality in bulimic individuals (Dym, 1985; Rizzuto, 1985). Jones (1985) described bulimic women she encountered in therapy as 'calm', 'poised', 'well-mannered', 'accomplished', 'compliant' and 'cooperative' (pp. 305–6, 312). Russell (1979) also asserted that bulimics tend to be more out-going socially. In sum, clinical reports paint a picture of the bulimic's public self – a self which appears competent and successful in academic, professional, social and personal realms. Such observations suggest that the bulimic is a relatively well-adjusted individual, suffering only from what Boskind-White (1985) has described as 'a learned habit' (p. 115).

However, initial views that bulimia is nothing more than a bad habit – the latest fad among college women – have given way in light of evidence of the intractability of bulimic symptoms. Pyle, Mitchell & Eckert (1981), using a clinical sample of 34 bulimic women found that all of their subjects reported attempts to stop binge-eating on their own, although none were successful. Commenting on bulimic behavior, Abraham & Beumont (1982) reported that '. . . it is often extremely difficult to help patients relinquish it' (p. 634). Similarly, Rosen, Leitenberg, Fisher & Khazam (1986) characterized binge-eating accompanied by vomiting as a 'severe and recalcitrant disorder' (p. 257).

The discrepancy between the competent public self, first observed by clinicians, and the recalcitrant and disturbed private world of bingeing, purging and negative affect suggests the importance of looking at the ecology of the daily life of bulimic patients. In this paper we will show how the collection of information on the hour-to-hour experience of bulimics begins to clarify the organization of symptoms associated with the disorder. By plotting out the affect and behavior of these patients by daily contexts we are able to sort out how features of affective disturbance are interrelated with the bulimic's unique symptoms surrounding food, an understanding which in turn provides a framework for diagnosis and treatment.

A study of the daily experience of bulimic patients

In collaboration with Craig Johnson, a researcher who has used a range of methodologies to study eating disorders, the first author employed the Experience Sampling Method (ESM) to investigate the daily experience of 15 bulimic patients. These patients, all women, were recruited from a larger study of bulimia that Johnson was carrying out through Michael Reese Hospital in Chicago. All reported episodes of uncontrolled eating as defined by DSM-III at least once weekly and use of self-induced vomiting following these episodes.

The average rate of bingeing during the week of the study was 1.4 per day, with a range from 0.4 to 2.6. Rate of purging during the week of the study averaged 1.3 per day, with a range from 0. to 3.0.

The average duration of the illness had been five years and while some had been as much as 15% below ideal body weight, none had ever met the criteria to be diagnosed with anorexia nervosa. All were of normal body weight for their height as defined by the Metropolitan Life Insurance Tables (1959). In short the sample met the criteria for bulimia as defined by DSM-III.

These bulimic patients carried electronic pagers for one week and provided self-reports on their experience in response to signals. They received seven signals per day with one occurring at a random time within every two-hour block of time between 8:00 a.m. and 10:00 p.m. Respondents completed a total of 672 self-reports, an average of 44.8 per person.

These women's reports on daily experience were compared to those provided by a 'normal' control sample of 24 young, single women from a study of adult workers carried out by Csikszentmihalyi & Graef (1980). This comparison sample was approximately matched on average age (24 vs. 23 for the bulimics), current employment (95% were employed vs. 86% of the bulimics), and living situation (29% lived alone vs. 40% of the bulimics). The bulimic sample was somewhat more educated (83% had college education compared to 50% of the comparison sample) and more likely to be currently married (27% vs. 0%). ESM procedures with the comparison sample were similar to those used for the bulimics, with seven signals per day between 8:00 a.m. and 10:00 p.m. The comparison sample provided a total of 1,117 self-reports, an average of 46.5 per person.

Preliminary findings: bulimia as an affective disorder

In the first analyses of these data, we accumulated a number of findings that lead us to support the categorization of bulimia as an affective disorder (Johnson & Larson, 1982). To begin with the baseline mood state of the bulimics was substantially lower than that of the comparison sample.

On each ESM sheet, participants rated their mood using seven-point semantic differential scales. We computed mean scores for each person's responses to these items across all of her ESM sheets. These means scores were found to be significantly lower for nearly every mood item. The bulimics reported feeling less cheerful, happy, sociable, active, strong and free (Table 14.1).

It was clear that the bulimics experienced fewer occasions of positive affect and many more occasions of negative affect. Figure 14.1 shows the overall frequency of states reported for the item sad–happy. One can see that the experience of feeling 'very sad' was reported for 8% of the time by the bulimics and only 1% by the comparison group. Likewise, the bulimics reported many more occasions of feeling milder degrees of sadness. In contrast, the

Table 14.1. *Differences between normals and bulimics in average self-reported moods[1]*

	Bulimics (N = 15)	Normals (N = 24)	t-value
Cheerful/irritable	4.00	4.75	4.14[2]
Happy/sad	4.11	4.93	4.66[2]
Sociable/lonely	3.76	4.74	4.12[2]
Alert/drowsy	4.69	5.00	1.68
Active/passive	4.08	4.54	2.40[3]
Strong/weak	3.79	4.70	4.21[2]
Excited/bored	4.06	4.17	0.71
Free/constrained	3.66	4.56	3.54[2]

Note: From Johnson & Larson, 1982.
[1]The Table gives the average means for each group on a scale of 1–7, with a value of 7 corresponding to the most extreme positive state.
[2]$P<0.001$; [3]$P<0.01$.

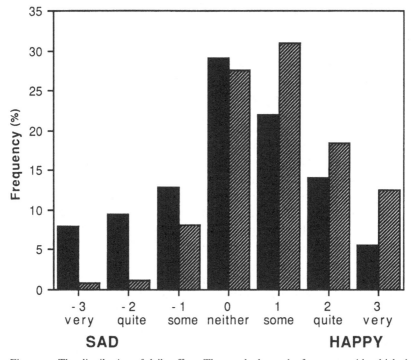

Fig. 14.1. The distribution of daily affect. The graph shows the frequency with which the bulimic patients (■) and normal controls (▨) reported levels of sadness vs. happiness during their daily lives. Percentages for the bulimics are based on 672 self-reports; for the controls, on 1,117 self-reports. (Modified from R. Larson & C. Johnson, *Psychosomatic Medicine*, 1982, **44**, 4, 341–51).

comparison group reported more occasions when they experience their affect to be on the 'happy' gradations of the scale.

It is important to note, however, that the bulimics did experience positive states. There were times when they felt 'very happy' and they reported feeling 'quite happy' and 'somewhat happy' more often than they reported feeling 'quite sad' and 'somewhat sad'. They did not show the pattern of pervasive negative affect that we might expect among depressed patients. They did not show anhedonia. Rather their moods oscillated back and forth between positive and negative.

Evaluation of the variance of bulimics' reported mood states confirmed this impression that their moods were highly variable. The average standard deviations for the bulimics were significantly higher on nearly every mood item (Larson & Johnson, 1985). Using one-time questionnaire measures, others had found evidence that bulimics experience lower and more variable mood states (Garfinkel, Moldofsky & Garner, 1980; Russell, 1979). Our data, obtained with a more ecologically valid methodology, confirmed this conclusion.

This first set of analyses also indicated other features of depression among the bulimic sample. They reported being alone significantly more often than the comparison sample, indicating a pattern of social isolation. They were alone for an average of 49% of the random signals compared to an average of 32% for the comparison sample ($t=3.29$, $P <0.01$). The bulimics also reported other subjective states associated with depression: guilt for 59% of occasions, shame for 80%, and vulnerability for 67%. In sum, these findings began to define a picture of global affective disturbance among the bulimics, including not only lower mood, but behavioral and cognitive features as well.

One additional set of findings suggested the association between bulimia and affective disorders. Within the sample of 672 random self-reports, there were 17 instances when they reported a binge in process and 12 occasions when they were purging. By looking at the moods reported before, during and after these occasions, we were able to reconstruct the emotional sequence associated with this symptomatic behavior. This reconstruction, shown in Fig. 14.2, shows relationships between affective states and the occurrence of bingeing and purging.

These data indicate that bingeing was preceded by lower-than-average mood states, as well as greater hunger, low sense of self-control, and feelings of inadequacy. This finding, replicated by Davis, Freeman & Garner (1988) with a similar methodology, and by Cooper and associates (1988) using retrospective reports, suggests that the cycle of bingeing and purging is elicited by a negative mood state – that bulimics binge and purge in response to dysphoric affect, perhaps in an effort to regain a sense of control. This conclusion, that bingeing is elicited by negative affect, is consistent with Carroll & Leon's

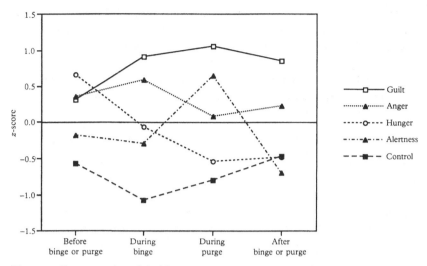

Fig. 14.2. Reconstruction of the binge–purge sequence, (Adapted from Johnson & Larson, 1982.)

(1981, cited in Johnson & Connors, 1987) finding that 86% of bulimics report that they first began bingeing while experiencing an upsetting life event.

Unfortunately, the binge only makes these women feel worse (Fig. 14.2). In our 1982 article we argued that, after the cycle of bingeing and purging becomes habitual, it is the purge rather than the binge that offers some relief from the negative affect. While in the initial stages of the disorder, the binge may have been soothing, as the behavior becomes established the purge becomes more significant. It is during the purge that there is a discharge of anger, increased alertness, and some restoration of a sense of control (Fig. 14.2). Research done since this study has corroborated the significance of the purge (Cooper, Morrison, Bigman, Abramowitz, Levin & Krener, 1988). Abraham & Beumont (1982) also found that patients who did not vomit after bingeing were more likely to report negative moods and anxiety.

But, while the purge brings some relief, after the purge our bulimics reported feeling no better. The entire sequence appeared to have had little net effect on their internal state (Fig. 14.2). The only significant difference between before and after is a diminution of hunger, a finding which was not replicated by Davis, Freeman & Solyom (1985). Thus, while bulimic behavior may be an attempt to regulate negative affect it is not very successful. Bulimics remain depressed afterwards, and, in some cases, may repeat the cycle of bingeing and purging over again.

All of these findings were consistent with the view of bulimia nervosa as similar to depression. Bulimics experienced more dysphoric moods, frequent guilt, more negative feelings towards the self, and a pattern of social isolation. Negative affect appears to trigger the symptomatic behavior. A second set of analyses, however, provided a more differentiated picture of the daily lives of bulimics which leads to some major qualifications of that conclusion and illustrates the importance of an ecological approach to psychiatric disorders (Larson & Johnson, 1985).

A contextual analysis of bulimics' affect and behavior

In the DSM-III-R criteria for depression, the subjective symptoms are defined to be 'relatively persistent, that is, they occur for most of the day, nearly every day' (p. 218). We have already seen that bulimics are not pervasively depressed, rather they experience wide fluctuations in mood and do experience occasions when they feel 'quite' and 'very' happy. The striking finding of our reanalysis was that these fluctuations in mood were not random, but rather were highly context-specific (Larson & Johnson, 1985).

We examined the average moods reported by the bulimics and the controls in six contexts of daily life. In order to avoid confounds, all occasions when individuals were in the process of bingeing or purging were eliminated. Our mood scale is computed from the eight items identified in Table 14.1.

The findings of this analysis, summarized in Fig. 14.3, indicate that the average mood states reported by the bulimics were not significantly different from the controls in many of these contexts, particularly at work and in public. The low moods of bulimics occurred when they were at home, especially when they were at home alone. It was in the private, solitary part of their waking experience, a context in which they spent much more time (32.4% of waking hours, vs. 18.7% for the controls), that their dysphoria was concentrated.

We found also that when they were alone at home they experienced higher levels of other symptoms. They reported significantly greater vulnerability, guilt and shame; they felt more ugly and confused than in any other context (Larson & Johnson, 1985). They also were much more preoccupied with food in this context. For 46% of the times they were alone at home they were either eating, preparing, or thinking about food. This compares with 23% of the times when they were at work and 35% of the times when they were in public. Time alone at home appears to be a focal context for the manifestation of their disturbance.

A further finding that reinforces this conclusion was that the severity of the disorder was closely related to how they felt alone at home. Johnson & Conners (1987) reported that frequency of bingeing and purging is a good criterion of severity; therefore we divided the bulimic sample according to these rates. Again cases when bingeing and purging were in process have been removed from the analysis to eliminate a potential confound. As Fig. 14.4 shows, there

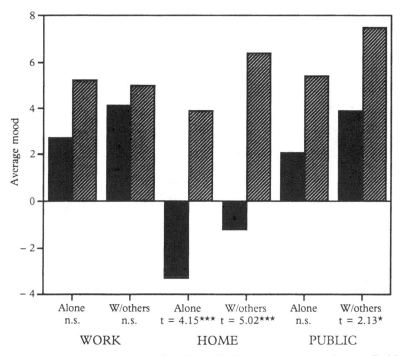

Fig. 14.3. Mood states by context. The figure displays average raw mood scores. Positive values indicate positive moods, negative values indicate negative moods. Bulimics, ■; controls, ▨.

is a strong relationship between this severity index and how they feel when alone at home. The more an individual binges and purges, the worse she feels when in this context. The correlation between a bulimic patient's average mood when alone at home (relative to her moods at other times) and rate of bingeing and purging is $r=-0.55$ ($P <0.01$).

A very similar graph could be made for the experience of control. Amount of 'control of the situation' experienced alone at home (again, relative to other times) is highly correlated with an individual's rate of symptomatic behavior ($r=-0.62$, $P <0.01$) (Larson & Johnson, 1985). It is those individuals who fall apart when alone – who experience the most negative moods and the greatest discontrol – that are most caught up in the cycle of bingeing and purging.

There is another important finding to be noted in Fig. 14.4. It shows that there is little relationship between the severity of bulimia and how people feel at other times in their lives – when they are not alone at home. Indeed the most frequent bingers and purgers are quite similar to the controls in what they feel outside this one context. In short, the lower moods that we originally attributed to the bulimics are due almost entirely to this one segment of their

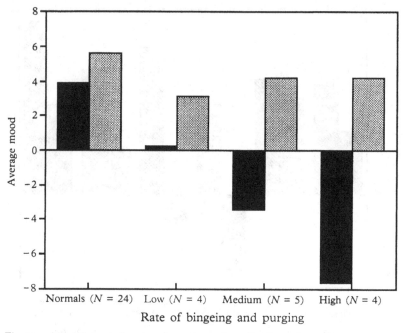

Fig. 14.4. Mood state as a function of symptomatology. ■, alone at home; ▨, all other times.

experience. The pathology they experience is concentrated in this one part of their lives.

Solitude and bulimia

The localization of bulimics' low moods to one segment of their experience brings together a number of pieces of the puzzle. First, it explains why bulimics are successful in their jobs and give a first impression of positive adjustment to psychotherapists: this is the public side of their lives. Their job is carried out in a structured, public environment. The therapist first sees the public self the bulimic patient presents to others. Our ESM data indicate that in this part of their lives bulimics experience subjective states consistent with a display of competence and normal adjustment. In these public contexts their mood states do not greatly differentiate them from others. While one could hypothesize that they experience latent or masked depression in this setting, they report the conscious experience of feeling happy, cheerful and motivated.

For coworkers, friends, even spouses and therapists, the private, depressed part of their lives may be opaque. There is an epistemological barrier that screens off this segment of their experience – if any of these people are present one sees only the competent public self. This barrier is fortified by the secretiveness of bulimics and their strong investment in presenting a favorable public facade (Jones, 1985). The solitary experience of bulimics, however, is a domain of depression, worry, and self-abasement.

The solitary part of their lives, of course, is also the segment of their experience in which the great majority of bingeing and purging occurs. In our study we found 88% of the binges and 92% of the purges occurred when alone (Johnson & Larson, 1982). Others have also found a strong preference among bulimics for bingeing and purging alone at home (Davis, Freeman & Garner, 1988; Abraham & Beumont, 1982). Pyle, Mitchell & Eckert (1981) concluded that 'all 34 of the patients in our series preferred to binge eat alone . . . Most preferred to binge eat at home'. The dysphoria of being alone and bulimic symptoms appear to be linked.

One can, however, question our earlier supposition and the conclusion of others that the cycle of bingeing and purging is triggered by low moods. The data could as easily be interpreted as showing that both the bulimic behavior and the low moods are *a result* of being alone, that it is separation from others that brings a state of discontrol leading to both aversive affect and impulsive bulimic behavior. In this interpretation, the fundamental problem of bulimics is not negative affect, but an inability to maintain self-regulation when they are alone. And the more they are alone and succumb to guilt-inducing bingeing and purging, the more they may experience dysphoria, low self-evaluation, helplessness, and impulsiveness in this context.

The findings, then, suggest that bulimics have two selves: one a competent, moderately happy public self, the other an uncontrolled, depressed private self. The public self expresses the perfectionism and high achievement strivings found to typify bulimics. Often devaluing their own needs, these patients are found to direct their energy towards meeting the needs of others (Johnson & Conners, 1987). They over-extend themselves in attempts to be amicable, well-mannered, cooperative, and compliant. Beneath this public facade, however, is often a sense that this is a false, inauthentic self. Jones (1985) and Johnson & Connors (1987) reported that many bulimics perceive their public self as fraudulent and unreal, a perception they attribute to bulimics' experience of having deliberately constructed this self in childhood to cover for an inner sense of emptiness created by distant, unresponsive and unsupportive primary caretakers.

The truer private self of bulimics, which they fall back upon when they are at home alone, is experienced as needy, frighteningly dependent, uncontrolled, and insubstantial. Jones (1985) and Johnson & Connors (1987) hypothesize that these patients never received the empathic encouragement in childhood that leads to the development of a strong, autonomous sense of self. Along with a feeling of insubstantiality, the private self lacks the sureness in its own powers that is necessary for self-regulation. A number of personality studies have shown that bulimics rely on external rather than internal cues to orient themselves (Garner, Garfinkel & O'Shaunnessy, 1985; Hood & Garner, 1982). Thus, when apart from the external structure imposed by others and the demands of the public facade, bulimics lack the ego resources to regulate their affect and control their impulses. Having denied their needs and over-extended themselves when they were with others, they feel empty, drained, and exhausted when alone. The bulimic cycle, then, is triggered (just as other impulsive behaviors might be for other individuals) as a desperate attempt to impose structure upon feelings of emptiness and disorganization. Once this response to being alone is established, it is self-reinforcing because the guilt and shame it creates increase the discrepancy felt between public and private self, making it harder to reach out to others. Their sense of shame may inhibit initiative to maintain interactions with others, leading to a life style of social withdrawal.

Conclusion

Our findings, then, show bulimia nervosa as a disorder that is highly situated within the contexts and rhythms of daily life. While we would not conclude that the problem could be eliminated by persuading patients to avoid being alone at home, it is clear that this one segment of their lives is critical to the disorder, and must be a focus of attempts at understanding and treatment.

The localization of bulimic symptoms to one segment of patients' lives certainly weakens the likeness between bulimia and affective disorders. The DSM-III criteria for depression specify that the symptoms pervade most or all of a person's waking experience and ESM studies of depressed patients confirm this picture (deVries, Delespaul & Dijkman-Caes, 1987; Larson, Raeffaelli, Richards, Ham & Jewell, 1990; Merrick, 1987). For bulimics the dysphoric affect is not pervasive, but highly localized. Attempts to relate bulimia to cyclothymia also are unpersuasive given an absence of evidence that the mood fluctuations of bipolar patients are so closely tied to daily contexts – nor has anyone described the positive moods of bulimics as manic-like. Rather than fitting existent nosology, bulimia nervosa clearly appears to present a unique constellation of symptoms, requiring separate classification and a dif-ferentiated approach to treatment.

Therapy for bulimic patients must include a focus on the daily experience of the painful, solitary part of patients' lives. Approaches which fail to acknow-ledge the context specificity of the symptoms may be counterproductive. The use of antidepressant drugs to treat dysphoria which occurs in only one seg-ment of a patient's life is rather like the use of an axe when a surgical scalpel is required. Jones (1985) argued that if the therapist responds to the patient's wish to strengthen the competent but false public self, she or he colludes with the pathology and may make matters worse.

Treatment for a bulimic patient requires breaking down the barrier that separates the public and private selves. This may involve compromising some of the high and unrealistic standards of the public self. Most importantly it involves fortifying the private self, strengthening its resources for self-regulation, impulse control, and maintenance of self-esteem. To accomplish this a therapist must penetrate the barrier that hides a patient's painful and chaotic experiences of being alone, a process likely to bring out the masked dependency and autonomy needs which may be very frightening to the patient and possibly to the therapist as well (Jones, 1985). Self-monitoring, such as was used in the study reported here, might provide a means of bringing these experiences to the fore (Johnson & Connors, 1987; Massimini, Csikszentmihalyi & Carli, 1987). Group therapy can also provide a context in which it is easier for patients to share their private experiences (Jones, 1985).

Broughton (1981) has suggested that most adolescents undergo a split between a truer painful private self and a more tentative public self. With the entry into adulthood most people learn to reconcile these two selves and achieve an integration between their daily experiences with others and their time alone (Larson, 1990). For adolescents as well as adults of all ages, however, time alone is a time of greater loneliness, greater dysphoria, and uncontrolled thoughts (Larson, 1990). The task of bulimics is to learn to accept and strengthen this private self, to learn what Winnicott (1958) refers to as the 'capacity to be alone', an ability to maintain ego-relatedness without the immediate presence of others. For bulimics, who may have lacked support and reinforcement of individual initiative in childhood, this may be a long and difficult process.

15

Alcohol and marijuana use in adolescents' daily lives[1]

REED LARSON,
MIHALY CSIKSZENTMIHALYI
and MARK FREEMAN

Introduction

Most researchers would agree that use of alcohol and marijuana, particularly by adolescents, must be understood in terms of the social and psychological context in which these drugs are taken. Pharmacologists have concluded that 'set and setting' play a decisive role in shaping drug experiences (Jones, 1971a, b; Weil, 1972; Weil, Zinberg & Nelson, 1968). Sociologists have described how effects of these drugs are related to the milieu in which they are used (Becker, 1963; Orcutt, 1972). There can be little question that social and contextual factors influence when these drugs will be taken and how they will be experienced. It is astonishing, then, how little is known about the actual circumstances surrounding their use.

A primary constraint on knowledge about the circumstances surrounding drug use has been methodological. Nearly all attempts at gaining systematic information have relied upon survey methods, despite recognized problems with this approach. Surveys typically gather information from people in settings far removed from the actual contexts of drug use; hence they depend upon people's ability to remember and reconstruct past experiences accurately. Artifacts due to selective forgetting, demand characteristics, and response sets can be substantial (Eichberg, 1975; Goodstadt, Cook & Gruson, 1978; Hochhauser, 1979). This was dramatically illustrated in a study of adult alcoholics in which the experience of intoxication was remembered as exactly opposite from what had been reported at the time (Tamarin, Weiner & Mendelsohn, 1970). Survey methods may be useful for studying rates of use and how these relate to well-established sociological and psychological variables (e.g. Kandel, 1978). But, in order to learn how drug use is embedded within ongoing lives it is necessary to have more direct information.

This paper reports on the use of a new technique (ESM) to study adolescent drug use. This involves having people carry electronic pagers (the kind that

[1] Previously published in *The International Journal of the Addictions*, 1984, **19**, 4, 367–81. Reprinted by courtesy of Marcel Dekker Inc.

doctors sometimes carry) for a week and filling out self-reports when they receive randomly scheduled signals (Larson & Csikszentmihalyi, 1983). By this means participants provide 30 to 60 self-reports on random moments in their daily lives. Because they report on experience as it occurs, the information is not dependent on recall. Because the signals are scheduled randomly across all hours of the day, reports approximate a representative sample of daily lives, including drug use. This Chapter is based on research with a randomly selected sample of 75 adolescents, many of whom reported alcohol and marijuana use as a part of their daily activity. The data allow examination of this drug use in relation to the rest of their lives.

A first concern is with external circumstances of adolescent alcohol and marijuana use. Survey research has linked adolescent drug use to peer association (Gorsuch & Butler, 1976; Jessor, Jessor & Finney, 1973; Kandel, 1973, 1987), suggesting that much drug use takes place with friends. But information is lacking about the time of day, the environment, and the social composition of gatherings at which these drugs are taken. The ESM provides a means for obtaining this kind of data.

A second concern is with the subjective, internal side of adolescent alcohol and marijuana experience. It is generally held that these drugs have a 'recreational' purpose, that they bring about a more favorable psychological state (Blum, 1969; Forslund, 1978; Shick & Freedman, 1975), or alleviate a negative one (Bracht, Brakarsh & Fellingstad, 1973; Paton, Kessler & Kandel, 1977). However, little evidence exists as to how regularly alcohol and marijuana actually have these effects. An extraordinary range of phenomenological effects have been attributed to marijuana (Grinspoon, 1977; Tart, 1971), but little is known about the frequency with which each is experienced, or even how often the drug is experienced as positive versus negative. ESM offers a means for obtaining this kind of data by securing reports on subjective states during daily drug use. It allows consideration of drugs states in relation to the baseline of daily states in people's lives.

Method

The data set used in this report is a subset from an experience sampling study of 75 White adolescents, conducted in 1977 (Larson, 1979; Larson, Csikszentimihalyi & Graef, 1980). These teenagers were selected from the student body of a large and diverse suburban high school bordering the city of Chicago. Sampling followed a stratified random procedure, designed to obtain equal numbers of boys and girls; equal numbers of 9th, 10th, 11th and 12th graders; and equal numbers of students from lower-middle-class census tracts (having an average family income of $14,000) and upper-middle-class census tracts (having an average family income of $25,000). The final sample included 69% of the girls and 45% of the boys initially invited to take part.

181

Participants in the study carried pagers for one week and filled out self-reports in response to signals they received. The signals, sent by a radio transmitter with a 60-mile radius, were scheduled randomly within every two-hour block of time from 7:30 a.m. until 10:30 p.m. on weekdays and until 1:30 a.m. on Friday and Saturday nights. Participants were asked to fill out self-report forms in response to each signal, with the understanding that they retained the right not to respond. Sixty-nine percent of the signals were followed by self-reports, providing a total of 4,489 time samples. Missed self-reports were due to mechanical failure of the pager, to respondents going to bed (in which case they were told to turn off the pager), to respondents unintentionally leaving the pager at home or deciding they wished not to be disturbed, and to a range of other reasons. In a debriefing interview, the students reported lower response rates when with friends and on Friday and Saturday nights.

The data considered here are from the 19 of these 75 students who indicated use of alcohol or marijuana on at least one self-report form. It should be noted that the self-report form did not ask about drug use; rather this information was volunteered in response to questions about activity at the time of the signal. Therefore it is probable that some instances of drug use, particularly those occurring in the intervals between self-reports, went undetected.

These 19 teenagers reported 25 occasions of alcohol use, 19 occasions of marijuana use, and four instances when both drugs were being used at the same time. Alcohol use was reported by 17 of the students (11 boys and six girls); marijuana by seven (three boys and four girls). The average age of these students was 17.1 (SD=0.9). Nine were from lower-middle-class census tracts, and 10 were from upper-middle-class census tracts. Because the research was not initially designed to investigate drug use, no information was obtained on these students' prior drug experiences.

The information obtained on the self-report form includes where students were and who was with them at the time of the signal. It also includes ratings of their subjective state, made on a series of standard psychometric scales. Among these are semantic different ratings of mood, scaled self-assessments of cognitive state, and ratings of motivation and the social situation at the time of the signal. In addition, students were asked about their thoughts at the time of the signal and were provided with space for additional comment.

Results

The objective circumstances of alcohol and marijuana use

The sample of ESM self-reports made during alcohol and marijuana consumption provides an opportunity to determine the 'objective' context under which these drugs are typically used. Figure 15.1 shows that all but four of the 29

WEEKDAYS (3:31 p.m. Sunday to 3:30 p.m. Friday)

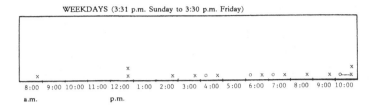

WEEKENDS (3:31 p.m. Friday to 3:30 p.m. Sunday)

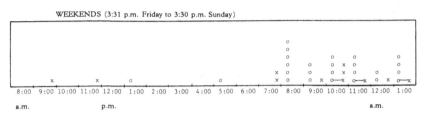

Fig. 15.1. ESM self-reports made during alcohol and marijuana consumption. o, alcohol; x, marijuana; o-x, alcohol and marijuana.

instances of alcohol used occurred on weekends, and nearly all of these on weekend evenings. There are no instances of drinking during the school day. Marijuana use, in contrast, was reported across all parts of the week, including school hours. One student reported herself to be 'smoking a joint' at 8:00 a.m. before going to school in the morning. On two other occasions students reported marijuana use during lunch time.

There are corresponding differences in where students reported using the two drugs (Table 15.1). Alcohol was used primarily at friends' homes; it was used five times in a public restaurant or bar (the legal drinking age at the time of the study was 18) and only three times at home. In contrast, virtually all of the marijuana use was reported either at home or in non-commercial public settings, while walking (two instances), in a car (three instances) or in a park (one instance).

A further difference in context involves the number of companions. For the great majority of times, students were with friends when using either substance. However, the two drugs differed substantially in the number of friends involved. Table 15.2 shows that alcohol was usually consumed in groups of four or more people, whereas marijuana use typically took place with only one other person.

To summarize, alcohol use was reported primarily on Friday and Saturday evenings, at friends' homes, with large groups of people; in other words, in the context of 'parties'. Marijuana use, in contrast, was reported over a broader range of contexts, occurring at all times during the week and in multiple environments. Whereas alcohol was clearly associated with social gatherings,

183

Table 15.1. *Locations in which drug use was reported*[1]

Location	% of time teens spend in this location[2]	Number of occasions		
		Alcohol	Marijuana	Both
Home	40	2	7	1
Friend's home	5	15	1	3
School	33	0	1	0
Public place	22	8	10	0
Total	100	25	19	4

[1] Significance test for comparison of alcohol and marijuana columns: $\chi^2 = 15.4$. $P = 0.0015$.
[2] Estimates based on ESM data for the entire sample of 75 adolescents.

Table 15.2. *Number of companions reported during drug use*[1]

Number of companions	Number of occasions		
	Alcohol	Marijuana	Both
0	0	2	0
1	5	10	2
2-3	2	3	1
4-6	3	1	0
7+	11	0	1
Total	21[2]	16[2]	4

[1] Significance test for comparison of alcohol and marijuana: Kendall τ B = 0.60; $P = 0.0001$.
[2] Subjects failed to report number of friends for several occasions.

marijuana use appeared associated with intimate interactions among one or two friends.

Subjective states during alcohol and marijuana use

The sample of self-reports also provides a record of adolescents' subjective experiences at the time of alcohol and marijuana use. To compare these ratings to the rest of daily experience, they were converted to z scores, for which a value of 0.0 corresponds to each individual's mean rating for that item across all of his or her self-reports. An interval of 1.0 corresponds to an individual's

Table 15.3. *Reported state when drug use was reported*[1]

	Mean z score		
Self-report item	Alcohol ($N = 25$)	Marijuana ($N = 19$)	Both ($N = 4$)
Mood items			
Affect			
happy (vs. sad)	0.61***	0.37	1.09
cheerful (vs. irritable)	0.52**	0.19	1.22**
Friendly (vs. angry)	0.56**	0.09	1.13**
sociable (vs. lonely)	0.76**	0.29	1.30**
Activation			
alert (vs. drowsy)	0.01	−0.38	0.08
strong (vs. weak)	0.22	−0.27	0.40
active (vs. passive)	0.42*	−0.20	0.05
Other			
involved (vs. detached)	0.56**	0.20	0.52
excited (vs. bored)	0.91***	0.57*	1.46**
free (vs. constrained)	0.71**	0.55**	0.73
open (vs. closed)	0.70**	0.27	0.57
clear (vs. confused)	−0.06	−0.40	0.21
Cognitive and Motivational States			
Cognitive			
concentration	−0.45*	0.34	0.15
ease of concentration	0.03	−0.29	−0.75
self-consciousness	−0.26	−0.16	0.43
Motivational			
control of actions	−0.87**	−0.76**	−1.61*
do you wish you were doing something else?	−0.40*	−0.64**	−0.96
Social Interaction			
Is talk joking (vs. serious)?	0.79***	0.27	−0.49
Are the goals of others the same As yours (vs. different)?	0.18	0.47*	0.32
Do you expect to receive positive feedback (vs. negative feedback)?	0.44*	0.32	0.50

[1] Significance tests of deviation from zero: *$P<0.05$; **$P<0.01$; ***$P<0.001$.

standard deviation. Table 15.3 shows the average reported states when using alcohol and marijuana, as compared to the overall average state, or baseline, of 0.0.

It is apparent from Table 15.3 that the experiences associated with alcohol use are substantially different from the normal state. For nearly all the mood items the students indicated feeling significantly more positive than usual, with the largest deviations on the dimensions Excited, Sociable, Free, and Open. The mood items dealing with activation (Alert, Strong, and Active) show the least elevation. On the cognitive state items, students reported levels below average when using alcohol. Concentration and Control of Actions were rated significantly lower than baseline, with Control nearly a full standard deviation below normal. Lastly, on the item dealing with motivation ('Do you wish you were doing something else?'), the students reported being favorably disposed to the situation they were in.

During marijuana use, changes in experimental state were not as evident. Whereas reported moods during alcohol use were clearly positive, during marijuana use the averages for several items were actually in a negative direction. Only two mood items, Excited and Free, showed significantly positive levels. Reported cognitive states were lower than baseline, only Control of Actions differed significantly from the mean.

Across all items, changes in state associated with marijuana appeared to be weaker than those associated with alcohol; it is striking then, that on the one motiviation item, students reported a stronger wish to be doing what they were doing during marijuana use. This drug is not markedly associated with positive moods; nonetheless the students indicated positive motivation when they were using it.

Case study: a heavy marijuana user

In order to examine more closely the pattern of drug experience among adolescents, it will be useful to look at the reports of one individual. Rick Marelli (pseudonym) was a high school senior of average intelligence, the youngest of four in a suburban middle-class family. Figure 15.2 shows the moods he reported during a follow-up conducted two years after the original study. The mood scale used in the graph is based on the first 10 semantic differential items from Table 15.3. Alongside these values is a summary of the situations he reported for each pager signal. In total Rick provided 46 random self-reports; 15 of these (one out of every three) involved consumption of either alcohol or marijuana, or both.

Rick received the first signal at 12:45 p.m. on a Monday, when walking home from school with a couple of friends. His mood was relatively positive, but it was substantially lower when he filled out a report later, 6:42 p.m. In the debriefing interview, he said he and his friends had been carrying some beers, which they drank in the afternoon, and the alcohol, he felt, had had a depressing effect on his mood. On the 6:42 p.m. pager sheet he added the comment: 'Should not have

186

got so buzzed. Delays school work'. His mood recovered later, but there was no indication that he got to the school work. At 8:40 p.m. he reported listening to the radio and tapping with drumsticks on a back-gammon set ('There was nothing better to do'). And at 10:24 p.m. he was cooking popcorn and drinking beer with his father.

On Tuesday Rick reported no alcohol or marijuana use, and his moods were as positive as on any other day. In English class feelings were low, but in Biology they were better, partly because he was think-ing about girls. At 12:45 p.m. he was riding a motorcycle with friends, and at 7:35 p.m. he was playing basketball and reported the highest moods of the week. It appears he was able to have a good time without drugs.

Nonetheless, when the pager signaled on Wednesday morning at 10:30 a.m., he reported taking a break from school with friends and that they had 'just finished getting high' and were walking down the street listening to the Grateful Dead. Feelings were positive, but it is not clear whether this was because of the drug, the music, or the reprieve from school. He also reported feeling less in control than usual and was concerned about getting caught.

For the rest of the day his mood appeared to be dominated by pain from dental braces, inflicted during his visit to the orthodontist at noon. The marijuana in the morning did not keep him from feeling low. When signaled at 4:24 p.m., he was playing softball and smoking more mari-juana, which temporarily lifted his mood. But during the next two reports that day, Rick was alone, walking in the rain with a low mood and sore teeth.

Thursday evening at 6:00 p.m. his mouth was still sore, but he was attempting to overcome the pain with improvised meditation tech-niques. He got stoned, put on 'Jesus Christ Superstar', and (as he described it later in the interview) was 'trying to absorb energy from the situation'. On the self-report form he reported very high Concentration and very high Control. However, Concentration, Control, and Positive mood all deteriorated by 7:05 p.m. when he was eating supper with his parents. And they were still low at 10:00 p.m. when he was watching TV and again getting high.

Friday turned out to be a day of extensive alcohol and marijuana use. About noon a group of friends started drinking beer and smoking pot. When Rick was signaled at 3:20 p.m. he was feeling quite good. But then he and his friends separated for a while, and at 3:40 p.m. he described himself as 'dulled out'. He was watching TV alone and drink-ing another beer. Later in the afternoon, at 5:00 p.m., he was again with his friends, was selling some joints, and his mood was up slightly. In the

Mood State

negative   neutral   positive

Monday

12 : 45 p.m. — Walking home from school with friends

6 : 42 — (Drinks beer) Resting & listening to music, in bedroom alone

8 : 40 — Listening to music & drumming, in bedroom alone

10 : 24 — Drinking beer / Eating popcorn with father in kitchen

Tuesday

8 : 45 a.m. — Thinking about lines from a Tennyson poem, in English

11 : 00 — Thinking about asking a girl to prom, in biology

12 : 35 p.m. — Getting on motorcycle, with friends

7 : 35 — Playing basketball with friends

Wednesday

7 : 35 a.m. — Taking a shower

10 : 30 — Just finished getting high / Skipping school with friends

12 : 16 p.m. — Paging through a magazine, at orthodondist / Checking the mail, at home alone

1 : 34 —

4 : 24 — Passing a joint / Playing basketball with friends

6 : 05 — Walking in the rain, thinking about a girl, alone

8 : 55 — Walking in the rain, alone

Thursday

8 : 50 a.m. — Listening & thinking, in English

9 : 40 — Discussing the 40's, in American History

6 : 00 p.m. — (Smokes marijuana) Meditating on mouth pain, in bedroom alone

7 : 05 — Talking with parents in kitchen

10 : 00 — Getting high / Watching T.V., in bedroom alone

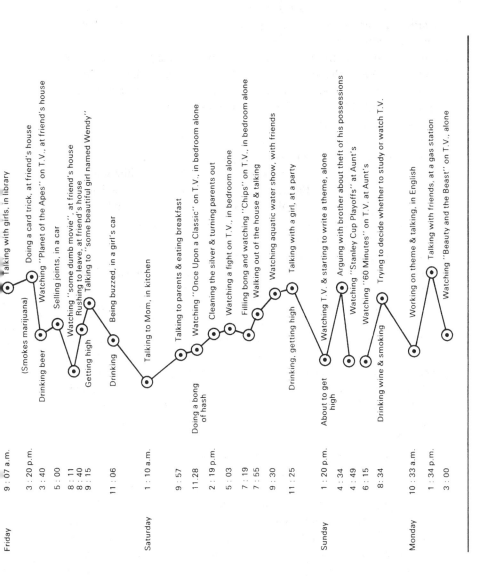

Fig. 15.2. Circumstances of alcohol and marijuana use in one case study.

debriefing interview he described it as what might be called a 'do or die' situation: 'You gotta keep partying. If not, you're just going to get tired'. He was trying to get a 'second wind' but instead was crashing. As the evening continued he and his friends continued to drink beer, smoke marijuana, and go from place to place looking for a good party; but on the self-report form he wrote, in an increasingly scrawling hand, that he felt very out of control as well as 'weak', 'passive', and 'bored'. For he and his friends, the party spirit had devolved into aimless driving around. The last report of the day (at 1:10 a.m.) showed him talking amicably with his mother about 'how rotten the night was'. In the interview Rick explained that he had not had fun; he 'just got drunk'.

The following morning at breakfast he was still thinking about what a 'rotten time' he had had and was feeling low. His mood had risen a little at 11:30 a.m. when he was smoking a bong of hashish while watching 'Robin Hood' on TV. Bored in spite of the hashish, he said in the interview, 'I'd rather be high and bored than not high and bored'. Marijuana and hashish were not necessarily elevating for Rick, yet he persisted in taking them.

Most of Saturday afternoon was spent cleaning silverware in preparation for his aunt's visit. Resentful of the work and the hypocrisy he saw in these special preparations, he wrote a string of obscenities on the self-report form. To deal with the situation, he smoked more marijuana, which evidently helped him to feel free. In the evening he did some more bongs, watched 'Chips' on TV, and again became angry about his obligations. Later he went out with friends, reported drinking and smoking again, but indicated having a much better time than the night before.

But Sunday was Mother's Day, which brought more conflict with his family. At 1:20 p.m. he reported he was getting high in order to write a theme. Later he had a fight with his brother and then got trapped at his aunt's house where all he could do was watch TV.

This narrative account suggests how drug use fits into Rick's life. The reports show him smoking marijuana to enjoy times with friends and times by himself. He used it in attempts to kill pain, cope with his family, and do homework. It appeared to be a part of nearly all social occasions, as well as something to do while alone. Yet there is no clear suggestion in these data that it had a positive influence on his mood; as often as not it left him feeling out of control. Alcohol appeared to be consumed in a narrower range of circumstances and appeared to be related to a more consistent change in state. Except for the miserable experiences on Friday, drinking alcohol was nearly always associated with a positive mood. Clearly Rick is an example of a heavy drug user;

nonetheless his experiences during the week exemplify the pattern for the entire group.

Discussion

The findings of this study are of a preliminary nature, but they do suggest basic patterns in how use of alcohol and marijuana fits into adolescents' daily experience. For this sample, alcohol was clearly a social drug, used almost entirely in a specific social context: Friday and Saturday night parties. The associated subjective state was one of high gregariousness, including feelings of cheerfulness, openness, and joviality. Alcohol and this sociable mood appeared to be an almost inseparable part of this social context. Rick Marelli's self-reports provided several examples of how alcohol use occurred as a normative part of such gatherings.

Marijuana, in contrast, appeared to be more of a private drug, most often used with one or two friends. Whereas alcohol use was reported by many individuals in a specific social context, marijuana use was reported by fewer individuals but across a wider range of contexts. It was reported at large social gatherings and solitary occasions, at home and in public, and across all hours of the week. In contrast to alcohol, marijuana use was associated with few changes in emotional or cognitive state. Notably, it was not related to positive affect, a finding that contradicts information from survey and laboratory research indicating positive or even 'euphoric' moods as a frequent product of marijuana (Grinspoon, 1977). This suggests that adolescents' memories of drug use, as reported afterward, may be much more positive than is actually the case in immediate experience.

If only minimal emotional or cognitive benefits are being derived from marijuana, it becomes essential to examine other, perhaps more subtle, motivating factors related to its use. In addition to the variety of social and symbolic factors described by others (e.g. Dembo et al., 1976; Kandel, 1978), it seems important to consider the particular ends that marijuana use may serve in relation to other routine tasks and activities. It is striking to us that the pattern of states reported during marijuana use is exactly opposite to that reported by these same adolescents during school classes. Whereas marijuana use is characterized by significantly high feelings of excitement, freedom, and wishing to be doing what one is doing, the experience of class is characterized by significantly high boredom, constraint, and wishing to be doing something else (Csikszentmihalyi & Larson, 1984). This pattern suggests that the drug serves as a response to feelings of boredom and constraint induced by the school experience. Rick Marelli certainly appeared to be using it as an antidote to school as well as the oppression he experienced at home on Saturday and Sunday. The use of alcohol and marijuana might be motivated less by the positive state they produce and more by the fact that they keep in abeyance the sense of constraint and boredom that might otherwise permeate teenagers' consciousness (Creason & Goldman, 1981).

The contribution of the ESM to the study of substance abuse lies in its capacity to obtain detailed information about how drug use fits into daily lives. In addition to the study of adolescents, it would seem to have potential for investigation of amphetamine use among housewives, alcohol use among business persons, and stimulant use among college students. The contextual analysis of drug taking could provide detailed knowledge about the daily conditions eliciting use, knowledge that might be extremely valuable to efforts at treatment and prevention, as Kaplan and his associates have shown elsewhere in this volume.

16

Drug craving and drug use in the daily life of heroin addicts
CHARLES D. KAPLAN

Introduction

In the field of drug and alcohol addiction, a renewed interest in clinical diagnosis has emerged. From an epidemiological viewpoint this interest has been stimulated by a convergence of clinical populations. There is increasing evidence that significant proportions of the psychopathology population have a high prevalence of drug and alcohol addiction and, concomitantly, increasing numbers of drug and alcohol addiction clients seem to present relatively high rates of psychopathology. This convergence in psychiatric epidemiology has resulted in the emergence of 'dual diagnosis' as a clinical and research problem (Wallace & Zweben, 1989; Hesselbrock et al., 1985; Rounsaville et al., 1982; Khantzian & Trece, 1985; van Limbeek et al., 1986; Bukstein et al., 1989; Jaffe, 1984; McLellan et al., 1980, 1983). In this regard, critical remarks have been addressed toward the simple reliance on specific psychiatric diagnosis and far more attention to the *severity* of psychiatric problems (Stoffelmayr et al., 1989). These criticisms underline a general need throughout psychiatry – the need to refine existing psychiatric diagnostic conceptualizations with data reflective of subtle temporal and contextual variations that contribute to the severity and intensity of these disorders.

Methodologically, the refinement of diagnostic categories can take place in various ways.

Apart from clinical research the refining of existing diagnostic categories can be accomplished through biobehavioral investigations in laboratory and naturalistic settings. These investigations both complement clinical knowledge and, at times, challenge its validity. Over the last decade supplementary methods have been developed for the understanding of certain fundamentals of mental disorders. Largely, these advances have been stimulated by the creative application of new technologies. For instance, in the field of biological psychiatry CATT and NMR scans as well as EEG monitoring have been used to obtain new and novel data bases to evaluate existing clinical diagnoses. In the field of social psychiatry, a parallel development incorporating electronic ambulatory signaling technology is being experimentally tested. M. deVries

(1987) has been vocal in calling for more attention to the investigation of mental disorders in their natural settings using this new research technology in time allocation and experience sampling methodology (ESM) designs. These naturalistic investigations point to the relevance of 'thick' description, ethnomedical designs and microbehavioral data sensitive to diurnal and environmental variations in refining diagnostic classification. The introduction of time-sampling data can significantly alter the diagnosis of anxiety and panic disorders (deVries et al., 1987; Dijkman & deVries, 1987. Margraf et al., 1987). The ESM functions as the Holter Monitor does in cardiology. Assessing functions and symptoms outside the laboratory, it provides a report of experience and illness that goes beyond the interconnections that a patient is ordinarily able to provide in an interview or clinical diagnostic setting. The ESM techniques have demonstrated the variability and patterning of mental states over time (deVries et al., 1986; deVries, 1987) and have proven capable of producing ecologically valid and replicable descriptions of illness and human behavior (Csikszentmihalyi & Larson, 1984, 1987).

In the addiction field, there is a long tradition of animal and human experimentation where various elements and processes are studied by the manipulation of experimental conditions (Meyer & Mirin, 1979; Wikler, 1973). Paralleling this tradition have been investigations conducted by social scientists of addicts in their naturalistic settings (Lindesmith, 1968, 1975; Preble & Casey, 1969; McAuliffe & Gordon, 1974, 1975, 1980; Agar, 1973; Biernacki, 1986). These studies often provide a conflicting view of addiction when compared to the clinical studies. They have emphasized the addictive behaviors and the determining effect of socially defined contexts on the course of addiction. Both the laboratory studies and the naturalistic investigations provide converging evidence that there is considerable variation in the existing diagnostic criteria that are attributable to conditioned and learned responses that function within specific contexts, time-frames and microbehavioral rhythms. Within psychiatry, there have been calls for a more dynamic approach to addiction that emphasizes the social ecology, natural history and interaction of 'drug, set and setting' (Zinberg, 1984; Shaffer & Zinberg, 1985; Shaffer & Jones, 1989; Vaillant, 1983; Zinberg & Shaffer, 1985).

Beneath dependency: syndrome intensity, craving and the experience-sampling of addiction

This chapter presents a state-of-the-art report of the application of ESM in concert with ethnographic interviewing (Spradley, 1979) to better understand the functioning and contexts of the daily lives of 20 Dutch heroin addicts. This study directly complements the research conducted in the WHO/ADAMA 'Classification and Diagnosis' addiction research program by following the recommendation that 'The present research suggests that the DDS (Drug

Dependence Syndrome) concept may have merit as a theory of drug and alcohol dependence, but should be subjected to a more rigorous program of research aimed at better operational measures and more intensive hypothesis testing, especially in samples of drug users (Babor et al., 1988:38) (see also Edwards & Gross, 1976; Edwards et al., 1981; Skinner & Goldberg, 1986).' One way of bettering the measurement of the DDS is to develop operational definitions that may be applied in natural settings.

Based on a social psychiatric perspective, this chapter addresses the limitations of prior clinical research (see Kosten et al., 1987a). Although the study reported here involves only 20 cases, the sample size in terms of observations is relatively large (over 600 complied to self-reports in addition to case description and demographic data). Data have been collected in a distinct cultural setting (Holland) with a very different set of political and treatment service conditions than is normally encountered in other countries (Engelsman, 1989). The study involves a community sample and avoids some of the self-selection bias of clinical populations seeking psychiatric and/or substance abuse treatment (see Rounsaville & Kleber, 1985). Especially designed to measure the real-time allocations and variations in symptom presence over the course of a week, this study provides a rather unique view of the correspondence between time-frames and syndrome assessments at a microbehavioral level of polydrug addicts.

The study of Kosten et al. (1987a) in a sample of psychiatric patients has demonstrated both the validity of the 'dual diagnosis' concept for clinical epidemiology and the DDS for clinical diagnosis. Using the DSM-III-R instrument, they found that the 10-item substance dependence criteria formed internally consistent, unidimensional Guttman scales across drug of abuse categories. These unidimensional scales were highly robust and relatively independent of medical and psychosocial problems. They indicated that higher scores were congruent with more severe syndrome representation within each type of drug, but, interestingly, the order of the items differed across the drugs.

The discovery of Kosten and his associates of a unidimensional scale of drug dependency has some important implications for the diagnosis and classification of addiction. The unidimensionality of the DDS supports the idea that drug dependency is not an all-or-nothing phenomenon and that conceptual matching of the DDS with the DSM-III-R substance abuse criteria (Rounsville et al., 1986) has been fruitful. That the DDS forms a unidimensional scale also suggests further theoretical issues. The theory of Guttman scales contends that the directionality formed by a unidimensional scale is indeed the first principal component of the scale, but other components also exist (Guttman, 1954). The second component Guttman terms 'intensity'. This component of the scale determines a zero point. The intensity of the attitude measured by the scale is indicated by the deviation from this zero-point representing the scale's 'entry point'.

Given this theory of scaling, the experience of *craving* can be conceived as the indicator of intensity and an analytic substrate 'beneath' the DDS. Recent efforts to find an adequate human model of drug-seeking behavior have been focusing on the concept of craving. Thus, Edwards et al. (1981) have concluded that addiction neuroadaptation in human subjects is much more sensitively measured by subjective reports of craving than by physiological or behavioral measures. If this view is valid the criterion of craving would have more general utility than that of withdrawal and tolerance in diagnosis, especially in cases of polydrug abuse. Kozlowski & Wilkinson (1987) have critically re-evaluated the concept of craving, precipitating a lively debate on its definition and applicability. They posit a cognitive model of craving with an emphasis on the subjective experience. Methodologically, this conclusion requires some innovations. Kozlowski & Wilkinson (1987:35) write

> if craving is viewed as a subjective state associated with specific introceptive or exteroceptive cues, it makes little sense to subject persons to quesionnaires on craving unless the cues are deliberately manipulated or unless subjects were asked to monitor variations in the presence and absence of craving over time . . . As we have indicated earlier, we think that the proper basis for the development of such hypotheses lies in the careful phenomenological description of the subjective state.

In order to measure craving by use of the ESM for self-monitoring subjective experience, a 'craving module' of items was constructed. The hypothesis guiding this research has been that, in addition to specific pharmacological effects on craving, set and setting factors would also be significant (Zinberg, 1984). This hypothesis is based on the axiom 'that not only must the drug and personal need of the user be taken into account but also the subtleties of history and social circumstances' (Zinberg & Shaffer, 1985:72).

Methods

Procedures

Because of the illegality, rarity and social undesirability of heroin use, it is often difficult to locate cases in a community. Furthermore, insofar as the self-report is often the only way of obtaining data, the reliability and accuracy of measurement is a persistent problem (Rouse et al., 1985). It is generally understood that the sole reliance on clinical populations of heroin addicts biases generalization (Rounsaville & Kleber, 1985). Furthermore, insofar as craving functions as a dependent variable determined by environmental, internal and pharmacological factors, retrospective research designs may not be appropriate for studying this phenomenon. ESM provides a technique of self-monitoring and has been employed in a longitudinal, prospective design of this sample of heroin addicts. Repeated measures were taken of a self-report questionnaire that monitored experience. Subjects were instructed to fill out these questionnaires 10 times a day, at preselected random moments, when the electronic signaling instrument prompted the subject with a beep tone. The signaling device was a Seiko RE-1000 wrist terminal that has the appearance of a digital watch. The questionnaires included Likert-type scales about: the quality of thoughts, mood, individualized complaints, anxiety/panic symptoms (based on DSM-III criteria), motivation in relation to performance of current activities, physical wellbeing and disturbance caused by the wrist terminal. The instrument also contained open-ended questions and additional codings of thought content, goofs (quality of thoughts; pathology), social contact (with whom?), spatial context (where?), activity (what are you doing?), use of drugs and posture. In addition, consistent to standard ESM designs, a 'pathological module' has been formulated consisting of five Likert seven-point scales indexing subjective elements theoretically associated with craving. The items composing this 'craving module' included: are you thinking about using, do you have yourself under control, do you feel yourself restless, do you need dope in a hurry, do you need money quickly. The module's content and wording were created in dialogue with street drug users and the community field worker research staff to increase the construct validity of the self-reports. The module is thus designed to stand up to both ethnographic (member) and psychometric construct validity (see Mehan & Wood, 1975). Parenthetically, this validation procedure is made possible by the commitment of the study to the organization of a 'research alliance' with the subjects, a fundament of the ESM methodology.

Subjects

Subjects consisted of a snowball sample of 20 active heroin addicts (Kaplan et al., 1987). The 20 subjects were recruited through the intensive case-finding of two community field workers. They were contacted a week prior to being included in the study and asked formally for their consent and explained the aims and protection procedures. Two subjects were 'run' each week for a total of 10 weeks. The inclusion criteria were a community status of a known heroin addict as verified through chain referrals and a current pattern of 'daily use' (at least three days in the last week of heroin use). One exception to the criterion of daily use was allowed because of a special opportunity. The subject, a woman, was a known heroin addict in the community. The week prior to her participation in the study she found out that she was five months pregnant. She then made the decision to try to stop taking heroin and methadone the following week. She was included anyway in order to study craving in this 'transition' situation. Contacts with these subjects were made solely through the snowball method and not through treatment or counseling institutions.

The mean number of lifetime drug treatments for the sample was 5.1 (SD=1.1). This is characteristic of Dutch heroin addicts in general – a relatively high frequency of treatment contacts and experiences. Some subjects were currently enrolled in 'low-threshold' methadone programs, but were contacted through street referrals and were using heroin daily. All subjects were also currently using methadone and cocaine. Sixteen were current users of tranquillizers, 12 alcohol, and five amphetamines. There was only one clearly documented refusal to participate in the study. This refusal was because of an involvement in heroin dealing and a concomitant fear of discovery. There were two additional cases where agreement was obtained, but because of contingencies related to the pressures of working in drug dealing functional compliance was impossible or too low. In one case, a number of valid reports were obtained, but because the subject was occupied as a 'doorman' at a dealing address constant interruption made compliance difficult. The subject was able to comply acceptably to 16 of 56 beeps. His girlfriend, also a subject, was only able to comply to 25% of the signals. In the debriefing she mentioned her difficulty in filling out the reports accurately and honestly because of her dependency on her partner for money, drugs and housing. This, however, did not affect the accuracy of her craving, mood and environment module responses, but mainly the open-ended self-reports. She was afraid that her partner would read negative reports about himself. In another case, the normal daily routine was interrupted by a day in jail. In two cases, a day was interrupted in a cocaine 'binge' when the beeper-watches were given as a deposit to a dealer. They were later recovered through the negotiations of the field workers and the sampling routine was resumed.

For the remaining subjects compliance was high. Missing signals were because the subjects were sleeping. There is no indication that activities were not reported: drug use, criminal acts and prostitution were all recorded. A special code was used in the self-report book to assure some protection on sensitive items. Some subjects expressed fear that the books could be used by the police as evidence against them. This suggests that there still may be some under-reporting of criminal activities. Nevertheless, the overall compliance level was 63% (1022 signals; 647 reported and verified for reliability through time-checking answers). Given the special pressures on the sample, especially those involved in drug dealing, the compliance level is comparable to the 70% level reported in blue-collar and student samples (Csikszentmihalyi & Larson, 1987).

Further demographic and background characteristics of the sample support its representativeness for the population of chronic Dutch heroin addicts. Fourteen (70%) are male and six (30%) female. The mean age is 27.0 years

(SD=3.38). Geographic residence is 12.8 years in the city (SD=2.2). Sixteen (80%) are single, two married and three divorced. Six (30%) live alone, nine with a partner (45%) and five (25%) have no fixed living arrangement. Five did not complete the lowest education, six only the lower education, five had some middle school and three some higher education. Ten (50.0%) are unemployed, one works at home, five (25.5%) are officially unfit for work and four have another work status (e.g. criminal). Twelve (60%) mentioned social security/welfare as their source of income and eight had a combination of income sources. Ten (50%) originate from complete families and eight (40%) from broken families (two cases' data are missing). Five (25%) had some former psychotherapeutic treatment, five had a history of suicide attempts and seven (35%) some history of somatic medical problems. Nine reported no medical problems related to their drug use, while 10 reported some medical problems related to drug use. The mean age of first use of heroin was 17.5 years (SD=2.56) and the mean years of heroin use is 9.25 (SD=3.45). The mean number of years using methadone is 6.21 (SD=2.90), cocaine 4.95 (SD=3.35), amphetamine 5.0 (SD=5.61), tranquillizers 4.0 (SD=4.49) and antidepressants 0.82 (SD=2.43). Eleven smoke heroin (chasing the dragon) and 11 inject heroin indicating some overlap of heroin smokers and injectors (missing data are four and two respectively). In terms of involvement in the drug world as measured by a 'strength of addiction' scale (Kaplan, 1977; Kaplan & Wogan, 1978), 14 (70%) reported that they could 'score' drugs in a strange town, three (15%) identified themselves as a 'junkie', one (5%) never tried to 'kick' voluntarily the addiction and three (15%) had had five or more overdose experiences while 12 (60%) never had a drug overdose. The mean number of weeks spent in jail was 20.88 (SD=29.95).

Data analysis

Data analysis was conducted on the 647 answered self-reports, the sociodemographic and drug history questionnaire and the fieldnote protocols of the debriefing sessions of the 20 subjects. The complexity of ESM datasets is well recognized. Analysis proceeded in accordance to Larson & Delespaul's (this volume) recommendations for an emphasis on description and deeper levels of understanding. They warn that ESM analysis must be careful not to confound questions about *situations* with questions about *persons*. In this light, the dependent variable, craving, can be conceived as both a property of situations and characteristic of persons. Along with this critical analytic distinction, Larson & Delespaul also introduce the critical relevance of the distinction between *trait* and *state*. Operationally, *between* subject or situation variance would define stable traits while *within* subject or situation variance would define state descriptions. The data analysis in this study, therefore, has been designed by crossing the situation/person levels with the trait/state levels. Four distinct analyses have been conducted: (1) within situation (situation-dependent states); (2) between situations (situation traits); (3) within subjects (person-dependent states); (4) between subjects (person traits).

The Likert scale items of the ESM self-reports were factor analyzed for interdependence by an initial principal components extraction. All factors extracted with an Eigenvalue greater than one were varimax rotated in order to facilitate interpretation. The extracted factors provided the basis for constructing a craving score for each situation and subject. These craving scores were computed by multiplying each Likert item by its respective factor loading and summating across these adjusted scores. Further analysis examined the patterns of subject variation by means of a one-way analysis of variance. The assessment of subgroup differences defined by the craving score criteria was undertaken through Scheffé tests. These tests are designed to verify the significance of post-hoc comparisons between the craving groups. For the within-situation analysis, craving scores have been analyzed by means of a one-way analysis of variance of drug, set (mood module), and setting factors (home, company). A two-way analysis of variance was conducted to test for the interaction of individual variation on the factors. The between-situation analysis examined the craving scores by means of a two-way analysis of variance of independent factors of drugs taken and home setting. The weights of these factors were in turn evaluated by means of a multiple classification analysis. The within-subject analysis relied upon the qualitative analysis of a single case inspecting for variations in drug and social environment aspects. This analysis was supplemented by non-parametric statistical analysis (Friedman two-way ANOVA; Kruskal-Wallis one-way ANOVA) testing for significant differences in the variation of Likert craving module items over the course of the week and for each separate day. For the between-subject analysis, two matched cases were systematically compared qualitatively with reference to life-event data drawn from the debriefing protocols. The qualitative analysis was supplemented by a non-parametric testing (Kolmogorov-Smirnov two-sample test) of the differences in craving items between the subjects. All statistical analysis employed the SPSS X program. SPSS X conventions for the reporting of results have been retained, e.g., degrees of freedom reported as a single parameter value rather than a ratio.

Results

Craving factor analysis

The factor analysis of the craving module items results in the extraction of two factors with Eigenvalues greater than one. Table 16.1 presents the loadings of the craving module items on the two factors and the summary descriptive statistics of each factor. The summary statistics indicate that across the entire

Table 16.1. *Craving item loadings and summary statistics of acquisition (dope-money) and loss of control factors*

Item	Acquisition	Loss of control
Thought about using	0.58854	0.38733
Was in control	0.01804	−0.84049
Felt restless	0.30796	0.74388
Needed dope quickly	0.80671	0.38605
Needed money badly	0.83655	−0.12650
explained variance	46.8%	20.5%
mean	7.26	−0.51
standard deviation	3.98	3.03
median	6.20	−1.31
mode	2.67	−4.49
minimum	2.56	−5.25
maximum	17.89	9.65
skewness	0.80	0.64
n of cases	631	631
missing cases	16	16

sample of 631 beeps, both factors are slightly skewed and show considerable variation as evidenced by standard deviations of 3.98 for the acquisition factor and 3.03 for the loss of control. The first factor explains 46.8% of the total variance and the second factor adds another 20.5% of explained variance. The total variance explained by this two-factor solution for the craving items is 67.3%. The first factor loaded high on the items 'needed money badly' (0.83655) and 'needed dope quickly' (0.80671) and also somewhat on 'thought about using' (0.58854). The second factor loaded negatively high for the item 'was in control' (−0.84049) and positively high for 'felt restless' (0.74388). Interpretation of these two factors is consistent with the multidimensional representation of craving in the literature first distinguished as 'symbolic' craving and 'physiological' craving (Jellinek, 1960; Rankin et al., 1979). The first factor reflects a dimension that varies from low to high. The dimension can be conceived as an *acquisition* subsystem that is constituted by thinking about using in a means/ends relationship with needing dope (the end) *quickly* and money (the means) *badly*. The second factor has been interpreted as the 'loss of control' dimension of craving, varying along a negative and positive axis. The dimension reflects the malfunctioning of a *control* subsystem and the associated feelings of restlessness that are commonly reported symptoms of withdrawal. This factor is interpretable whereby, if subjects are in control, they are likely not to feel restless and, conversely, if they are not in control, they are likely to feel restless. Thus, a 'high positive' rank on the dimension would satisfy the conditions of not being in control and feeling restless while a 'high negative' rank satisfies the conditions of being in control and not feeling restless. Since both positive conditions of the dimension are associated *with not* being in control, the factor is termed *loss of control*.

Factor scores have been computed by adding the subject's scores on the five craving module items multiplied by the item's loading on the factor. Separate factor scores for the acquisition factor and the loss of control factor were computed for each subject. Since all the loadings of the acquisition factor are positive, possible factor scores can only be positive, ranging in value from 2.51 to 17.90. The loss of control factor had a combination of positive and negative loadings and therefore possible values ranged from −5.25 to 9.45. The computed factor scores for each subject functioned as dependent (i.e. criterion) variables in subsequent analyses as has been proposed in the literature (see Hughes, 1987).

The means and standard deviations of the acquisition and loss of control factor scores were computed for each subject. The results are compiled in Table 16.2. Subjects have been ranked from low to high according to their score on the acquisition factor. For the total sample, the grand mean on the acquisition factor is 3.98 (SD=7.26) and for the loss of control factor −0.51 (SD=3.03). The low compliance indicated by relatively low numbers of beeps (<20) can be seen in subject 18 who had been occupied with the dealing role and subject 15 who had the week interrupted by a day in jail. Inspection of the distribution of both means and standard deviations of both factors across subjects suggested a significant amount of inter- and intrasubject variation in craving. Further support of this hypothesis was obtained through the oneway analysis of variance of an aggregate 'subject factor' which took each individual subject as an exclusive factor level. Hays' (1973: 483–4) recommendation of non-robustness of homogeneity of variance tests for problems of the equality of means was followed suspending their application in this analytic situation. Significant between-subject differences in means were found for the acquisition factor ($F=14.11$; d.f.$=19$; $P <0.001$) and the loss of control factor ($F=9.32$; d.f.$=19$; $P <0.00$).

To explore further the craving score data, post hoc comparisons between subjects were made using Scheffé tests set at a $P<0.05$. The post hoc comparison analysis supported the validity of the two factor solutions for the craving module items. The extreme highest (subject 11) and lowest cases (subject 10) were internally consistent in their extreme ranks across both factors. Further face validity of the craving factors was obtained upon examination of the qualitative data obtained in the debriefing sessions. Subject 11, Janny, is the one who had decided not to use heroin following the news of her pregnancy. High acquisition and high loss of control experiences are

Table 16.2. *Mean scores and standard deviations on acquisition and loss of control factors by subject*

	Acquisition		N	Loss of control	
10	3.08	3.09	29	−2.91	1.83
17	4.26	1.67	25	−1.12	1.70
20	4.80	2.21	50	−0.22	2.32
18	5.05	2.17	19	−2.27	1.57
15	5.44	2.46	18	0.76	2.21
19	5.52	3.72	54	−1.65	2.95
5	6.46	2.69	25	0.52	3.70
12	7.03	3.39	27	0.20	2.31
9	7.06	4.42	34	−0.92	3.16
13	7.07	3.29	34	−1.95	2.01
8	7.61	5.12	42	−1.11	3.56
4	7.63	3.36	39	0.07	1.58
16	7.73	3.81	20	2.91	3.15
7	7.76	3.53	24	0.84	1.90
14	8.20	3.30	30	0.68	2.85
3	8.21	2.40	37	−1.91	2.10
2	9.17	3.88	36	−2.41	2.81
6	10.35	3.83	34	0.90	2.47
1	11.12	3.70	34	−0.39	4.01
11	12.87	2.92	20	3.18	3.52
Total	7.26	3.98	631	−0.51	3.03

predictable in a situation of sudden self-induced detoxification. In contrast, subject 10, Bowie, reported the lowest score on both craving factors. He was described in the debriefings as a controlled user of small quantities of heroin, 30 years old with a relatively high education level and a middle-class background. Most of his friends were not heroin addicts and he was actively interested in art and politics. He had chosen his friends carefully, on the basis of 'self protection' against escalating drug use. Although using daily, he does not define himself as addicted saying: 'If I have the feeling that I can feel good without dope, well . . . then I don't feel addicted.' He reported that he does not get really sick without methadone although he complains of tiredness, cold shiver, slight sleeplessness and a light 'flu. He does not want to have anything to do with drug care institutions or methadone programs saying: 'all the fuss around it, have to go everyday, intakes, etc., etc.' He would rather take care of his drug-related problems by himself, buying heroin and methadone on the black market.

Within-situation analysis

Given the significant effect of individual subject differences, two-way analysis of variance models were tested for main drug, set, and setting factors and the interaction effect of these factors with the subject factor. Table 16.3 presents the results testing the null hypothesis of equality of means between the levels of the positive mood (set factor), cocaine, heroin and combinations of cocaine and heroin taken before the beep (drug factors) and the company the subject is with (setting factor).

On the positive mood factor significant differences are found between the below-moderate, moderate, and above-moderate levels on both the acquisition factor ($F=38.36$; d.f.$=2$; $P <0.00$) and the loss of control factor ($F=123.52$; d.f.$=2$; $P <0.00$). A statistical criterion was used to define the cutting points of this trichotomized factor. A moderate positive mood level was obtained in the interval where approximately 60% of the total valid Likert observations fell. The remaining 20% of the observations that fell below this interval were defined as below moderate and those 20% that fell above the interval were defined as above moderate.

Higher craving occurs when the positive mood is below moderate while, conversely, lower craving exists when the positive mood is above moderate. This relationship is consistent across both craving factors. On the acquisition factor a mean craving score of 9.71 is found at the below-moderate level, dropping to 7.01 at the moderate level and further decreasing to 5.57 at the above-moderate level. This inverse relationship between craving and positive mood is also seen in the loss of control factor with a positive score of 2.23 at the below-moderate level (high restless; not under control), a slightly negative score of -0.68 at the moderate level and a clear negative score of -2.95 at the above-moderate level. Individual subject differences are also significant suggesting a trait effect involving a subject by mood interaction for both the acquisition factor ($F=2.85$; d.f.$=30$; $P <0.00$) and the loss of control factor ($F=2.01$; d.f.$=30$; $P <0.00$).

Turning to the drug effects, a mechanism can be observed whereby specific drugs effect specific craving components independent from subject differences. In contrast, however, combinations of drugs seem to have more diffuse effects and are interdependent on individual subject differences. Thus, there is no significant effect of cocaine use on the acquisition factor, but there is a highly significant effect on the loss of control factor ($F=25.91$; d.f.$=1$; $P <0.00$). Loss of control increases when cocaine is taken (0.53) and decreases significantly when it is not used (-0.87). For heroin the inverse results are found. If no heroin is taken, the mean score on the acquisition factor is significantly higher (7.63) than if heroin is used (6.75) ($F=7.31$; d.f.$=1$; $P <0.01$). There is no significant difference in the loss of control factor scores

Table 16.3. *Mean factor scores on acquisition and loss of control craving by mood, drugs taken and company*

	Acquisition		Loss of control
Mood			
below moderate	9.71	(*n* = 122)	2.23
moderate	7.01	(*n* = 375)	−0.68
above moderate	5.57	(*n* = 117)	−2.95
Cocaine taken			
no	7.29*	(*n* = 455)	−0.87
yes	7.49*	(*n* = 155)	−0.53
Heroin taken			
no	7.63	(*n* = 378)	−0.50*
yes	6.75	(*n* = 247)	−0.58*
Polydrug/monodrug taken			
heroin only	6.28	(*n* = 105)	−1.79
cocaine and heroin	7.35	(*n* = 126)	−0.48
cocaine or heroin	7.60	(*n* = 349)	−0.60
cocaine only	8.07	(*n* = 29)	0.77
Company			
alone	7.57	(*n* = 221)	0.07
one other	6.29	(*n* = 254)	−1.06
more others	8.54	(*n* = 151)	−0.46

* = Not significant; $P>0.05$.

whether heroin is used or not. For both the heroin and cocaine effect, there are no significant individual subject interactions. In comparing the effects of a monodrug (heroin or cocaine) with both a polydrug (heroin and cocaine) and a no-drug situation, significant differences on both the acquisition and loss of control ($F=13.34$; d.f.$=3$; $P <0.00$) craving factors have been found. The highest acquisition craving scores are associated with the cocaine only (8.07) and no-drug situation (7.60). The lowest score is for the heroin-only situation (6.28). This effect is not interdependent with subject differences. While taking heroin seems to dampen acquisitional craving, the taking of cocaine seems to have the opposite effect, elevating the need for dope and money above the no-drug 'abstinent' level. A complementary effect can be seen on the control craving factor with the cocaine situation associated with a positive score (0.77) on loss of control and heroin with a relatively higher negative score (−1.79). In contrast to the acquisition factor, the loss of control factor shows a significant interaction effect with individual subject differences ($F=12.09$; d.f.$=33$; $P <0.00$). Parenthetically, the apparent discrepancy between the significance of the 'cocaine only' situation on the acquisition factor and the non-significant difference on the cocaine-taken factor is related to the definition of the cocaine-taken factor to include *both* situations when cocaine is taken alone or with heroin.

The setting effect indicates certain subtle relationships. Significant differences on both the acquisition craving factor score ($F=16.82$; d.f.$=2$; $P <0.00$) and the loss of control craving score ($F=8.45$; d.f.$=2$; $P <0.00$) can be observed. On both these factors there is no significant interaction effect of individual differences. The highest score on the acquisition factor occurred in the situation of the company of two or more others (8.54), and the lowest in the situation of one other. In this regard, the saying 'two is company while three is a crowd' has some meaning insofar as the 'intimate' company of one other seems to lower the need for dope and money, while the dynamics of a larger group tend to increase it. This proposition is supported by the differences found in the variations of scores on the loss of control factor. In the 'intimate' situation, the craving score is negative and at its lowest level of intensity (-1.06). The 'crowd' situation also seems to 'absorb' some of the loss of control craving with a negative score of -0.46. The craving in terms of the control criterion is highest and becomes positive in the situation when subjects are alone.

Between-situation analysis

Because of the relative independence of the drug and setting effects in the within-subject analysis, a more detailed analysis of the drug effect hierarchically compared between the setting situation of 'at home' and 'not at home' was conducted. This setting factor has been selected to better observe the functioning of the 'intimacy' and 'crowd' situations.

Being 'at home' is seen as a basic ecological situation that should produce an effect comparable to being with one person. The within-situation analysis showed the relative independence of the drug and setting factors from individual subject interaction. A related question is whether these two factors are independent or whether they interact to effect craving.

The two-way analyses of variance showed that there were significant main effects of the drug taken and the setting on both the acquisition and loss of control criteria. There were no significant interaction effects between the drug taken and setting factors on either of the craving measures. Because no interaction between the drug and setting factors was found the variation of the two craving scores could be conceived as a linear function of the two factors.

Tables 16.4 and 16.5 present the results of a multiple classification analysis (MCA) of the mean variations of the acquisition and loss of control scores within and between the drug and setting factor. A beta weight statistic could be specified to assess the contribution of each factor to the total variation. For the acquisition score the setting (beta$=0.29$) proved more important than the drug used (beta$=0.14$). For the loss of control factor the pattern was reversed with

Table 16.4. *Multiple classification analysis on the acquisition craving score*

Variable & category		N	Adjusted for independents deviations of grand mean	β
Drug used				
	nothing	345	0.24	
	heroin only	100	−1.13	
	coke only	29	1.14	
	coke & heroin	122	−0.03	
				0.14
Setting				
	not at home	197	1.61	
	at home	399	−0.79	
				0.29

Multiple R, 0.316
Multiple R squared, 0.100

Grand mean = 7.31.

Table 16.5. *Multiple classification analysis on the loss of control craving score*

Variable & category		N	Adjusted for independents deviations of grand mean	β
Drug used				
	nothing	345	−0.06	
	heroin only	100	−1.35	
	coke only	29	1.48	
	coke & heroin	122	0.92	
				0.26
Setting				
	not at home	197	0.63	
	at home	399	−0.31	
				0.15

Multiple R, 0.289
Multiple R squared, 0.083

Grand mean = 0.56.

the drug (beta=0.26) being more important than the setting (beta=0.15). Examination of the Multiple R Squared statistic indicated that the model of the drug and setting factors explained 10% of the acquisition score and 8.3% of the loss of control score. For simple two variable explanatory models this is judged as acceptable.

Further inspection of the Tables shows that the stereotypical view of the heroin addict as constantly on the streets in search of dope is not the case in this sample. Fifty-eight per cent (345/596) of the total time of the sample was spent without drugs and 67% (399/596) of the time at home. When the subjects were using drugs they were most likely to be using heroin only (17%) or using a cocaine-heroin 'cocktail' (20%) – the most frequent drug situation. The rarest situation was on cocaine alone (4%). Clearly, the sample were not preferring any single drug, but choosing a polydrug (cocaine-heroin) pattern.

Considering the MCA of the acquisition score, the subjects are slightly more elevated from the grand mean (7.31) in their craving in the nothing situation (0.24) and slightly less elevated in the cocaine-heroin situation (−0.3). A dramatic elevation occurs in the situation of cocaine only (1.14). Conversely, a dramatic decrease can be observed in the heroin-only situation (−1.13). Turning to the setting factor, being at home is slightly more conducive to lowering acquisition craving (−0.79) while being not at home elevates craving to the highest level (1.61). Inspection of the relationship of the drug situations with the loss of control score reveals a similar pattern. In the situation of using cocaine only the craving score is the most elevated from the grand mean (1.48). Conversely, in the heroin situations, the lowest level of craving is found (−1.35). The cocaine-heroin cocktail also increases the loss of control score. Furthermore, the effect of being in the not-at-home situation (0.63) elevates loss of control.

In summary, Figs. 16.1 and 16.2 graphically represent the pattern of differences of the acquisition and loss of control scores between the drug and setting situations. Figure 16.1 shows that acquisition craving is lower across all the drug situations in the situation 'at home' compared to being 'not at home'. The 'intimate' setting effect can be clearly seen in comparing the heroin situation at home with the heroin situation not at home. In the difference between the loss of control craving scores, Fig. 16.2 provides supporting evidence for the dampening effect of the at-home situation on craving. The highest loss of control is experienced in the not-at-home situation when only cocaine is being used. Cocaine use at home (with or without heroin) does not result in an elevation of loss of control craving much above the zero point. The dampening effect of the home situation is most clearly seen by the negative scores in the situations of no drug use.

Finally, in a situation of heroin use alone, loss of control scores are negative

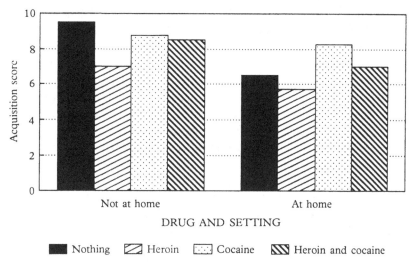

Fig. 16.1. Acquisition craving score by drug and setting.

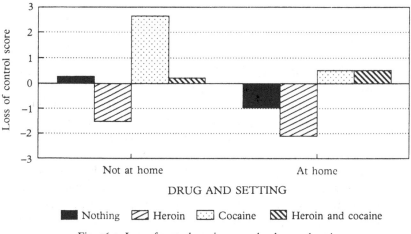

Fig. 16.2. Loss of control craving score by drug and setting.

in both setting situations. Nevertheless, the 'at home' situation decreases loss of control even more in the heroin situation.

Within-person analysis

The relatively large standard deviations in both craving factor scores and the significant effect of individual subject differences call for an idio-

209

graphic level of analysis producing a microscopic view of persons. For these purposes, Bob (subject 9) has been selected as typical of the sample on both craving factor scores and demographic variables. Bob is 30 years old, white and unemployed. His family is working class and he is one of eight children. Along with three of his brothers, he spent much time in a children's home as his parents could not support so many children. He has been using heroin for 10 years and is registered as a client in a 'low threshold' methadone program. Despite participating in the program, he was still using heroin and had added cocaine forming a characteristic polydrug pattern. In order to finance his polydrug use Bob had done some small-scale dealing in the employment of large dealers.

The non-parametric Kruskal-Wallis test showed no significant differences between Bob's days for either the 'control' item or the 'dope' item. However, the Friedman two-way test showed a significant difference for each item score over the course of the entire week of beep times ($\chi^2 = 15.56$; d.f. $= 1$; $P < 0.00$). This analysis indicates that the significant differences in craving are the result of diurnal variation.

Figure 16.3 plots Bob's Likert scores on two highly loading craving module items representing the two acquisition and loss of control factors (need dope quickly and have yourself under control) during the course of day 1 of his week.

The y-axis represents the Likert-scale range from 'not' to 'very' while the x-axis depicts the beep-time (time 1, time 2, etc.) and the drug used preceding the beep. Inspecting Bob's first day, the association of the use of cocaine with a higher level of need for dope can be seen. Control is maintained at a moderate level over the first two time-beeps. Suddenly, control drops at T3 as the need for drugs continues to accelerate. Although Bob is still taking only cocaine, he records in his ESM self-report that he is thinking of 'smack?' (heroin). Bob has learned that he can use heroin to regain a sense of control. This cognition alone seems to have an effect in lowering the need for dope and heightening the sense of control. At beep-time T4, a homeostasis is reached (the slopes of the curves intersect) even though cocaine is still the only drug being used. The mere anticipation of 'self-medication' through heroin has an homeostatic effect. Finally, at T5, Bob substitutes heroin for cocaine and achieves a state of calm with a very low need for dope and a high sense of control. This state continues to be maintained by the heroin at T6 as the day ends.

A further inspection of Bob's week reveals a patterned relationship such that when the need for dope is high, the sense of control is lowered. Inversely, when the sense of control is high, the need for dope is low. For example, Bob's second day is characterized by relatively high con-

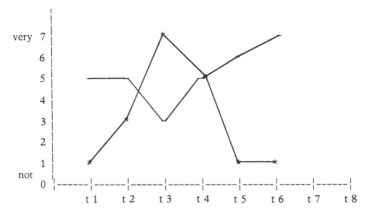

Fig. 16.3. Craving module item Likert scores by beep time over day 1 for Bob (subject 9). Drug used: C, cocaine; H, heroin. Items:– [ ] Were you in control of yourself? *[ ] Did you need dope quickly?

trol and low need of dope. Heroin is taken throughout the day having the effect of keeping control at a constant level while lowering the need for dope. As the need for dope stabilizes at a low level, control increases to a high level. This optimal state is maintained throughout the day. In addition to this drug effect, there is a setting effect. During the day Bob is visited by close relations. He takes a walk with his brother and sees his girlfriend. This human contact seems to reinforce the stable state brought about by the heroin 'self-medication'. Bob has noted that loneliness and addiction are his main complaints. Both are relieved somewhat by the visit of close relations. As Bob describes it:

'(loneliness and addiction) they have a lot to do with each other. I'm living alone in this house, my girlfriend lives in another town. The only thing I got outside is the methadone program. It breaks my day; I meet people down there. For the rest, I'm mostly at home watching television. And I really feel bad about that. You can see it in the book (NB – the experience sampling diary) that when somebody is coming by I feel better right away. I would like to have my girlfriend around more. When I'm lonely I use more too.'

Later in the week the destabilizing effect of cocaine on Bob can be further observed. When alone, he uses cocaine. He also uses cocaine at times in the company of others. In this social setting, the need for drugs is dampened. Bob's diurnal variations can be understood as a persistent attempt to control his cocaine addiction by the use of heroin and the intimate, negative reinforcement provided by his girlfriend. He says:

211

'Last year on my birthday I stopped dealing. I couldn't let my hands off the coke. Well you know how it is when you are in a coke binge, you can hardly stop then. One moment I really spit on it and said to myself, 'Knock it off, quit with that stuff'. My girlfriend didn't want to see me anymore because I was dealing. Not for the dealing itself, but because she can't accept that I earned money like that on other people. I offered her a trip to Paris and she said she did not want to go with me the way I was now. She then went with a friend and paid me one ticket back.'

Between-person analysis

In the within-person analysis, a typical subject has been selected. In contrast, the two extreme high subjects on the acquisition craving score have been chosen for the purposes of between-person analysis. Both subjects are women. In the weeks prior to data collection each subject experienced dramatic life events. Linda (subject I) obtained the results of an HIV-test and was informed of a seropositive result. Janny (subject II) found out she was five months pregnant.

Linda is 30 years old. She works as a streetwalker prostitute. She has been greatly disturbed by the positive results of her HIV test. Her main complaints are a 'continuous craving for heroin' and 'depression'. Her seropositivity compels her to give up prostitution because of her fear of infecting others. However, her drug craving exerts a counterpressure on her to work. She is quite open about her test results talking about her feelings with others in the hope that she will be cheered up. She maintains a good contact with her mother and is open about her problems. Her mother is very worried about the additional burden of the test results. In the course of the debriefings, Linda expressed the lack of control she has over her cocaine taking. In connection with this, she uses many pills, mostly Valium and Rohypnol. Her mother regularly provides her with these pills. Linda sells a part to obtain money. During the week of data collection, she was arrested by the police for shoplifting, but was released a few hours later. She lives in a comfortable, well-decorated apartment with a male prostitute who is also an addict. At times, they have allowed their apartment to be used by a drug dealer for selling.

Janny is 31 years old. She considers herself not to be a big user, smoking on the average between 0.1–0.2 g per day. When not taking heroin, she uses small doses of methadone. Her main complaints are 'loneliness' and 'having to lie all of the time through leading a double life'. She originates from a provincial town from a large, traditional family. Her family and friends know of her history of addiction, but think she has been clean for the past two years. She maintains this lie because it requires less explanation. Many of her friends are ex-heroin addicts and would have difficulty seeing a person who is still using. This lying gives her the motivation to cease heroin use. Janny does volunteer work helping foreigners and has a qualified education as a social worker. She has a work history in her profession. During the week of data collection, she was able to keep to her decision to stop using both heroin and methadone. She defined her withdrawal symptoms as a common 'flu. Her decision has been reinforced by a fear that she will get the 'junkie treatment' in the hospital as a pregnant addict. She is aware that kicking off use of heroin during pregnancy is not without risk, but she is optimistic. During the week of data collection, she was very busy arranging for the birth. She is aware that there is not much time. She has pride in her house and of being a modern woman. Her current house is too small for a baby, so she will have to move. The father is her ex-boyfriend. She informed him of the pregnancy, but she does not want him to be involved. There is some conflict over this and she feels threatened.

The results of the Kolmogorov-Smirnov Two-Sample tests comparing the Likert scores on the highly-loading craving module items of the acquisition and loss of control factors over the course of the week between the two samples of beeps ($N=70$) of Linda and Janny are significant. On both the items 'need dope' (K-S $Z = 1.54$, 2-tailed $P <0.02$) and 'in control' (K-S $Z = 1.76$, 2-tailed $P <0.00$) significant differences have been found. Figure 16.4 plots the need dope score for Janny and Linda by the beep-time over the course of the week.

For Janny, the need for dope score drops to a weakly low level in the middle of the first day, but climbs to a high level by the end of the day. A sort of 'minicrisis' presents itself with the dope score at a high level (the corresponding control item score not plotted was at a low). The second day, stabilization at a high level of needing dope occurs. This stabilization seems to have been aided by a self-medication intervention. Janny reports taking Rohypnol and an antihistamine in the morning. This leads to a drop in the need for dope towards the end of the day. On the third day, the need for dope increases again despite the taking of a sleeping pill and alcohol at the beginning of the day. By the end of the third day, stabilization returns. The fourth day shows a decrease in the need of dope. Janny reports a steady intake of alcohol. On the fifth day, Janny takes paracetamol. Despite this self-medication, the need for dope increases. She takes another paracetamol which lowers slightly the need for dope. Unfortunately, the data on the remainder of the day are missing as Janny had placed the wrist terminal in her handbag and could not hear the signal. On the sixth and last day, Janny begins at a relatively moderate level of need. She takes an antiflu tablet and maintains a moderate state of dope need.

The weekly profile of Janny shows a relatively high state of need for dope. This is indeed expected in that she has self-consciously decided to quit using both heroin and methadone in light of the life event of the news of her pregnancy. However, she is able gradually to stabilize her fluctuations in the need for dope through a substitution regime which includes pharmacological means of pills and alcohol and behavioral means of a busy schedule of activities in preparation for giving birth. Indeed, the life event of pregnancy has provided a new impulse for quitting her opiate use. Janny is engaged in a self-conscious and voluntary process of managing her need for dope. First she tries will power alone and when this coping strategy fails she self-employs a medication and behavioral modification regime.

In contrast to Janny, the case of Linda illustrates a very different pattern. The profile of Linda's week is that of a highly unstable pattern in her need for dope. Although the overall level of need for dope is lower than with Janny, the relatively continual vacillation between high and low levels of need indicates an extremely labile state. Among the determinants of this vacillation seem to be both the pattern of prostitution and the heavy use of benzodiazepines.

On the first day, the need for dope starts at a moderate level and drops steadily over the course of the day. Toward the end of the day, Linda begins a night of prostitution. The craving for dope is suppressed in the middle of the day to low level by the self-administration of three (10 mg) Valium. The low level of needing dope induced by the Valium is maintained during work by taking one (2 mg) Rohypnol. On the second day, there is no pressure for working. The need for dope is suppressed in the morning by taking three Valium. This low level of need is maintained until toward the end of the day. Then, the need for dope starts to rise to a moderate level. This rise is suppressed by the administration of one Rohypnol. The need for dope then returns to a low level. On the third day, the need for dope starts at a moderate level. The usual morning dose of three Valium is taken. This does not seem to work at suppressing the need for dope. In response, one Rohypnol is taken which temporarily lowers the need for dope. However, the need for dope rises to a new high and Linda goes out to work. Her need for dope increases to a high level as she works. The next morning she supplements her normal 'wake-up' dose of three Valium with an additional Rohypnol. This allows her to manage her need for dope which rises to a moderate level, but falls at the end of the day. She does not work on this day. On the fifth day, she begins at a high level of need for dope, despite her morning dose of three Valium. Although her need drops in midday, it rises to a relatively high level as the day proceeds. Linda goes out to work and by the end of the night her need for dope has gradually declined. She begins her sixth day at a low level of need for dope, taking her daily three Valium 'wake-up'. By midday her need has risen to a

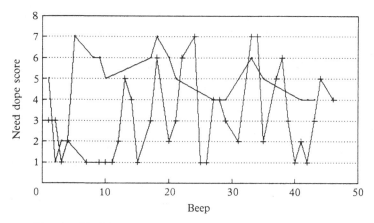

Fig. 16.4. Need dope item by beep and subject. ◆, Janny; +, Linda.

moderate level and remains there for the rest of the day. She neither works nor takes additional pills.

The debriefing of Linda indicates a weekly process of negative reinforcement. The news of her seropositivity has established a new existential condition of fear. Now her states of vacillating need for dope and loss of control are joined by the fear that she may both infect her clients and die. On one of the nights of prostitution this became terribly apparent when she pleaded with a client to use a condom and he refused. She felt extremely guilty that her need for dope had overcome her good intent. The guilt was further reinforced when the client revealed he was married with several children. Linda feared that she would be responsible for his infection. Clearly, the life event of seropositivity has added a severe psychological burden to an already difficult life.

Discussion

The results of this study demonstrate the utility of using ESM as an operational measurement of craving and as a criterion for investigating the relationship of certain situational determinants of addictive behavior. In line with Kozlowski & Wilkinson's (1987) critical re-evaluation of the craving concept a cognitive model has been shown to be a valid representation of this subjective state. The 'classic' distinction of Jellinek (1960) between 'symbolic' and 'physiological' craving has been supported in the dual factor structure of the craving module used in this study. It may, however, vary as to which factor is more heavily weighted in a particular complex of addictive behavior. The results show clearly a high correlation between money and drug need that leads to a strong acquisitional behavior complex. It may be that the 'drug-seeking' component represents the specific animal model effect while the 'money-seeking' is the specific human model effect conditioned by specific socio-economic factors. In this regard, Marlatt (1987: 42–3) has proposed that the definition of craving be moved away from its earlier physiological somatic roots to a conception of 'a form of psychological attachment, based on the individual's cognitive capacities to anticipate, expect, and desire the effects of a given activity or substance that has yet to occur'.

The craving module used in this study supports the view that craving is partially constituted by purely symbolic cues such as money as well as physiological symptoms such as restlessness. Recent research on cigarette addiction has concluded that '. . . the most consistent withdrawal symptom is craving, by which we mean a preoccupation with, thoughts about, or an urge for, the habituating substance, not necessarily associated with any physical distress . . . It is unnecessary to limit this craving model to habituating substances. Behaviors that reduce tension and noradrenergic activity, such as binge eating, could be habituating because of a similarly learned craving for the behavior' (Glassman et al., 1984: 866). That the seeking of money has become an essential element in the illicit drug subculture and lifestyle would explain its bond with drugs themselves as a part of the symbolic craving component. Further support of this view can be found in the literature on the management of craving and relapse prevention. Biernacki (1986: 121), for instance, concludes that 'in any event, the symptoms must be *interpreted as craving for drugs* before they can direct or guide behavior toward the use of drugs'. In addition, craving has been seen in this ESM study to be linked to specific temporal contexts. The microscopic, idiographic analysis has revealed significant fluctuations of craving over the course of hours and days. This critical linkage of craving with time has also been found in the Biernacki (1986) research. He found that the duration of a craving experience is approximately twenty minutes. The frequency of this experience as well as its intensity can be greatly diminished over time. After about one year of abstinence, significant readaptations as a function of memory and cognitive strategy can be observed.

Following the suggestion of Hughes (1987), the ESM operationalization of craving has been used as a dependent variable in models constructed from factors indicating drug, set, and setting. In general, specific situational circumstances and psychological states were correlated with modulations of craving supporting the guiding hypothesis of the study. An important finding has been that there seem to be specific pharmacological mechanisms associated with heroin and cocaine that are independent of individual subject differences. Heroin has been shown specifically to effect the acquisition dimension of craving while cocaine has been seen to effect the loss of control dimension.

Considering these results in light of the increasing trend of polydrug use, it is plausible to see the cocaine-using heroin addict involved in a complex spiral of self-medicating side-effects of various drugs alternating over the course of time (Khantzian, 1985). The need for drugs and money may be a way of producing arousal to compensate for the depression that results from a maintenance opiate addiction lifestyle. The introduction of cocaine into this delicate loop seems to have the effect of accelerating feedback and resulting in a panic and loss of control that in turn must be treated by either more heroin or money (see Gawin & Kleber, 1986). In any case, the relationship between panic and cocaine has been recently documented (Aronson & Craig, 1986). In heroin addicts who are in the maintenance phase of their addiction, the introduction of cocaine would be expected to increase panic and loss of control as it changes the very function of heroin itself.

Apart from generally independent 'drug' effects, specific 'set' effects can be distinguished. A low positive mood is clearly correlated with high craving. This lends credence to the 'temperamental traits' theory of the vulnerability to addiction (Tarter et al., 1985). In this theory, the emphasis has been placed upon certain specific 'set' variables such as speed and strength of response, quality of prevailing mood and lability of prevailing mood. This trait explanation is supported by the ESM data where there is persistent interaction effect of the mood factor with individual subject differences across both craving dimensions. In addition to this 'set' effect, an independent 'setting' effect having to do with the social company and environment has been correlated with craving. Higher craving seems to be associated with 'crowd' or isolation situations and negatively related to 'intimate' ones. This finding is supported by animal experiments whereby a negative social environment has been found to be a key determinant in drug self-administration behavior (Alexander & Hadaway, 1983).

The finding of this study, that in contrast to the 'set' effect, both the 'drug' and 'setting' effects on craving are relatively independent of individual subject differences, has certain important implications. Whereas a growing body of neuropharmacological evidence has been accumulating in the addiction field, there has been less progress in specifying the social facts that may be intrinsic to the addiction syndrome and not merely preconditions or consequences. The finding that situational variables as well as social intimacy have been observed in this microscopic study to be correlated with craving is supported by other studies. For example, extensive documentation exists of the cessation of addiction by American soldiers on their return home from Vietnam (Robins et al., 1974; Ingraham, 1974). Furthermore, the ESM study has been able to specify that the 'setting' effect has more influence on the acquisition dimension of craving while the 'drug' effect has more weight on the loss of control dimension. The idiographic case studies presented in this Chapter support a revised 'sociobiological' view of craving whereby persons are clearly engaged in persistent attempts to implement coping strategies of adjusting and adapting to a changing situations of drug, setting and life historical events (see Alexander, 1990; Newcomb & Harlow, 1986).

In conclusion, the results reported in this Chapter have more general relevance for psychiatric classification and diagnosis. In terms of the DSM-III-R, craving has only been formulated as a criterion for smoking tobacco disorders. By use of the ESM methodology, craving has been postulated as a potential criterion across a range of drugs. Furthermore, craving has been identified with another formal component of addiction, intensity. This component has not been recognized in the current work in the DSM-III-R which has tended to focus upon severity (e.g., Kosten et al., 1987a, b; Rounsaville et al., 1987). By employing an ESM design, it has been possible to highlight analytically certain 'biopsychosocial' variables such as 'lack of intimacy' and 'homelessness', that could be candidates for future diagnostic systems. Further research along this line should potentiate a true synthesis of the disease and adaptation models of addiction, thus overcoming the current tensions of a paradigmatic dispute (see Miller & Gold, 1990). Systematic description in natural, ecological situations should be relevant for the development of future diagnostic systems by documenting new facts. The measurement of craving by ESM illustrates new situational variables. The conclusions of Frances et al. (1989: 375) may thus be facilitated in that 'It is in fact possible that the major innovation of DSM-IV will not be in its having surprising new content but rather will reside in the systematic and explicit method by which DSM-IV will be constructed and documented'.

17

Stress, coping and cortisol dynamics in daily life

NANCY A. NICOLSON

Introduction

Psychosocial stress is thought to play an important role in the development and course of many psychiatric and psychosomatic disorders. Major life events, such as the death of a family member or recent unemployment, have long been implicated as precipitating factors in illness (Dohrenwend & Dohrenwend, 1974). More recently, attention has shifted toward the possible impact of minor stressors or 'daily hassles' (Kanner et al., 1981). An inability to cope with the demands of everyday activities might contribute to the development of disorders or to the exacerbation of existing symptoms.

A wide range of physiological changes occur in response to stress. In most cases, these reflect normal, adaptive processes which prepare the body to cope with the situation by active behavioral strategies (for example, 'fight' or 'flight' reactions). However, when adequate behavioral or cognitive solutions to the problem are not available, physiological responses may be so exaggerated or prolonged that pathological processes are set in motion. One major impetus for research in stress psychobiology is to clarify the role stress reactivity plays in the pathophysiology of cardiovascular disease, diabetes, and aging, among others. Knowledge of the way in which physiological stress reactions might contribute to the development of psychopathology is currently limited, although promising theoretical models have been advanced (e.g., Anisman & Zacharcko, 1982; Ehlers et al., 1988). Apart from their possible causal role in psychiatric disorders, however, physiological responses provide a window on the nature and adequacy of psychological responses to the stresses of daily life. Regardless of an individual's ability to deny, repress or otherwise defend against emotional distress, as revealed in self-reports or interviews, or the level of behavioral function, if physiological indicators of stress fail to return to normal, we can conclude that the coping process is incomplete and the individual remains at risk.

Both stress and coping are currently conceptualized as dynamic processes, which change over time and in relation to the environment. Individuals respond to the situation at hand in terms of the degree of threat or challenge it poses, the stakes involved, how much control can be exerted over the outcome, and what personal skills or resources are available (Folkman & Lazarus, 1980, 1985; Frankenhaeuser, 1986). In order to clarify the relationship between psychological processes and physiological response patterns, it is therefore necessary to include measures of emotional state, coping mechanisms and appraisal of the situation (Mason, 1975; Frankenhaeuser, 1980). Ideally, these relationships should be studied in naturalistic settings and over time, so that we can begin to understand how adaptation occurs in response to intermittent daily hassles as well as to major life events, in individuals who are observed in their normal social networks, settings, and activities (Dimsdale, 1984). A major drawback of laboratory experiments is that they do not evoke the intensity of emotions or richness of coping strategies observed in daily life; this may be one reason why real life stressors appear to induce physiological responses more consistently than experimental tasks (Weiner, 1985). Not surprisingly, perhaps, studies of neuroendocrine responses to laboratory stressors have produced only modest results, with great variability both within and between individual subjects (Berger et al., 1987). Moreover, we do not know to what extent laboratory findings are generalizable to real-life stress (Marschall, 1987).

The studies reported below take advantage of two relatively new techniques, Experience Sampling and ambulatory monitoring of salivary cortisol, to assess the relationship between an individual's affective state and neuroendocrine changes over time in response to potentially stressful naturally occurring activities and situations. The choice of cortisol as a physiological stress index is based on both theoretical and practical considerations. Studies since the 1950s have clearly demonstrated that the adrenocortical system is sensitive to psychological stimuli (Mason, 1968; Hennessey & Levine, 1979; Rose, 1984). Cortisol secretion appears to increase specifically in response to distress, as opposed to effort or general arousal (Lundberg & Frankenhaeuser, 1980; Delahunt & Mellsop, 1987). In addition, cortisol activity is thought to reflect the adequacy of coping behavior (Wolff et al., 1964; Ursin & Murison, 1984; Vickers, 1988); that is, effective coping results in a faster recovery of cortisol to normal basal levels following a stressor. The persistence of high cortisol levels, on the other hand, is asociated with poor adjustment to chronic stress (for example, in Iran hostages (Rahe et al., 1990) and in residents of Three Mile Island (Schaeffer & Baum, 1984)) and may be predictive in psychiatric disorders of poor follow-up outcome (Steiner & Levine, 1988).

Given that cortisol levels parallel increases in anxiety and distress in healthy individuals undergoing acute stress, one might expect to find cortisol hypersecretion in psychiatric disorders in which these emotional states are prominent. The pioneering psychoneuroendocrine studies of Edward Sachar indeed suggested that acute distress might be the link connecting endocrine disturbance in psychiatric disorder with normal responses to stress in healthy individuals. Based on longitudinal case studies, Sachar documented cortisol hypersecretion not only in depression but also in other psychiatric disorders, coinciding in time with phases of agitation or acute distress (e.g., Sachar et al., 1963, 1967). Over time, it has become clear that chronic disturbance of the hypothalamic-pituitary-adrenal (HPA) axis is common only in major depression and cannot be adequately explained by the stress of the illness alone. The anxiety disorders and post-traumatic stress syndrome are generally characterized by normal HPA activity. At this point, it remains unclear whether anxiety and distress in these disorders are qualitatively the same states as those experienced in response to stressful events (Mason et al., 1986; Cameron & Nesse, 1988; Kathol et al., 1988).

In depression, challenge tests such as the dexamethasone suppression test (DST) have identified feedback deficits in HPA axis regulation, which appear at first sight to argue for a biological rather than a psychosocial interpretation of the neuroendocrine abnormalities. Evidence that real-life stress can result in DST non-suppression in healthy individuals (Rose, 1987; Frecska et al., 1988), however, suggests that stress could still play a role in the development of HPA irregularities, which might then persist independent of further environmental input. Psychosocial factors might, for example, be involved in the initial disregulation of diurnal rhythms in depression (Ehlers et al., 1988). Repeated diurnal measurement of HPA activity is more likely to reveal synergistic or other effects of stress than simple procedures such as the DST (Rose, 1987). While some promising efforts have recently been made to link intra-individual fluctuations in cortisol and symptoms in depressed inpatients (Blackburn et al., 1987; von Zerssen et al., 1987), additional insights could be gained by extending psychobiological research on depression and other disorders to the natural environment.

In short, cortisol continues to offer a theoretical bridge between psychosocial and biological approaches in contemporary psychiatry. From a practical viewpoint, cortisol is one of the few hormones that can be measured repeatedly and non-invasively in real-life settings. Until recently, psychoendocrine studies in daily life were hampered by methodological obstacles. The measurement of hormones in blood requires interruption of ongoing activities and is often stressful in itself. While these problems can be solved, for example by sampling blood through indwelling catheters during public speaking (Dimsdale & Moss, 1980), repeated sampling of blood over periods of ambulatory monitoring longer than a few hours or a day does not appear feasible with currently available technology. Urine collection is relatively stress-free, but because the level of a hormone determined in urine represents its integrated excretion over a period of hours, this method gives a more global measure of response to specific events. Collection and storage of urine presents additional practical problems for ambulatory subjects. Recent developments in immunoassay techniques, however, have made it possible to measure a number of hormones, including cortisol, in saliva (Vining & McGinley, 1986). Saliva samples can be reliably collected and stored by subjects themselves, enabling them to carry out their daily routine without undue interference. Cortisol concentrations in saliva have been shown to be highly correlated with the plasma 'free' fraction, which is considered to be the biologically active hormone, and are independent of the flow rate of saliva (Vining et al., 1983). Also advantageous is the fact that cortisol responds within minutes to acute stressors (Hellhammer et al., 1987) and has a half-life in blood or saliva of approximately an hour (Frederikson, Sundin & Frankenhaeuser, 1985), which provides an appropriate time frame for studying its relationship to mood and symptom fluctuations and to stressful events in daily life.

Studies of acute stress in healthy subjects

We have combined ES with salivary cortisol sampling in healthy young adults to address three fundamental questions about the psychobiology of stress. Firstly, are naturally occurring daily events of sufficient intensity to activate the pituitary-adrenal system? In three related studies, we examine cortisol responses to anticipated events varying in severity from mild to moderate. Saliva samples obtained at frequent intervals allow us to describe the cortisol responses over time, from anticipatory through recovery phases. The second question focuses on the meaning of individual differences in cortisol reactivity. As Mason stated (1968, p. 594), 'The relevant question is "Do those individuals who become emotionally upset in this situation show significant hormonal response?" rather than "Do most people show hormonal responses in this situation?" ' In laboratory studies, the failure to find consistent associations between self-reported distress and cortisol reactivity has cast doubt on the usefulness of cortisol as an index of psychological state (Bossert et al., 1988). Naturalistic studies have not always produced clearer results. In studies of examination stress, for example, cortisol reactivity has often shown no association with psychological measures (Allen et al., 1985; Herbert et al., 1986; Jones et al., 1986; Kahn et al., 1991; but see also Hellhammer et al., 1985). Thirdly, we ask whether coping behavior influences the cortisol response to stress. Theoretically, effective coping should result in a more rapid termination of the hormonal response.

Subjects and methods

In order to maximize chances of obtaining data relevant to these issues, we have included 'natural experiments' in the design of the ES studies described below. That is, we selected three groups of subjects who had already been scheduled to undergo similar types of potentially stressful events (examinations) during the sampling period. The first group were 28 first-year university students who took a minor multiple-choice test on the 4th day of the six-day sampling period. The second group was comprised of 13 third- and fourth-year medical students, who were also sampled for six days; here, the potential stressor was a major examination (demonstration of clinical skills under time pressure, while being rated by a unfamiliar observer) lasting an hour on each of two consecutive days. The 10 subjects in the third group were candidates for a driver's license and took the practical driving examination on the second day of a three-day study. Participation was voluntary, and subjects were completely unrestricted in their daily activities.

ESM, as developed for use in psychiatric and psychosomatic research (deVries et al., 1987; Delespaul & deVries, 1987), was used to collect self-reports from subjects at selected moments during their normal daily activities. Subjects received signals via a preprogrammed wristwatch, after which they filled in a questionnaire concerning both objective aspects of the situation at that moment and subjective reactions to it. The ESM form contained open-ended questions concerning thought content, the physical and social context (where and with whom), and what the subject was doing. The forms also included seven-point Likert-type scales grouped into modules for the evaluation of thoughts, mood, the presence of individually defined somatic and psychologic stress symptoms, evaluation of the present activity, and physical wellbeing. The mood items, in particular, provide a means of distinguishing emotional distress from general arousal or effort. Items from the activity evaluation section measure the subject's appraisal of his skills in relation to the perceived demands of the situation at that point in time and aspects of control and desirability. Additional items were included to evaluate the level and kind of stress experienced and to help interpretation of the hormonal data; these asked the subject to indicate the occurrence and intensity of physical exertion, distressing or arousing events, and any ingestion of food, coffee, alcohol, medications, or smoking which may have taken place since the last signal. Finally, the subject was asked to describe stressful events or situations which might have taken place in the interval since the last ESM report.

Subjects received a beep signal 10 times each day between 7:30 a.m. and 10:30 p.m., with an average interval of 90 min between consecutive beeps. The intervals were programmed so that the exact signalling times would be unpredictable but would still approximate a fixed time series. In the current studies, beeps were randomly distributed around fixed time points (e.g., 8:15 a.m., 9:45 a.m., and so on throughout the day), with a maximum deviation of 20 min. As soon as possible after each beep, subjects filled in an ESM form and simultaneously collected a saliva sample by holding a cotton dental roll in the mouth for one minute. Saturated dental rolls were then placed in a capped plastic vial ('Salivette', Sarstedt), labelled with the time of day, and stored with the ESM booklet in a specially designed wallet. Subjects placed saliva samples in their home freezer compartments within 12 h. We found no change in cortisol levels in uncentrifuged samples stored at room temperature for up to 24 h (Nicolson et al., 1991); other experiments indicate that cortisol is stable at room temperature for as long as 30 days (Kirschbaum & Hellhammer, 1989). At the end of the sampling week, Salivette vials were frozen at −20°C until assayed.

Compliance with the above procedures has been good, with 74% of the ESM forms and 74.5% of the saliva samples completed, including occasions when the watch failed to beep or was not heard. As in most ESM studies, data loss was greatest in the early morning, when subjects tended to be still sleeping. In general, subjects reported that ESM and saliva collection procedures caused only minimal disturbance of ongoing activities and rarely resulted in any change in the daily routine (Nicolson et al., 1991).

In addition to the ESM procedure, subjects took saliva samples immediately before and after the examinations and rated their mood on 15 Likert scale items, with subscales representing emotional responses to 'threat' (anxious, fearful, worried), 'challenge' (eager, hopeful, confident), 'benefit' (relieved, happy, pleased, exhilarated), and 'harm' (disgusted, guilty, angry, sad, disappointed) (Folkman & Lazarus, 1985). All subjects completed the Spielberger State-Trait Anxiety Inventory (Dutch version ZBV, van der Ploeg et al., 1979), the Test Anxiety Inventory (van der Ploeg, 1988), and the Zung depression scale (Dutch version, Dijkstra, 1974). The Utrecht Coping List (Schreurs & van de Willige, 1988) was administered at the end of the study to assess coping strategies used in dealing with the examination situation from preparation through recovery phases. Scores were obtained for the scale's seven factor-analytically derived coping styles, namely 'problem-oriented', 'palliative behaviors/distraction', 'avoidance', 'seek social support', 'expression of emotions/anger', 'comforting cognitions', and 'depressive reaction/giving up'. Additional questionnaires were designed to assess individuals' appraisal of the situation in terms of the stakes involved, expectations of success or failure, preparation, and actual performance.

Analysis

Cortisol levels were determined in duplicate by direct radioimmunoassay, by Dr. J. Sulen, University of Liège (for details, see Ansseau et al., 1984). The lower detection limit of the assay was 12 ng/dl, with a mean intra-assay coefficient of variation of 4.7%. All samples from one individual were analyzed in the same assay to minimize variability of results.

Cortisol response, or reactivity, to the testing situation was defined as the absolute change in salivary cortisol measured immediately before and after the examination, relative to the individual's mean level in time-matched samples on non-examination days ('baseline'). For analyses in which we are primarily concerned with the relationship between stress and cortisol fluctuations *within* individuals, we have standardized cortisol values for each subject for each of the 10 diurnal sampling times. This method controls for the strong diurnal pattern of cortisol secretion and for individual differences in baseline levels, thus making it possible to analyze morning and evening values, for example, either together or separately (see also Nesse et al., 1985). Unless otherwise indicated, all statistical tests are two-tailed. Significance levels are indicated as follows: $P \leq 0.05^*$, $P \leq 0.01^{**}$, $P \leq 0.001^{***}$.

Results

Cortisol reactivity in relation to type of stressor, subjective experience and coping

Summarizing results of the three studies, in which each group of subjects underwent a different potentially stressful event, we find evidence that both characteristics of the situation and of the individual influenced cortisol reactivity. Firstly, group mean salivary cortisol levels rose in anticipation of all three examination situations. As shown in Fig. 17.1, however, there were differences among the studies in the magnitude of the pre-examination cortisol response and its duration, as reflected in post-examination levels.

In general, the higher the stakes involved in passing the examination, the greater the pre-examination hormonal response. Students taking the minor university test, for example, showed elevated cortisol levels in the hours preceding the test (data not shown), but by the time the test was about to begin cortisol was only moderately elevated relative to baseline. The medical skills examination, which took place on each of two consecutive days, brought about more pronounced pre-examination cortisol responses on the first day; here, too, post-examination cortisol recovered quickly in the group as a whole, with no significant difference from baseline. All of the driver's license candidates showed a pre-examination cortisol increase, and for nine of the 10 cortisol remained elevated after the examination, suggesting that this situation was particularly stressful.

Secondly, in each of the three studies we found large individual differences in cortisol reactivity. A significant percentage of this variability could be explained by differences in the degree of subjective distress individuals experienced in relation to the potential stressor. Table 17.1 presents the correlations between measures of emotional state, appraisal of the situation and cortisol responses right before and again after the examinations, for the combined university ($n=15$) and medical ($n=13$) student groups. For the medical students, only the first of the two examination days is included in the following analyses.

As predicted, subjects who experienced the greatest distress immediately before the examination showed the largest increases in cortisol. Similarly, subjects who reacted to the impending examination as a threat showed

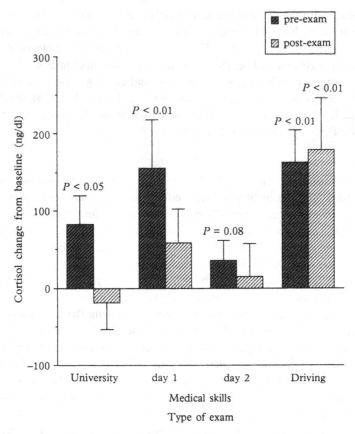

Fig. 17.1. Salivary cortisol responses before and after examinations (mean + SEM). A response is defined as the change from an individual's mean level at the same time of day on non-exam days. Significant changes from baseline are indicated on the figure (Wilcoxon matched-pairs signed-ranks test). Pre-exam responses for the medical exam-day 2 approached significance ($0.05 < P < 0.10$). Dark columns, pre-exam; lighter columns, post-exam.

increased cortisol levels, whereas subjects who regarded the impending examination as a challenge had even lower cortisol levels than on non-examination days. Pre-examination cortisol responses were also correlated with subjective appraisal of the examination situation, both in terms of its anticipated difficulty and how certain the individual felt of performing well. In contrast, post-examination cortisol responses were not significantly correlated with any subjective measure of distress rated at that moment, but continued to reflect the *pre-examination* mood states.

Finally, we examined the relationship between cortisol levels and coping style (see Table 17.2). While not associated with either pre-examination

Table 17.1. *Spearman rank correlations between psychological state measures and cortisol responses*

State measures	Salivary cortisol response	
	Before exam	After exam
Before exam		
state anxiety	0.52**	0.60***
threat	0.53**	0.53**
harm	0.38*	0.25
challenge	−0.64***	−0.29
benefit	−0.25	−0.36
expect test will be difficult	0.48**	0.30
confident will perform well	−0.47**	−0.36*
feel well prepared	−0.12	−0.07
After exam		
threat		−0.05
harm		0.02
challenge		−0.16
benefit		0.14
test was difficult		0.10
confident performed well		0.17

Significance levels for two-tailed tests: *$P<0.05$; **$P<0.01$; ***$P<0.001$ ($N=28$).

A cortisol response is defined as the exam-day change from the individual's mean level at the same time of day on non-exam days. Pre- and post-exam responses were negatively correlated with baseline levels ($r_s = -0.43$** and -0.61***, respectively) and positively correlated with each other ($r_s = 0.39$*).

Table 17.2. *Spearman rank correlations between cortisol responses and coping style*

Coping style	Salivary cortisol response	
	Before exam	After exam
Problem-oriented	−0.28	−0.37*
Palliative/distraction	−0.04	0.45*
Avoidance	0.13	0.18
Seek social support	−0.11	0.28
Express emotions/anger	0.02	0.23
Comforting cognitions	0.16	0.39*
Depressive reaction	−0.02	0.35*

Significance levels for two-tailed tests: see Table 17.1 above ($N=28$).

distress or cortisol reactivity, coping appeared to play an important role in terminating the hormonal stress response after the examination. That is, although group mean post-examination cortisol levels had returned to baseline, individuals with persisting high cortisol tended to be those who employed less-effective coping strategies. Post-examination cortisol responses were positively correlated with the coping subscales 'distraction', and 'comforting cognitions', with 'depressive reaction' approaching significance. 'Problem-oriented' coping, on the other hand, was associated with low post-examination cortisol levels. In summary, it appears that emotional distress was an important determinant of cortisol reactivity to the impending stressor and that effective coping helped bring about faster post-stress recovery.

Stress, distress and cortisol dynamics throughout the week: a case study   As noted previously, we chose to sample individuals who had a scheduled examination during the week in order to have a more or less comparable stressor for all subjects. We have seen that the individual experience of this event was highly variable. In fact, for a surprising number of subjects, the most stressful experiences of the week were *not* related to the examination situation. Although the mean severity of stressful events reported on examination days (4.2) was higher than that on non-examination days (3.5), only 74 of the 244 reports in which recent stress was rated as moderate to severe (4 or greater on a 7-point scale) took place on an examination day. Examples of the types of stressors described include a narrow escape from a traffic accident, public speaking, and the death of a friend's parent.

The case study of a subject who happened to have a very stressful week provides a clear illustration of the relationships between two discrete events (both anticipated), anxiety, somatic symptoms, and cortisol. A 19-year-old university student R. began the ES procedure on the Tuesday of a week in which she was scheduled to take a driving examination on Wednesday (2 p.m.) and a university test on Friday (10 a.m.). She had already failed the driving examination on two previous attempts. The university test was the first one of the academic year, so while the stakes were low, the situation was somewhat novel and unpredictable. Scores on trait anxiety and depression scales were in the normal published ranges and were also close to the medians for our combined sample ($n=42$). In contrast, R. scored extremely high on trait test anxiety, specifically on the emotional subscale (total score: 53, emotional subscale: 26, worry subscale: 13); for comparison, group median scores were 33, 15, and 12, respectively. State anxiety measured immediately before the university examination was also much higher than average (68

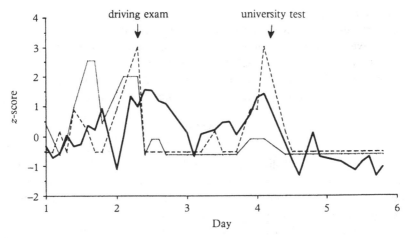

Fig. 17.2. Case study: Cortisol (–), anxiety (---), and somatic symptoms (...) over a period of five days. Cortisol z-scores have been calculated separately for each diurnal sampling interval. Z-scores for anxiety and somatic symptoms (stomach ache) are based on the total of 38 ESM ratings.

in comparison to a group median of 49). With respect to coping style, R. scored high relative to published norms on the factors 'depressive reaction' and 'seek social support' and low on 'palliative behaviors/distraction'. During the briefing session, R. identified a feeling of restlessness as her primary psychologic stress symptom and stomach aches as her somatic stress symptom.

Figure 17.2 shows fluctuations in anxiety, stomach complaints, and cortisol levels for R. over the five-day sampling period. Anxiety increased in anticipation of both of the two scheduled stressful events. Stomach complaints were more severe in the hours before the driving examination than before the university test. Cortisol peaks are also evident in relation to both events. In the case of the driving examination, post-examination cortisol levels remained high for the rest of the day, even though R. knew she had passed the examination and reported no lingering anxiety or stress-related symptoms. As mentioned earlier, we have observed the same pattern of cortisol elevation following driving examinations in other subjects, which suggests that aspects of this type of stressor (for example, the high stakes or the unpredictable behavior of the driving examiner) might be involved. For the 38 measures obtained from R. over the five-day period, cortisol z-scores were associated with self-reported anxiety ($r_s=0.30$, $P=0.07$), loneliness ($r_s=0.32^{\star}$), current symptoms (somatic: $r_s=0.37^{\star}$; psychological: $r_s=0.32^{\star}$), and symptoms in the preceding interval (somatic: $r_s=0.45^{\star\star}$; psychological:

$r_s = 0.44^{**}$). The remaining ESM mood items (tense, sad, discontent, angry, unsure) showed the same pattern of positive correlations with relative cortisol levels, but were not significant. The fact that correlations with cortisol are slightly higher for recent than for current symptom levels provides evidence for a temporal delay in cortisol response to distress, as would be predicted on theoretical grounds.

Discussion

In summary, analysis of measures of salivary cortisol and mood in relation to acute, anticipated real-life stress revealed clear and robust associations between subjective experience and intra-individual changes in cortisol secretion before and after examinations. Individuals who appraised the impending examination as threatening showed elevated cortisol; those who responded to the situation as a challenge, in contrast, showed no increase in cortisol. After the examination, only problem-focused coping was effective in reducing cortisol levels, whereas depressive reactions and emotion-focused coping strategies were associated with a delay in cortisol recovery to baseline. Given that similar studies of examination stress have failed to find these predicted associations between cortisol, distress and coping, it may be useful to speculate on the factors that may have contributed to our positive results. Firstly, both the frequent sampling procedure and the choice of salivary instead of plasma hormone measures may have resulted in more reliable individual baseline cortisol estimations. Secondly, the timing of psychological state measures appears to be important. If we had only measured anxiety or distress after the examinations, for example, no correlation with cortisol responses would have been found. Lastly, the psychological variables which were most closely related to cortisol activity (distress, appraisal, and coping measures) were all formulated as state measures; trait measures are, as a rule, much less effective in predicting cortisol responses in a particular situation.

A case study was used to illustrate how mood, symptoms and cortisol levels fluctuate in relation to stressful events. It is important to note that not all subjects showed significant correlations between mood and cortisol measures. In subjects like R. with multiple stressors, correlations between cortisol and ESM stress, anxiety, and psychosomatic symptom items were higher in general than in subjects who simply did not experience any stress, whether by chance or through more effective coping. Furthermore, the ESM items which were associated with cortisol differed from one subject to the next, probably reflecting idiosyncrasies in how subjects interpreted their emotions in terms of the questionnaire items. Person-specific correlations between physiological measures and perceived symptoms have also been found in within-subject studies of blood pressure and blood glucose fluctuations (Pennebaker et al., 1985).

The study of cortisol dynamics in daily life necessitates a willingness to sacrifice much of the experimental control possible in laboratory settings in order to gain ecological validity. Some level of control can and should be exerted in selecting subjects; habits or conditions which are known or strongly suspected to affect cortisol levels (e.g., endocrine disorders, major weight loss, alcoholism, use of benzodiazepines in high dosages, opioid use) require the establishment of exclusion criteria. On the other hand, there are happily no sex differences in baseline cortisol levels in humans (Forsman & Lundberg, 1982) and no changes in cortisol over the menstrual cycle (Ablanalp et al., 1977; Collins, Eneroth & Landgren, 1985). From our own studies as well as controlled experiments elsewhere, it appears that contraceptive pill use has either no effect on salivary cortisol or, at worst, a slight elevating effect limited to morning samples (Guechot et al., 1982; Kirschbaum & Hellhammer, 1989; van Poll, Nicolson & Sulon, 1990).

The effects of commonly used substances such as cigarettes and coffee also appear to be slight at normal levels of intake (Cherek et al., 1982; Pincomb et al., 1987). Evidence that higher levels of intake may well have an effect on cortisol levels (e.g., Wüst et al., 1990), however, necessitates caution. In addition, some individuals exhibit increased cortisol levels in the hour following a meal, especially lunch (Quigley & Yen, 1979). While preliminary results indicate that food intake has no large systematic effects on cortisol in our ESM studies (Nicolson et al., 1991), the fact that subjects are free to eat whatever and whenever they want may introduce unavoidable 'noise' into the analysis. Exercise can clearly elevate cortisol secretion (Cook et al., 1987), but this effect is limited to prolonged strenuous exertion; normal daily activities such as bicycle riding or recreational tennis had no discernible effect in our studies. As a precaution, however, we have excluded cortisol values obtained within 90 min of self-reported strenuous activity (2–3% of the total responses in our student samples) from further analysis.

Even though we believe that salivary cortisol is a sensitive physiological index of psychological distress, one should not expect a one-to-one relationship between subjective experience and endocrine response. In addition to extraneous influences on cortisol levels, as described above, and the normal physiological secretory pattern of this hormone, our data suggest that there may be a threshold level of arousal which must be reached before the pituitary-adrenal system is activated. However, timing may also be important. Laboratory experiments indicate that cortisol levels peak approximately 20–45 min after the onset of an acute stressor and then begin to drop (Wittersheim et al., 1985; Hellhammer et al., 1987). It is thus possible that even minor increases in anxiety or distress produce a small rise in cortisol; given that the 90-min ESM sampling intervals are somewhat longer than the half-life of cortisol in saliva, however, these transient, low-level responses would have less chance of being recorded. Finally, the fact that cortisol levels often rise in anticipation of an event and may under certain conditions remain elevated for hours, days, or even weeks after a stressful event means that new methods must be developed to model the relationship between subjective experience and cortisol dynamics *in time*. Psychological states can also be expected to have distinct temporal properties, making it unlikely that simple correlation techniques will provide an adequate description of the relationships. Keeping these difficulties in mind, we believe that ES combined with simultaneous measures of salivary cortisol offers the potential for investigating adaptive and maladaptive responses to the full range of acute and chronic stressors encountered in daily life.

18

Vital exhaustion or depression: a study of
daily mood in exhausted male subjects at
risk for myocardial infarction
ROB VAN DIEST

Introduction

Many subjects, suffering from a first myocardial infarction (MI), describe a
lack of energy, excess fatigue, listlessness, a loss of libido and increased irritability as their most dominant feelings in the months prior to this cardiac event
(Appels & Mendes de Leon, 1989; Falger, 1989). A prospective study (average
follow-up period 4.2 years), in which the association of these feelings with
future MI was explored, showed that subjects, suffering from these feelings,
had at least a two-fold increase in risk for future MI (Appels & Mulder, 1988).
The aforementioned studies suggest that a lack of energy, excess fatigue,
listlessness, loss of libido and increased irritability are important premonitory
symptoms for MI.

These feelings reflect a state of exhaustion which people develop when their
resources to adapt to stress break down (Appels, 1989). These feelings are also
reported by subjects suffering from depression (DSM-III-R, 1987) leading to
the question whether exhausted subjects are also suffering from depression.
An association between depression and coronary heart disease has been
previously reported by Crisp, Queen & d'Souza (1984) and Booth-Kewley &
Friedman (1987). Current psychiatric consensus on depression is that depression is a complex of cognitive, behavioral, motivational and somatic symptoms
that manifest themselves around a core symptom of depressed mood (DSM-
III-R, 1987). The assessment of depression, however, is problematic
(Bouman, 1987) because both kind and severity of symptom components show
considerable inter-individual variability. Furthermore, depressed subjects
overestimate negative behaviors and underestimate positive behaviors (Roth,
Rehm & Rozensky, 1980) and emphasize somatic symptoms (Hamilton,
1982). Since retrospective bias is a widespread phenomenon, it may also play a
role in reports from exhausted subjects. The use of research approaches that
obtain better information about depressive symptoms (Bouman, 1987) circum-
venting bias is required.

To meet this requirement, two methods were used to investigate depression in exhausted subjects in this study. An adapted version of the Experience Sampling paradigm was developed to circumvent retrospective bias and explore feelings of depression, fatigue and vigour on a daily basis in the natural environment. Furthermore, the constituent symptoms of a depressive syndrome were assessed in retrospect by the Beck Depression Inventory (BDI) (Beck et al., 1979). The following question was explored:

Are exhausted subjects characterized by feelings of depressed mood or by feelings of a loss of vigour and excessive fatigue?

Method

Subjects

Sampling of subjects A random sample of 1,500 men (45–65 years old) from the city of Maastricht received a postal invitation to participate. Of the 471 volunteers who returned the Maastricht Questionnaire (MQ), that assesses the degree of exhaustion, 451 men were included in the study. Subjects from the exhausted group (158 men) and the control group (161 men) were telephoned at random and asked if they were willing to fill out a logbook six times a day for 21 days. Those who gave informed consent started the logbook study within five weeks after returning the MQ. The week prior to starting they were visited at home to discuss the questions and instructions involved.

From the above sample, 35 exhausted and 11 control subjects were asked to participate; 15 subjects were excluded, either because they did not fulfil the inclusion criteria (six men) or were not willing to participate (nine men). Twenty one exhausted men and 10 control subjects entered the study. The exploration of selection bias at the first selection step revealed that the 451 volunteers were not significantly different in age from the non-responding subjects. In addition to this, the 10 control subjects did not differ significantly from the subsample they were drawn from with respect to age, type A behavior or proportion of reported sleep complaints. The same is true for the 21 exhausted subjects except for their mean age which is slightly lower.

The 21 exhausted and 10 control subjects did not differ significantly with respect to age or type A behavior either. However, 61.9% of the exhausted subjects reported sleep complaints while in contrast 10.0% of control subjects had sleep problems.

Finally, non-participation occurred almost entirely in the exhausted group. There were no significant differences with respect to age, type A behavior or depression as assessed with the BDI between participants and non-participants.

234

Exclusion criteria   Subjects for the present investigation also participated in a study of sleep-physiological characteristics of exhausted men. They therefore met the following exclusion criteria: no sleep medication use, shiftwork or medical history of MI.

Instruments

Assessment of exhaustion   To assess a state of exhaustion, the 'Maastricht Questionnaire' (MQ) was used. This questionnaire consists of 21 items (Cronbachs' alpha 0.89) (Appels, Höppener & Mulder, 1987) which predicted future MI (Appels & Mulder, 1988). To maximize the contrast between exhausted and control subjects, those with scores in the highest tertial of the MQ distribution were assigned to the exhausted group while control subjects had scores in the lowest tertial.

Assessment of depression   Current affective, cognitive, motivational and somatic symptoms of depression were assessed with the 21-item version of the BDI (Beck et al., 1979) prior to starting the ESM part of the study. Subjects filled out the BDI which registered information about the occurrence of symptoms over the past two weeks including the 'present' day.

Profile of Mood States (POMS)   Depressed mood, vigour and fatigue were assessed in the natural context with three subscales of the Profile of Mood States (POMS) (Dutch version) (Wald & Mellenbergh, 1990). A depressed mood was assessed as: *Blue, Helpless, Sad, Lonely, Unhappy Unworthy, Gloomy* and *Desperate* (range 8–40: higher scores indicate depressed mood). Vigour was assessed as: *Active, Lively, Energetic, Cheerful* and *Clear-headed* (range 5–25: a higher score equals more vigour). Fatigue was assessed as: *Exhausted, Bushed, Fatigued, Listless, Worn Out* and *Weary* (range 6–30: higher scores register more fatigue).

Experience Sampling Method (ESM)   With an adapted version of ESM, subjects were signalled, during a 21-d period, to fill out the above items of the POMS (deVries, 1987). In its adapted version, the beeps were programmed in six consecutive blocks of 150 min each. To avoid expectancy effects, the beep in each block was given at random, although beeps of consecutive blocks were at least 60 min apart. Subjects were instructed to answer the POMS items according to how they felt at the moment they heard the beep.

The average loss of data was five beeps out of 126 (range 0–10); missing values were replaced by the mean values of the remaining beep scores. Intervals are relatively large (2.5 h) and will be treated as fixed intervals.

BDI item scores from every subject were totalled and averaged for the exhausted and control group separately.

POMS subscale scores were obtained for every beep and subject. Average diurnal course for depression, fatigue and vigour was then calculated for each subject by averaging of 'same time' beeps over the 21 days. The individual diurnal courses were analyzed in a two (group) by six (time) MANOVA of repeated measures design (O'Brien & Kister Kaiser, 1985).

Selection bias was studied with measures available at the various steps of the selection.

Results

Depression as assessed with the BDI   Current affective, cognitive, motivational and somatic symptoms of depression were present to a significantly greater extent in exhausted men (mean BDI=10.3; SD=8.8) than in control subjects (mean BDI=1.1; SD=1.0) (Mann-Whitney U=19.5; P <0.01).

Depression, vigour and fatigue as assessed with the POMS   The average diurnal courses of depression, vigour and fatigue are shown in Fig. 18.1.

A summary of a two (group) by six (time) MANOVA of repeated measures is shown in Table 18.1.

Exhausted men, on average, are significantly less vigorous and more fatigued during the entire day than control subjects. There was, however, no difference in disturbed mood. Furthermore, there is a significant time-of-day effect for vigour and fatigue but not for depression. Inspection of Fig. 18.1 shows that vigour declines and fatigue inclines during the day, while the daily course of depression is flat. This time-of-day effect appears to be the same for both exhausted men and control subjects because there is no significant group × time interaction for depression, vigour or fatigue. This is also readily seen from Fig. 18.1, which shows that the daily courses of these mood dimensions run almost parallel in both groups.

Discussion

Depressed mood, as assessed with the POMS using the adjusted ESM, did not discriminate exhausted subjects from control subjects. In fact, feelings of depressed mood were rarely experienced by any of the subjects. However, feelings of increased fatigue and diminished vigour were reported significantly more often by exhausted subjects. Furthermore, the respective daily course of fatigue, vigour and a depressed mood ran almost parallel in exhausted and control subjects. Throughout the day, exhausted subjects experience more fatigue and less vigour than control subjects. Retrospective assessment of

Table 18.1. *Summary of a two (group) by six (time) MANOVA of repeated measures*

	Between-group test		Time-of-day effect		Group × Time interaction	
	d.f. 1,29		d.f. 5,25		d.f. 5,25	
Depression	$F = 3.6$	n.s.	$F = 1.0$	n.s.	$F = 0.89$	n.s.
Vigour	$F = 5.7$	$P<0.02$	$F = 19.5$	$P<0.001$	$F = 0.55$	n.s.
Fatigue	$F = 6.1$	$P<0.02$	$F = 6.6$	$P<0.001$	$F = 1.27$	n.s.

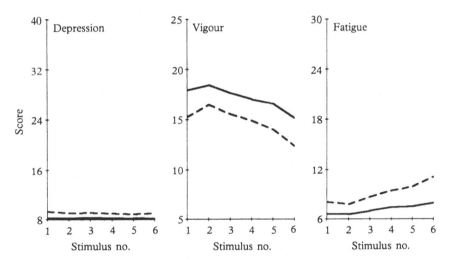

Fig. 18.1. Average diurnal course of depressed mood, vigour and fatique in exhausted (---) and control (—) subjects, as assessed with the POMS.

depression with the BDI, however, showed that exhausted subjects reported significantly more affective, cognitive, motivational and somatic symptoms of depression than control subjects. According to the cutoff scores used by Beck & Beamesderfer (1974), the group of exhausted subjects would be described as mildly depressed. Given that depression refers to a complex of cognitive, behavioral, motivational and somatic symptoms which manifest themselves around the nuclear symptom of a depressed mood, this finding contrasts the lack of depressed mood obtained with the POMS. Depressed mood assessed with the POMS was rarely ascertained.

One explanation of the difference is that the methods gather data within different time frames. The BDI asks subjects to rate the occurrence of symptoms during the preceding two weeks including the 'present' day. The POMS, on the other hand, asks subjects to rate how they felt at any of 126 moments over a three-week period. Since the two assessment periods essentially overlapped, it is unlikely that instructions only were the main reason for the contrasting results. Quite another explanation arises from what Mayer (1977) considers to be one of the major deficits of the BDI, the fact that the BDI is oriented more toward the assessment of cognitive symptoms of a depressive syndrome than to the affective and somatic ones. The POMS, on the other hand, is oriented towards the assessment of affective states, including the nuclear symptom of a depressive syndrome, a depressed mood (feeling blue, helpless, sad, lonely, etc.) (McNair, Lorr & Droppleman, 1971). The absence of any feeling of depression, as obtained with the POMS, suggests that the complex of complaints as assessed with the BDI does not refer to a mild depression in exhausted subjects. It is more likely that both the POMS and the BDI depict a state of exhaustion in their own way, the POMS showing that a state of exhaustion is more characterized by a 'loss of vigour' and 'excess fatigue' than by a 'depressed mood' and the BDI showing that a complex of cognitive, behavioral, motivational and somatic symptoms, characteristic for a depressive syndrome, are also characteristic for a state of exhaustion.

The present study therefore provides evidence that a state of exhaustion, characterized by increased fatigue and diminished vigour throughout the day, is not associated with depression. These results are probably not explained by retrospective bias, because subjects were signalled randomly six times a day for three weeks to report how they felt at that moment. There were also no strong arguments that selection bias would have influenced the results to any great extent. In particular the absence of a significant difference in depression between participants and non-participants makes it safe to assume that non-participation did not influence the results of the present study.

The present study is based on two small but carefully selected samples of exhausted subjects and control subjects, in which the ESM has been used in an attempt to clarify whether a state of exhaustion is characterized more by feelings of a depressed mood or more by feelings of a loss of vigour and excess fatigue. The ESM has been chosen because it circumvents retrospective bias and allows investigation in a natural context. The results suggest that, throughout the day, exhausted subjects experience increasingly more fatigue and lower vigour than control subjects without any concomitant increase in depressed mood. The results with the BDI, however, suggest that the difference between exhausted subjects and depressed subjects may be rather subtle. The ESM proved to be very useful in the detection of this difference with respect to a disturbed mood. In future research, given the relevance of these findings for understanding risk for myocardial infarction, it would be of great interest to apply ESM also to the study of the cognitive, behavioral, motivational and somatic symptoms in both exhausted and depressed subjects.

19

Blood pressure and behavior: mood, activity and blood pressure in daily life[1]

LAWRENCE F. VAN EGEREN
and SUTHEP MADARASMI

Ambulatory blood pressure monitoring (ABPM) has become a valuable tool for the evaluation of the borderline hypertension patient (Pickering et al., 1985; Weber & Drayer, 1984) just as the random daily monitoring of mood and cognitive states with Experience Sampling has provided insights into the experience of psychopathology (deVries, 1987). Ambulatory monitoring provides a glimpse of the circulatory system in dynamic action viewed from within the pattern of the patient's familiar daily life. Blood pressure readings taken in the unfamiliar setting of the physician's office are often unrepresentative of the patient's level of pressure outside the office (Perloff & Solokow, 1978). Perhaps for this reason, office readings are less closely related to target organ damage associated with elevated blood pressure than are ABPM readings (Perloff et al., 1983; Devereux et al., 1983).

Much of the variability in blood pressure in the active person is behaviorally induced (Pickering et al., 1982). These behavioral influences must be taken into account in interpreting BP readings. A systolic pressure of 150 mm Hg while climbing a flight of stairs is one thing. The same pressure while sitting quietly takes on a new meaning and appears in a new perspective.

Unlike ESM studies where behavior is recorded randomly throughout the day, in medical applications generally, fixed and physiologically linked monitoring sampling strategies have been the rule. In these studies, behavior is usually monitored by having the patient keep a behavioral diary on the day of monitoring. The patient is typically instructed to record all significant events immediately following each BP reading. The aim of the diary is to capture the 'when, where, what, and how' of each BP reading: *when* was the reading taken, *where* was the person located at the time of the reading (e.g., work, home, car, other), *what* was the person doing at that time (e.g., subject chooses one of 10 activities), *how* did the person feel (e.g., subject chooses one of three mood states), and *how* was the body positioned (sitting, standing,

---

[1] Appeared in the *American Journal of Hypertension*, 1988, **1**, 3, part 3, pp. 1795–855.

reclining)? When blood pressure is read every 15 min during 16 waking hours the diary described above will generate 21 (number of diary variables) × 64 (number of waking readings) = 1,344 scores. When the diary information is to be used in research or in a computer-generated clinical report the 1,344 scores must be entered into the computer manually from the keyboard.

The great volume of behavioral data in ABPM poses a major problem for both patient and technician or clinician. Patient acceptance of the diary is often far from ideal, and the quantity of information provided by the patient may vary from the obsessionally detailed to none at all, even when the diary format is standardized (Roffe et al., 1985). Chesney & Ironson review these and other problems associated with the construction and use of behavioral diaries in ABPM (Chesney & Ironson, 1989).

The gathering and processing of behavioral data are so time consuming as to pose a formidable barrier to wider use of ABPM. To lower this barrier, the method of logging behavior must be interesting enough to motivate the patient and simple enough to avoid disrupting the normal flow of patient activities. The information obtained must be easily accessible to the investigator for clinical report writing and data analysis.

With these thoughts in mind, we developed a computer-assisted diary (CAD). The CAD system enables the user to monitor the behavioral conditions surrounding ambulatory blood pressure readings, to extract critical features of the data, and to readily access and use the information. The system was designed to meet the specific performance criteria that it should (1) be clear and simple to use, (2) have good subject acceptance, (3) monitor activities that have been shown to be related to ambulatory blood pressure, (4) have a low user error rate, (5) provide automatic computer checks for errors, (6) be implemented on an IBM-compatible PC, (7) download diary information to the computer automatically rather than manually, and (8) yield quantitative diary information that is usable both for research and for clinical evaluation. The result is the computer-scorable diary card and the associated computer software described here.

Mark-sense diary cards

We initially considered using a small, hand-held programmable micro-computer to log diary information but abandoned the idea because the operation of these devices is too complex and the fear of computers on the part of some people too great to ensure reliable performance. Instead, we developed the mark sense diary card shown in Fig. 19.1.

Following each BP reading, the subject marks boxes on the card to indicate the time of the reading, his location (work, home, car, other), his body position (sitting, standing, reclining), his activity (working, watching television, reading, talking, walking, eating, talking on the telephone, drinking a

Used with permission.

Fig. 19.1. Mark-sense diary card.

caffeinated beverage, smoking, drinking an alcoholic beverage, and other), the number of people he is having a face-to-face interaction with, and his emotion or mood (happy, angry, tense, rushed, tired, feeling goals are blocked, and other). There are places on the card where the subject can write comments as well as locations, activities, and moods other than those printed on the card. It takes approximately 30 to 45 s to mark the diary card each time blood pressure is read.

The card is printed on both sides, with two diary records on each side, so that each card can accommodate diary information for four BP readings. When blood pressure is read every 15 min, the subject fills out one card per hour.

CAD procedure

Prior to a BP scan, the subject receives detailed written instructions describing the use of the diary and the operation of the BP monitor. The instructions define key variables and illustrate how the cards should be marked for many common situations. Instructions are reviewed with the subject in the laboratory prior to the BP scan. The person fills out a diary record immediately following calibration of the BP recorder and completes at least one additional record before leaving the laboratory. Any errors are discussed and corrected.

Upon returning to the laboratory following a 24-h BP scan, the person rates the scan (five-point scale) for the quality of sleep, problems with the BP recorder, problems with the diary cards, the extent to which monitoring interfered with the individual's customary routine, the level of stress on the day of monitoring relative to the usual level of stress, and the level of physical activity (body movement) on the day of monitoring relative to the usual level of activity. This information is transferred to a 'header' card (not shown in Fig. 19.1), along with the subject's age, sex, height, and weight. The back of the header card has boxes for additional scores and codes for the patient. The header card is placed on top of the stack of diary cards, the cards are placed into the hopper of a card reader, and the information is downloaded into a personal computer for automatic scoring, data storage, and clinical report writing.

Derived categories

Any practically useful behavioral diary is powerfully constrained by the need for economy of space and economy of time in marking the diary. Consequently, items printed on the card were carefully selected for their fertility as 'root' categories from which ancillary behavioral information could be generated. In addition to the aforementioned information, each diary record is computer-scored for the following ancillary or 'derived' activities: transportation (usually driving, derived from the 'car' location item); household chores (scored when the 'home' and 'work' boxes are both marked); desk work (scored when 'sitting', 'work' location, and 'work' activity boxes are marked, and the 'people with' box is marked as zero, indicating the person is alone); attending a meeting (the same as for desk work, except that the 'people with' box is marked as 2 or 2+, indicating that the person is actively interacting with two or more people); relaxing (scored when the 'recline' box is marked, the 'work' activity box is not marked, the 'tense' mood box is marked zero or 1, and the 'people with' box is marked zero); and sleeping (scored when during a period of at least 90 min there is a string of at least three BP readings for which there are no diary entries).

The following composite variables are also computed:

stress = angry + tense + rushed scores
frustration = (angry −1) × (tense + rushed −2) × (5 − accomplishing things)
efficiency = accomplishing things + (5 − tense)

The CAD computer program

The user options available in the CAD computer program are (1) read cards, (2) prepared BP report, (3) print BP report supplement, (4) check card reader, and (5) exit. The primary functional units of the computer software are subroutines for (1) reading cards, (2) checking data quality (diary card information is checked for accuracy and consistency, any errors discovered are flagged for operator inspection and correction, (3) scoring diary records (each diary record for a single BP reading is scored for 36 variables – four locations, three body positions, 17 activities, nine moods, one social behavior, one behavioral efficiency estimate, and one comments score), (4) matching diary records to BP readings (employing several rules and checks, the CAD program assigns each diary record to the BP reading which best matches it in time, making allowances for the possibility that the subject may have forgotten to record diary information for a particular BP reading or may have mistakenly recorded information for a faulty reading), and (5) creating a data file (blood pressures, heart rates, diary scores, and header card information are written to a data file, ready for statistical analysis and BP report generation).

The CAD system interfaces with manufacturer-supplied computer software for the Spacelabs ICR BP monitors. When the Spacelabs BP report program is executed CAD automatically inserts activity and mood labels into the report, obviating the need to enter them manually from the keyboard. CAD also creates a supplementary BP report, which can be printed at the end of Spacelabs' standard report. The supplementary report includes (1) a table containing the average systolic BP, diastolic BP, and heart rate for each of ten activities and five moods, (2) a table listing the five highest systolic pressures and five highest diastolic pressures during the BP scan, and (3) a summary description of the behavioral conditions under which the patient's blood pressure was monitored.

The results of an application of the CAD system will be presented to illustrate the system. The purpose of this study was to examine the subject's acceptance of the system and to determine the relationship of activities and moods (monitored by means of CAD) to blood pressure changes during the course of a routine day.

Procedures

Subjects

Thirty-two healthy, normotensive Michigan State University employees, 16 males and 16 females, were monitored on a workday. The employees were primarily administrators, program managers, laboratory technicians, and secretaries.

Methods

Twenty-four-hour BP readings were obtained with the Spacelabs Model 5600 portable noninvasive monitor. The monitor was programmed to read blood pressure every 15 min from 6 a.m. to 12 p.m. and every 30 min from 12 p.m. to 6 a.m.

Subjects reported to the laboratory on the day of monitoring at 8 a.m. The monitor was applied and checked for accuracy. The hose of the cuff was attached to a mercury manometer through a Y connector. The subject's brachial pulse on the non-preferred arm was located. The microphone was taped directly over the pulse and the cuff was attached to the arm. Three calibration readings were manually triggered a couple of minutes apart. The operator read the blood pressure (diastolic pressure read as the fifth phase) with a stethoscope microphone placed under the cuff near the recorder microphone by checking sounds against the falling mercury column. The simultaneous recorder and operator readings had to agree within 5 mm Hg for both systolic and diastolic pressures for three consecutive readings in order for the recorder readings to be considered acceptable.

Subjects entered the time and their activity and mood state on a CAD diary card following calibration of the recorder. Instructions for marking the diary card were reviewed, and the subject filled out at least one additional diary record. Subjects were instructed to keep their cuff arm motionless during a BP reading and to mark the diary card immediately following each waking reading. Subjects were encouraged to follow their normal daily routine when they left the laboratory.

Statistical analysis

Because multiple readings were made on each employee the BP readings may be sequentially dependent. Sequential dependency complicates data analysis by reducing the effective degrees of freedom associated with statistical tests and introduces uncertainty into the confidence statements about the test results. The potential seriousness of the problem was examined by computing the first-order autocorrelation and Durbin-Watson D statistic (Draper & Smith, 1981) for the residuals of statistical models tested.

Before examining the effects of activities and moods on blood pressure the influence of differences between individuals in mean waking blood pressures was removed from the waking blood pressures by means of covariance adjustments. Failure to make this adjustment could give misleading results. Suppose that blood pressure during cigarette smoking was greater than blood pressure during watching television. Two interpretations would be equally plausible: (1) the momentary act of smoking a cigarette caused a greater increase in blood pressure than watching television caused, or (2) cigarette smokers as a group had higher overall waking blood pressures than did non-smokers; since only smokers smoked cigarettes, but both smokers and non-smokers watched television, cigarette smoking was associated with higher blood pressure than watching television merely because of overall group differences in blood pressure which were unrelated to the transient acts of smoking and watching television. We were interested in the acute effect of momentary waking states rather than in stable intersubject differences in blood pressure, and therefore partialed out intersubject variability in mean blood pressure before examining waking states.

Subjects rated their moods by marking one of five boxes for each mood scale on the diary card. The middle, or '3', box was a neutral category. A mark in the middle box indicated that the individual felt neither happy nor unhappy, neither tense nor relaxed, and so on. Discrete mood states were derived from the quantitative mood scales by scoring the person as either 'happy' or 'unhappy', either 'tense' or 'relaxed', etc., whenever he had marked a box above or below the middle box denoting 'affective neutrality'. If a single BP reading was associated with two or more mood states, e.g., the person reported feeling both tense and rushed when the reading was taken, the 'tie' between moods was broken by a computer program which randomly assigned the BP reading to one of the two mood states. Ties between activities were broken in the same way.

Results

The mean rating of severity of problems experienced in using the diary, which was made on a five-point scale (1 = no problem, 5 = very serious problem), was 1.06. The result indicates that subjects experienced few problems marking the diary cards.

Problems in using the diary were also studied by examining errors detected by the CAD computer program. Errors occurred on 9% of the 1,639 diary records for the 1,639 waking BP readings taken on the 32 subjects. A diary record usually required marking 14 boxes. Therefore, on the average, subjects made errors on only 0.6% (9%/14) of the boxes marked. The error rate per opportunity for error was very small. Most of the errors involved marking a card for a failed reading, failing to mark at least one activity box, or marking the time incorrectly, and were typically corrected easily by the technician who was informed by CAD about the location and nature of the error.

Subjects wrote comments on the 'Comments' line of the diary card on 24% of the diary records. The written comments provided specific qualitative 'coloring' to the coded quantitative information obtained from the boxes marked.

Blood pressures and activities which were excerpted from a sample BP report are presented in Table 19.1.

The report is for a man who weighed 270 lb and was marginally normotensive (BP slightly below 140/90 mm Hg) the day he was screened but was hypertensive the day he was monitored. The BP report was created by the Spacelabs computer program. The activity and mood labels in the 'Diary Activity' column were introduced by the CAD computer program. The activity and mood information indicate what the person was doing and how he reported feeling at the time each blood pressure was read. For example, information inserted by CAD indicates that when the person's systolic pressure peaked at 206 mm Hg at 4:59 p.m. he was driving home from work and feeling rushed. When his diastolic pressure reached 97 mm Hg at 1:29 p.m. he was at his desk at work and feeling angry.

The CAD computer program created the summary information appearing in Table 19.2.

The Table relates blood pressure and heart rate to major categories of activity and mood for the person cited above. It gives a synoptic view of the relationship between behavior and blood pressure for the particular person. It becomes clear, for example, that the person's blood pressure was higher at work than at home in the evening. Systolic pressure dropped slightly during sleep but was still unusually elevated (134 mm Hg). Systolic and diastolic pressures were noticeably higher when the man was angry, tense, or rushed compared to feeling happy or relaxed.

Using header card information, the CAD program constructed and printed the following summary of information about the conditions under which the man's blood pressure was monitored: 'On the day of the blood pressure scan the patient's stress level was slightly above average and activity level was average. The patient experienced mild problems with the blood pressure

Table 19.1. *Sample of patient's blood pressures and activities*

Time	Systolic	Diastolic	Mean	Heart rate	Diary activity
13:14	137	82	105	77	On phone, angry
13:29	162	97	108	78	Desk work, angry
13:45	142	78	116	72	On phone, tense
13:59	140	80	110	63	On phone
14:14	145	87	117	68	Desk work, rushed
14:29	155	91	106	80	Desk work, rushed
14:44	160	95	102	67	Rushed
14:59	150	83	110	74	Talking
15:14	160	83	106	80	Desk work
15:32	155	76	113	77	On phone, tense
15:44	166	92	115	73	On phone
15:59	176	88	118	77	Walking, tense
16:15	161	96	111	69	Desk work, rushed
16:29	161	100	107	94	Rushed, tense
16:44	122	81	85	81	Leave work, driving
16:59	206	92	111	80	Driving, rushed
17:14	145	76	98	73	At home, TV, talking
17:29	140	76	102	65	TV
17:44	130	83	98	68	TV
18:00	142	86	101	71	Eating, tense
18:14	152	90	108	75	Eating, TV
18:29	142	72	95	77	TV

monitor and no problems with the diary. The patient's normal routine was slightly disrupted by wearing the monitor and the patient slept poorly.'

The average 24-h blood pressure and heart rate for the 16 female employees were 114/73 mm Hg and 77 beats per min. The averages for the 16 males were 125/74 and 72. The values are similar to those reported by others (Wallace et al., 1984) for normotensive adults in the 20–50 years age range.

The average systolic blood pressures associated with the 16 activities coded by the CAD system are illustrated in Fig. 19.2.

The blood pressures are 'adjusted' blood pressures, i.e., the waking blood pressure measurements corrected for the individual differences in mean blood pressure by means of the covariance adjustment described above. The bar graph is based on all (1,639 waking, 310 sleep) BP readings of all employees. The number of times each activity was reported, and the number of subjects who reported it, are shown in the Figure.

The activities associated with the highest average systolic blood pressure

Table 19.2. *Average blood pressure during activities and moods*

	Systolic	Diastolic	Heart rate	Readings
Activity				
At work	151	86	76	32
At home	144	78	69	24
Sleeping	134	70	57	13
Walking	162	94	78	4
Talking	150	84	74	21
Driving	164	86	80	2
On telephone	147	82	73	6
Watching TV	144	76	68	19
Desk work	150	85	76	19
Meeting	NA	NA	NA	0
Mood				
Happy	142	74	66	13
Angry	149	89	77	2
Tense	152	86	79	16
Rushed	151	86	76	27
Relaxed	139	69	62	7

NA = Not available; blood pressure not read during activity or mood.

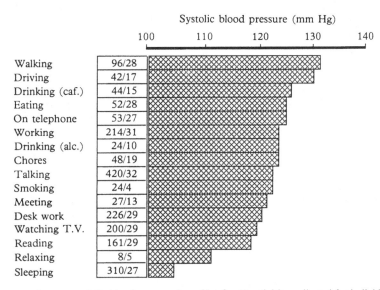

Fig. 19.2. Average systolic blood pressure (mm Hg) for 16 activities, adjusted for individual difference in mean blood pressure. The numbers inset in each bar indicate the number of times the activity was reported and the number of subjects who reported it.

were walking (131 mm Hg) and driving an automobile (130 mm Hg), followed by drinking a caffeinated beverage (128 mm Hg). Relaxing at home in the evening (110 mm Hg) and sleep (105 mm Hg) were associated with the lowest pressures. The CAD program scores an activity as 'relaxing' when the individual is reclining at home, is not socially interacting with anyone, and reports being in a relaxed mood. The activity of 'relaxing' is different from a 'relaxed' mood, in that the person must be behaviorally, as well as emotionally, quiescent.

The analysis of variance indicated that the 16 activities were significantly different in the adjusted systolic blood pressure, F (15, 193) = 33.59, P <0.001. The multiple correlation for the relationship between systolic blood pressure and the 16 activities was 0.46. Approximately 21% of the variability in ambulatory systolic blood pressure can be explained by the activity the individual was performing at the time the blood pressure was read.

The Durbin-Watson statistic, D = 1.63, indicated that there was statistically significant autocorrelation in the set of 1,949 adjusted blood pressures. However, the degree of first-order autocorrelation present was weak (0.18). Less than 4% of the variability in blood pressure can be accounted for by sequential dependency in adjacent BP readings. The test results suggest that while the BP readings were not strictly independent, they were nearly so. Such slight sequential dependency as probably exists in the population is unlikely to alter significantly the confidence level (P <0.001) for the decision that the 16 activities differed in the level of systolic blood pressure. However, because of sequential dependency in the BP readings, the confidence level should be regarded as being approximate.

Blood pressure levels were related to mood states coded by CAD, as illustrated in Fig. 19.3.

Figure 19.3 is based on 1,260 BP readings. On 379 of the 1,639 waking readings subjects had marked the '3' box on all mood scales. By the definition of mood states described above, distinct mood states were not identifiable on those 379 BP readings, so they were omitted from the analysis.

Systolic pressure was highest when employees reported feeling rushed (129 mm Hg) or unhappy (128 mm Hg). Feeling unrushed and tired (120 mm Hg) were associated with the lowest pressures.

The analysis of variance indicated that the 10 mood states shown in Fig. 19.3 differed significantly in adjusted systolic blood pressure. F (9, 1250) = 2.64, P <0.006. The multiple correlation between mood stated and systolic blood pressure was 0.14. Approximately 2% of the variability in blood pressure can be explained by the individual's reported mood states at the times the readings were taken.

The Durbin-Watson statistic, D = 1.67, indicated the presence of statistically significant first-order autocorrelation in the set of 1,260 BP readings.

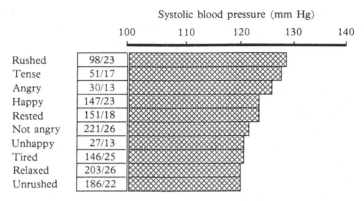

Fig. 19.3. Average systolic blood pressure (mm Hg) for 10 moods, adjusted for individual differences in mean blood pressure. The numbers inset in each bar indicate the number of times the mood was reported and the number of subjects who reported it.

However, once again, the degree of autocorrelation present was weak (0.17). Less than 3% of the variability in a BP reading can be explained by the reading immediately preceding it. This result indicates that the readings roughly approximated, but were not identical to, independent observations.

Discussion

The results indicate that the computer-assisted diary system met our most important performance criteria. Subjects made relatively few errors in marking diary cards. The low error rate (less than 1%) and frequent written comments suggest that subjects were willing and able to use the diary correctly.

The CAD system successfully (1) scored diary cards and stored the information in a computer file, which was immediately accessible for data analysis and for clinical reports, (2) automatically inserted activity and mood information into computer-generated clinical reports, (3) created useful summary tables, relating blood pressure to activities and moods, and (4) described conditions surrounding extreme BP readings and the BP scan as a whole. The system completely eliminated the need to manually enter diary scores, which numbered approximately 2,300 for each 24-h scan, into the computer, resulting in a substantial saving in technician time.

The observed relationship between systolic blood pressure and activities and moods confirms and extends findings of others (Pickering et al., 1982). The results demonstrate once again that moment-to-moment fluctuations in blood pressure are influenced by the pattern of daily life which is expressed externally in behavior and internally in mood states.

Existing diaries for ABPM lack adequate standardization (Chesney & Ironson, 1989). In the absence of standardization, making inferences about the effects of behavior on blood pressure will remain hazardous. Two people may differ in 24-h blood pressure because of a difference in behavioral activity or because blood pressure was maintained differently at comparable levels of activity. Currently, we cannot distinguish satisfactorily between these two important cases.

The use of computer-automated standardized activity diaries for ambulatory monitoring can potentially introduce the following benefits: first, better quantification of behavioral information; second, greater accessibility of this information for diagnostic and research purposes; third, greater comparability of data gathered at different centers; fourth, the possibility of developing activity-standardized blood pressure norms for use with patients; fifth, significant reductions in clinician and technician time. For these reasons, the use of a computerized activity diary for ambulatory blood pressure monitoring merits, as does ES research in general, further investigation and trial applications.

PART IV

Therapeutic applications of the Experience Sampling Method

20

The uses of the ESM in psychotherapy
MARTEN W. deVRIES

What clinician has not experienced with perplexity the chance meeting of a patient in a social or non-clinical setting when he or she appears remarkably different, more or less distressed or capable than the therapist expected from the previous clinical encounter? This experience may relieve or shock the therapist. We are likely to be philosophical about the encounter or muse over the problems of diagnosis and the perplexing nature of man. We may also mention it to the patient depending on our therapeutic proclivity, but more systematic inquiries into the questions raised by the discontinuity of clinical perception are generally not considered. This situation is an understandable outcome of the assessment methods that we employ in psychiatry. Most often we rely on the clinical interview or at best a few observations to provide us with data about patients' lives. These standard psychiatric diagnostic instruments, however, provide neither sufficient access to the subjective experience of the patient nor to the context of his or her life. Yet, we do err, often fooled by the intimacy of our interaction with patients that we have accumulated such knowledge and undisturbed tend to carry on with our psychosocial formulations about the dynamics of patients' lives.

Recent diagnostic advances such as the ICD-10 and DSM-III-R (or IV) have attempted with multiaxial strategies to describe the patient more fully. But as clinicians know, diagnosis sets the frame for professional communication, but is not adequate for treatment. Treatment may only be constructed through psychosocial formulations about individuals' lives. But what is sufficient psychosocial reasoning? This varies across schools of thought from behaviorism to psychoanalysis. The authors in these chapters examine whether an integration of existing approaches is facilitated by ESM data. Since ESM elucidates dynamic properties of psychological state, the actual mental set, setting and variability of daily human behavior, it becomes easier to go beyond static descriptions of diagnostic trait. Clinicians may then be encouraged to gather and include more information about the ongoing reactive style of patients in their evaluations and ongoing treatment. While this new information is meant for general therapeutic uses, it is particularly useful during acute and reconstitution phases of severe illnesses where environmental interactions with the often-vulnerable, rehabilitating individual may play a dominant role.

The ESM research presented by the authors in this volume has attempted to correct this shortcoming by carrying out research that places the person within the space and time of his daily existence. The quantitative time-sampling data of diverse disorders provided in previous sections gives ample testimony that this is a feasible and useful adjunct to current psychiatric evaluations ranging from drug abuse to schizophrenia. The ESM studies into mental disorders provide powerful descriptive tools for future taxonomic purposes. They further serve as background for clinical application in the day-to-day care of patients. ESM is here, I think, most dramatic. This power is derived primarily from ESM's capability of describing the individual in detail within specific contexts which have hitherto been hidden from the eyes of the therapist. Accommodating these new data clinically, requires careful thought and systematic study. In this Section a number of cases and theories are offered; they represent the beginnings of systematic work in this field. Data are promising that ESM is useful for guiding more realistic psychotherapeutic approaches and interventions as well as in evaluating their efficacy. This is clearly illustrated by articles where ESM was used to sample the subject repeatedly throughout the course of treatment and the various phases of therapy, recovery and rehabilitation.

Since, in the treatment of mental disorders, we wish to help suffering individuals achieve a way of functioning that is subjectively, interpersonally, and socially more satisfying, or at least more tolerable, the power of ESM in psychotherapy to help should be judged on its capacity to fulfil these goals.

What makes ESM relevant for mental health treatments and what ingredients are particularly active in influencing the treatment processes?

Clinically, however, we still need to concern ourselves with the value or power of basic ideas such as what makes interpersonal influencing processes like psychiatric treatment effective and what is actually meant by improvement or change. The papers in this Section highlight processes such as bringing extra-therapeutic life into dyadic therapy (Donner, this volume), increasing the opportunities for optimal experience (Massimini et al., this volume) and facilitating activities that achieve this (Delle Fave, this volume), evaluating responses to therapeutic interventions for use in rehabilitative, personalized case management (van de Poel & Delespaul, this volume) and examining the role of self-awareness in psychopathology and therapy (Figurski, this volume). These are but beginnings. They cover a range of activities from self-help to dyadic therapeutic approaches to case management strategies. All require a different level of intensity and involvement of both the individual and the therapist.

Certain common ingredients are involved in the use of ESM, regardless of the approach taken. The first aspect is the effect of actively carrying out the self-evaluations from hour to hour. Here, consciousness of behavior and experiences develops. In a motivated individual who is guided by a specific goal this potential increase in self-awareness can be a powerful stimulus to change. For such people, the ESM procedure alone functions as a learning experience from which they can draw the necessary conclusions to make changes in their lives.

The second ingredient is found in the process of giving feedback to the patient about his ESM data. Providing feedback involves an interpersonal process of constructing an integrated and shared view of a patient's life and mental state. ESM helps here with the detection of persistent and maladaptive behavior and the subsequent activation of various alternative mental states and settings. The activation of alternative modes of thought, behavior and feeling potentially promotes experiential learning which leads to psychological change and experienced wellbeing, as exemplified in the chapters by Donner and Delle Fave. Within the context of clinical care, the briefing and debriefing processes of ESM, and research alliance required becomes an integral part of the therapy. Since the goal is to obtain a complete set of reports about a person's mental state and context, considerable new previously undisclosed information becomes available to the therapeutic relationship. This is particularly true at the end of the week when the therapist can sit down with each subject and review the period, discuss how the sampling went, highlight problems, and focus on particularly relevant aspects of experience. In therapy, such disclosures may have great impact on therapist and client alike.

The third ingredient is the case-management approach. Here, the therapist takes a directive role in actively advocating alterations in life style, environment and social relationships, based on ESM data about the occurrence of symptoms or wellbeing. Simple advice may be given so that negative situations are minimized or avoided and positive situations, particularly those with which the person has had previous positive experience, are optimized (Delle Fave et al., this volume).

The therapeutic effect of ESM may be summarized at a number of levels:

(1) The effect on the person as he evaluates his own experience and activities in the walk of life. His own shift in consciousness and behavior.
(2) The effect of more or less interpretive feedback by the clinician based on the accumulated self-reports.
(3) The effect of ESM information on organizing the mental health worker's care planning, view of the patient, treatment approaches and specific interventions.
(4) The effect of suggesting direct changes in life style and activities of the patient: 'case management'.

(5) The effect that this information has on the therapeutic relationship between the mental health worker and the client, in terms of transference, feelings of being understood, consensus, etc.

In the process of therapy, information functions as a videotape of daily life that the therapist and patient project and view together. The increased information may break through the high level of dependency between client and therapist. Viewing the week together fosters mutual respect and partnership. The detailed dimensions of a person's experience, visualized from the plots and frequency counts, averaged data, situational correlations, time-budgets, variability, stability and patterns in their self-reports, provide the material for a script immediately available for clinical use.

Time and place in psychotherapy

In addition to the practical processes described above another useful frame of reference for understanding the integration of time and place in psychotherapy is the existential psychoanalytic approach. In general, this holds that the psychotherapeutic process should 'temporalize' and 'historize' the person. The view holds that individuals are often incapable of using time and abuse it. They project onto it the current concrete distillations of past fear, anxiety and dread. This non-temporalized condition is marked by a sense of urgency in which the world is viewed within a context of projected dread. The various forms of psychopathology in this model are seen as mechanisms for dealing with this projection in terms of over-planning, over-organizing, or ritualizing, or worse by invoking random activities and alternate cognitive modes in an inane attempt to obliterate anxiety. A temporalized individual, on the other hand, has the capacity to observe, to make plans, and most of all, to stop for a moment and seek a way out. It is this process of stopping, evaluating, observing and 'making time', that is achieved by building up the capacity of an 'observer' in therapy who can plan, learn, and experience himself as an adaptive element in the real world, a temporalized person. This model uses a vocabulary that today may seem anachronistic but suggests that time and the evaluation of its use with ESM provide a mechanism for psychodynamic, ego-integrating therapy.

In addition, ESM is useful in evaluating the effectiveness of psychotherapeutic interventions. The repeated sampling of experience as demonstrated in the chapters by van de Poel & Delespaul and Delle Fave and Massimini, can monitor the effect of clinical interventions on variables not typically considered targets of treatment. Here, activities, alone time, work, leisure, flexibility of emotional reactions, time-budget allocations, percentage of time spent in social interactions, as well as the range of mental state reactions to life situations, are both therapeutically and evaluatively useful. In ongoing therapy, ESM also provides concrete milestones or end points for therapy that can occur outside the relationship between therapist and client. Again this window on the real world of the patient provides the therapist with a better perspective than the evaluation of the relationship with the client from the office alone. ESM is useful in short-term psychotherapy where specific treatment targets may be selected and guide therapy. Whether and when these goals have been reached is a useful adjunct to short-term treatment which is increasingly important in our often overburdened community mental health centers. The door is here again open for creative applications.

The chapters in this Section demonstrate that therapy, rehabilitation and evaluation may be facilitated by fine-grained ESM analyses of psychopathological experience. ESM introduces, more concretely than is typically done, aspects of a person's life that are often hidden from the therapist. This is therapeutically beneficial and may be accommodated within a variety of theoretical frames of reference from the psychodynamic to behavioral approaches. The strength of this claim is evaluated in the chapters that follow.

21

Expanding the experiential parameters of cognitive therapy

ED DONNER[1]

While the specific reasons vary widely, people generally seek therapy to relieve emotional distress or to modify troublesome attitudes or behaviors. The means by which therapists contribute to the accomplishment of these ends are as varied as the presenting problems. Still, a dual process takes place where on the one hand the patient brings his or her extra-therapeutic life into the therapy session, and on the other hand the therapist facilitates the exportation of therapeutic gains into the everyday extra-therapeutic life of the patient. The present chapter will explore the possible contributions of the ESM to this dual process of importing extra-therapeutic life into therapy sessions, and of generalizing therapeutic accomplishments to everyday life. While ESM may be useful within many different therapeutic programs, the therapeutic utility of ESM will be illustrated in the cognitive treatment of depression.

The cognitive treatment of depression assumes that clinical depression is the result of negative cognitive distortions (Beck, 1979; Diekstra, Engels & Methorst, 1988; Wright & Beck, 1983). In light of the presumed etiological role of negative cognitions in clinical depression, it is not surprising that the modus operandi of most cognitive interventions revolves around identifying and decreasing negative thoughts (e.g., Beck et al., 1979; Stravynski & Greenberg, 1987; Teasdale & Fennel, 1988; Teasdale, Fennel, Hibbert & Amies, 1984). Cognitive therapists may differ in the specific techniques they employ, but invariably they attempt to (1) identify the occurrence of negative thoughts in the everyday life of the patient, and (2) educate or train the patient in strategies which will undermine the incidence or power of these negative thoughts in their day-to-day life.

While the identification of negative cognitive bias takes various forms, generally the therapist guides patients in retrospectively examining their experiences when they were with particular social partners or in key targeted situations. The therapist and patient explore specific maladaptive thoughts and

[1] The author wishes to acknowledge the support provided by the National Institute of Mental Health, grant #PHS5T32MH17053-08, 'Research on the Delivery of Mental Health Services' during the preparation of this manuscript.

underlying cognitive assumptions and evaluate their impact on the patients' emotional experience and behavior (e.g., Beck, 1979; Marshall & Mazie, 1987). Cognitive approaches rely heavily on patients' reconstructions of past experiences but cognitive therapists view such exercises as the stuff of therapy. Any embellishments that might occur during the recall process are important intervening processes that merit therapeutic processing.

Once the patient and the therapist have identified maladaptive thought processes, effort is directed to 'correcting' these judgement errors. The therapist may offer specific alternative constructions, provide feedback to alternatives generated by the patient, redirect patients' attention away from their negative affect (Schmitt, 1983), actively criticize patients' negative approach (Beck, 1979; Gauthier, Pellerin & Renaud, 1983), or present more adaptive cognitive constructions (Beck, 1979; Ellis, 1962). Collectively, these cognitive interventions have been termed 'cognitive restructuring' (Gauthier, Pellerin & Renaud, 1983; Zettle & Hayes, 1987).

The appellation of 'cognitive restructuring' suggests the means by which intra-therapy experience is thought to generalize to extra-therapeutic situations. Maladaptive thought processes are considered to reflect relatively enduring constructs (Kelly, 1955) which can be reorganized into more-adaptive forms. The education that takes place within therapy transforms cognitive structures into new, enduring forms which presumably generalize to experience outside therapy. Some therapists may facilitate generalization to everyday life through cognitive or behavioral rehearsal within the therapeutic session (Gauthier, Pellerin & Renaud, 1983; Weiner, 1983). Others will encourage generalization by assigning homework tasks in which patients apply new cognitive interpretations (and the concomitant behavioral strategy) to specific distressful situations outside therapy (see Parsons, Burns & Perloff, 1988; Zettle & Hayes, 1987). Failures in application of the adaptive constructs, if they are important, will presumably be remembered and become the focus of further therapy.

Expanding the experiential parameters

While cognitive therapy has been found to be effective in the treatment of depression (e.g., Jarret & Nelson, 1987; Wright & Beck, 1983), over-reliance on patients' recollections and over-confidence in the generalizability of therapeutic experience may limit its effectiveness. Several authors have noted that patients displaying greater pathology are less responsive to cognitive therapy than are their more healthy counterparts (Fennel, Teasdale, Jones & Damle, 1987; Keller, 1983). The limitations of cognitive interventions with the depressed, and especially the severely depressed, are in large part a product of the very cognitive tendencies which are the focus of the treatment. Severely depressed patient's cognitive distortions limit the effectiveness of cognitive interventions, and necessitate the utilization of additional procedures. Experience sampling can be a useful adjunct in such cases.

Patients' reconstruction of past events may yield insights on the nature of their cognitive distortions, but their reconstructions may not, and in fact probably do not, accurately reflect the true nature of their moment-to-moment experience. Inaccurate recollection of past experience is not a phenomenon peculiar to clinical patients. Rather, it seems that recollections of experience tell as much about a person's self-concept as they do about the experience itself. For example, in the process of debriefing normal, non-clinical subjects who participated in ESM research on stress, inaccuracies in self-perceptions were quite common (Donner, 1989). During the debriefing, subjects' ESM response sheets were used to identify times that they felt at least a little tense. It was quite common for the subjects, all of whom were high level executives, to be quite surprised at how often they were tense. Once confronted with the 'evidence', they were able to incorporate the additional information into their self-perceptions.

People are often unaware of their experience at any particular time because attention is generally focused on other matters. People spend more time thinking about their activities than their *reactions* to the activity. Research on a wide variety of samples ranging from normal high school students (Csikszentmihalyi & Larson, 1984), talented high school students (Donner, Csikszentmihalyi & Schneider, 1987), young adults (Donner, Nash, Csikszentmihalyi & Chalip, 1983), middle-aged factory workers (Csikszentmihalyi & LeFevre, 1987), and executives (Donner, 1989) indicate that a person's attention is focused on the particular activity he or she is doing 50–60% of the time. Additionally, a significant portion of conscious thoughts is directed to matters which are outside the here-and-now domain. Thus, when they are not thinking about what they are doing, people have daydreams and fantasies which channel attention beyond the current situation.

The proportion of reported thoughts which are directed toward the self and the self's reactions is, on average, quite low. For example, in a sample of 49 executives, thoughts about the self and the self's emotions were reported only 1.3% of the time. A sample of 200 high school students did have a higher proportion of self-referential thoughts. Still, less than 9% of all reported thoughts were directed to the self. Of course, some proportion of these self-directed thoughts were in reference to situations that had already occurred or were expected to occur. Consequently, the amount of attention directed to examination of the self's response to the current situation is relatively small. The person who is at school listening, at work writing, at a store shopping, or at home watching television, will tend to be directing attention to things besides his or her reactions to that activity.

Thus, it seems that people tend to be rather unselfconscious while they go about their daily activities. They go from one situation to the next without giving much thought to how they feel at any given time. One ESM research subject exemplifies the lack of self-awareness which typifies most people. During a study debriefing, the researcher pointed out that most people tend to have a positive relationship between their mood and their motivation. That is, when people feel good, they tend to want to be doing the activity. When people are sad or unhappy, they will tend to want to be doing something else. Interestingly, this relationship did not hold true for this subject. The correlation between mood and motivation was around zero. Apparently, there were times when this person felt poorly, but he wanted to be doing what he was doing. Careful examination of those instances when mood was low but motivation was high revealed one consistent factor: the man was with his girl-friend. The subject confessed that the relationship was troubled. Although he knew the relationship was a source of distress, he was sincerely surprised to see how greatly and consistently his girl-friend affected his experience. He had thought that, although the relationship was a source of frustration, it generally made him feel good. His view of the relationship underwent a dramatic change when he was faced with the 'evidence' of his own experience. In a later follow-up, the man offered that after seeing the effect the relationship had on him, he let go of the seemingly hopeless relationship after having pursued it for over a year. Although he was grieving the loss, he had become receptive to other, hopefully more-rewarding relationships.

The above examples illustrate several important points for the present discussion. First, there are significant discrepancies between persons' immediate experience and their later reflections about that experience. Even when there is some general concept of how a particular situation is experienced, the precise nature of that experience is not easily reconstructed after the passage of time. Second, several factors contribute to the inaccurate recollection of past experience. Inaccuracies are due partly to the general tendency for attention to be directed to matters other than one's own responses. Notably, inaccuracies also result from limitations in individuals' interpretation and categorization of their experience. Finally, although the effect was inadvertent, the use of structured items on the ESM protocols provided a mechanism for the restructuring and refining of subjects' self-representation.

Aaron Beck (1979) has suggested that cognitive therapists 'take patients at their word'. To the degree that cognitive therapists accept patients' recollected representation of their experience in particular contexts, they are vulnerable to several errors. First, patients may consider particular situations to be the primary source of their distress, when in fact other situations are just as important. The executives described above who were unaware of the tension they experienced in their work-place could hardly be expected effectively to develop strategies to reduce their tension. Likewise, the depressed patient who attributes his angst to a particular source may overlook other important people or situations that would appropriately be dealt with in therapy.

Secondly, the therapist may lose access to potentially counter-balancing positive experiences. The negative cognitive distortion evinced by the depressed person will make it difficult for him to remember positive experiences. Further, the depressed patient may have some difficulty arriving at alternative views of situations when working with non-directive therapists. To the extent that a more positive reconceptualization requires the patient to draw on his own phenomenological world, he will be hampered by his negative cognitive distortions. Even if the patient is working with a more directive therapist who offers more positive reconstructions of experience, the patient is likely to be resistant. This is not necessarily because of transference issues, but because of the resiliency of his negative beliefs about the world and himself. Positive reframes will not resonate with the patient's views because they will not be grounded in his conscious phenomenological reality. The severely depressed patient will tend to view himself as a person who *is sad*, *has been sad*, and *will continue* to be sad. The hopelessness that characterizes his view of the future is rooted in his observations of his past and present experiences. These self-observations, of course, are biased by the negative distortions of the patient. Often, the depressed individual is unable to recognize his or her past positive experiences, even when others point them out. They might say their past observable positive affective state was an act in order to please others . . . They were not *really* happy . . . They were *acting* happy. Or they may undermine the validity of such positive experience and view it as a momentary lapse from their true normal state of depression. The depressed person who does recognize positive experiences may learn eventually to disregard them because the sadness inevitably returns. The return to sadness comes to signal the return to 'normal', and the fleeting excursion into wellbeing comes to be viewed as 'abnormal'.

Depressed persons' consistently negative view of their experience does not jibe with the results of research. Other research described in this volume suggests that even those who are severely depressed have some variability in their experience (Kraan et al., this volume; Merrick, this volume). Hospitalized depressed adolescents and depressed outpatients regularly reported occasions when they felt good. In short, the exclusion of these positive experiences from the person's self-concept helps perpetuate the depression and undermines the therapist's efforts to alter the patient's views of himself and his future.

The role of ESM in therapy

Experience sampling is effective in expanding patients' self-conceptualizations because it is derived from their own experience. The depressed patient increases his self-perception as someone capable of happiness with help from the therapist and the ESM sheets. He can see that at such and such a time, when he was with a particular person or doing a particular thing, he did indeed feel happy. Faced with his own report of feeling O.K., the patient can more readily believe that the possibility of feeling something besides sadness is more than the articulation of an insistent outsider. His feeling good is an empirical fact. The therapist can also legitimize the positive experiences as part of the patient's true self. The aim for the therapist is to help the patient obtain a more realistic view of himself, a view which includes the full range of felt experiences. As patients recognize that both positive and negative experiences are 'temporary', each passing into the other, they can tolerate the low periods more effectively.

Another strength of ESM in therapy is that the patient and the therapist can work together to identify empirically those activities and social contexts which are associated with more positive affect. Thus, the patient not only obtains a more realistic view of himself that includes both positive and negative experiences, but also becomes more aware of those conditions which enhance the quality of experience. The therapist can then encourage the patient to engage in those activities or contexts which bring about elevations in mood. The stated rationale for pursuing these actions is not because the patient may feel better if he indulges the therapist and tries the activity, but rather because when he is involved in activities like this he *does* tend to feel better. Inquiry into the specific aspects of the situation that elicited the patient's positive affect can thus provide empirically grounded leads for future action. The patient may then become more effective at identifying positive experiences and pursue the behavior that elicits them. A greater sense of control over his emotional life is thus possible. ESM within a cognitive therapy orientation appears to operate by introducing evidence which contradicts patients' negatively biased self-perceptions, and by facilitating efforts to have patients carry out mood-elevating behaviors.

ESM can also aid in the exportation of therapeutic strategies into daily life. Since people respond to the signal by filling out a short questionnaire, the signal can serve as a focus for intervention or a reminder to alter thoughts and behavior. For example, the therapist can encourage the patient to respond to the signal by screening his thoughts. Negative automatic thoughts can be targeted for specific interventions. For example, some patients contribute to the downward spiraling of their mood by repeatedly imagining upsetting scenarios. Such patients can be instructed to interrupt these self-defeating thoughts whenever the signal catches them. Similarly, the signal can prompt patients to reframe their circumstances in a more positive manner, or to take actions which generally elicit more positive affects from them. The ESM signal then may work primarily to help the patient's monitoring of self-destructive or inhibitive automatic thoughts, and to remind him to implement an intervention.

Conversely, patients can be instructed to attend specifically to their positive experiences when the beep goes off. Patients can take note of the circumstances surrounding their more positive experiences in an effort to identify why specifically they feel better at those times. Their attributions for the cause of their positive affect may be less important than the fact that they are directing attention toward their positive affect, and modifying their self-perceptions. On the other hand, insights may be gained as to what activities, contexts or aspects of situations contribute toward the patient's wellbeing.

A case study: Experience Sampling in cognitive therapy

Robert, a white, working class husband and father of two, presented with symptoms of major depression including early morning awakening, insomnia, anhedonia, feelings of worthlessness and hopelessness, guilt, psychomotor agitation and suicidal ideation. Although the onset of the depression could be traced back at least two years he had decided to enter therapy only recently because of his impending divorce. Married for 14 years, Robert had over a period of several years become socially withdrawn. He avoided interactions with his wife and children, had no active friendships and had only occasional contact with his family of origin.

After having made strong initial progress, by the third month Robert's therapy had stalled. His improvement in mood had leveled off. He saw himself as perpetually depressed, and his life as void of enjoyment. Robert's early efforts to reach out to social supports and to take an active approach to his problems had peaked. He became more withdrawn. His relationship with his children was, in his mind, very unsatisfying and associated with guilt and pain because he had 'failed' them by ruining his marriage. Attempts to identify activities which could distract him from his ruminations and which could provide some satisfaction, seemed fruitless. Robert was convinced that there were no activities he could ever enjoy.

It was at this point that the therapist discussed with Robert the use of ES as part of his therapy. Robert welcomed the opportunity. He carried the pager for three periods across a period of 10 weeks and responded to signals for a total of 54 days. He completed 141 ESM forms during this time.

Robert's experience sampling can be divided into three periods according to the central therapeutic issues he faced at that time. During the first three weeks of Robert's ES, the emphasis was on realigning his consciousness so that he could become more aware of his positive states and the circumstances associated with these positive emotions. This was accomplished through examination of his ESM protocols during therapy sessions. He learned that his best moods occurred when he was in the presence of and interacting with another person, particularly his children, his brother, and coworkers. He also learned that some of his more positive moods occurred while he was preoccupied with the demands of his job. Seeing that participation in activities and engagement with people elevated his mood, Robert finally responded to the therapist's urgings to engage in some leisure and social activities. As Robert started to acknowledge the positive pole of his experiences, he also started to evince a more realistic view of his present and past relationship with his ex-wife. He no longer shouldered all the blame for the problems in their relationship, and for the first time, he started to feel some anger toward his ex-spouse. Also, for the first time, he consciously admitted that perhaps there would be no reconciliation. The renewal of his hope for attaining some degree of happiness appeared to provide the strength he needed to acknowledge the reality of his marital situation.

During the second period of ESM it became evident that these gains had a price. Now that he was no longer denying the loss of the marriage and was acknowledging his ex-wife's role in their difficulties, both anger and grief set in with a vengeance. Robert reported fewer occasions of positive moods. His thoughts about his situation became far more obsessive. For example, he reported thoughts about his ex-spouse on 61% of his ESM protocols during this second period as compared to 45% during the first three weeks of ESM.

A dramatic effort was needed to interrupt Robert's depressive thoughts. While he could intellectually acknowledge that the therapist had predicted his current condition, he felt overwhelmed by the flood of emotions which had for so long lain dormant. The therapist worked with Robert to establish several replacement thoughts, including a reframe of his anger and sadness. Robert was instructed to think of these powerful feelings as predicted signs of progress that would indeed eventually wane. The validity of this reframe was established in Robert's eyes through a psycho-educational discussion of his ESM. Having seen his moods rise and then fall, only to rise again, Robert could believe the therapist's prediction that his mood would become better in the future. A second replacement thought was also established. Discussions of his ES revealed to Robert that he felt better when he was actively engaged in endeavors which could distract him from his preoccupations. Robert was instructed to interrupt and then replace his negative thoughts about his divorce or his ex-wife with thoughts about activities he could do that made him feel better.

Notably, the thought interruption and replacement required several weeks, with many repetitive reminders before it had any observable effect in Robert's daily life. These interventions were first initiated around the fifth week of experience sampling, but their effects were not observable until the third period of his ESM sometime around the seventh week. During this third period of Robert's ESM, he had more occurrences of positive moods, his negative moods were not as consistently extreme and he became less preoccupied. Robert's incipient belief that activity could serve to enhance his mood was reaffirmed during this third period. He began to pursue in earnest activities which had earlier been shown to be related to better moods. Review of the protocols confirmed for Robert that he was indeed having positive emotional responses to his activities. Having seen himself move beyond the angst of the middle period, Robert reaffirmed his belief in the cyclicity of his moods, and in the possibility of having positive experiences despite the recurrent presence of his depression. Continued thought interruption and replacement, and emphasis on the proactive attempts to improve his mood through action empowered Robert.

While the ESM stopped after the tenth week, therapy continued to focus on many of the issues which had been established during the ESM. The cyclicity of his moods, the power of action, the importance of social contacts, and the need to manage negative thoughts continued as therapeutic issues in the months that followed. Although he no longer carried the pager, the insights Robert gained during his ESM served as a catalyst to his continued improvement.

Discussion

Several factors contribute to the power of ESM as a therapeutic tool. The introduction of a relatively sophisticated technology into therapy creates a positive transference with a scientific mystique that secures patients' respect. From the perspective of the patient, the technology legitimizes the therapist's interpretations of the patient's experience. More importantly, interpretations are viewed as credible because the data are based on patients' own self-reports during their everyday life. Unlike observation-based interpretations, or interpretations which are derived from more standard psychological assessment tools, interpretations based on ESM are likely to resonate with a patient's everyday experience because it is based on that experience. Finally, despite the fact that the data are not generally a part of patients' consciousness, they are readily accessible even to those who are not psychologically minded or introspective. The therapist who comments on a patient's self-reports of daily experience is not perceived as a magician who offers mysterious incantations derived from ink blots or pictures. Rather, the therapist who employs ESM works as a consultant who helps refine patients' self-understanding by reflecting, clarifying and exploring the implications of patients' self-reported experiences.

From the perspective of the therapist, the technology of ESM can be a nuisance. The research procedures for ESM can be labor-intensive or costly. Therapeutically, shortcuts may be useful, since the aim of ESM in therapy is to obtain reports which are not self-selected. Any device which can generate signals randomly can be used to remind the patient to complete a questionnaire or to carry out a therapeutic intervention.

The use of ESM also presents some potential problems for the patient. Some effort must be taken to limit the intrusiveness of the ESM for the patient, including limiting the number of signals each day and the number of consecutive days the pagers are carried. The three periods described in Robert's ESM exemplify the periods during which some limited sampling of experience may be fruitful. In the first period, ESM was used to expand Robert's negatively biased self-concept to include his positive experiences. This first period also provided insights as to what kinds of thoughts, contexts and activities were associated with both positive and negative experiences. The next period affirmed Robert's incipient belief that even in the worst times, he was capable of having some positive feelings. It was during this second period, too, that the pager signal served as a reminder to implement therapeutic strategies, specifically thought interruption and replacement. The third period solidified the gains of the first two periods. Robert continued to interrupt his thoughts, and he was able to see the improvement in his mood and thoughts after having regressed. The catastrophic expectations associated with such regressions were effectively countered. These three purposes could have been served through a careful selection of three separate sampling periods.

The present emphasis has been on the use of ESM in bringing extra-therapeutic life into cognitive therapy, and on exporting cognitive therapeutic strategies into daily life. However, there is no reason why ESM should be restricted to cognitive therapy. Indeed the uses of ESM as a therapeutic tool are limited only by the imagination of therapists.

22

The monitoring of optimal experience: a tool for psychiatric rehabilitation[1]

FAUSTO MASSIMINI, MIHALY CSIKSZENTMIHALYI and MASSIMO CARLI

Unlike somatic medicine, psychology has failed to develop an adequate model of the healthy individual and particularly of the range of variations of normal experience in daily life. Consequently, psychiatry lacks what physiology contributes to pathology in medical sciences. The task of studying normal consciousness should be the concern of psychology, so that a theoretical discipline could become available to psychiatry in the same fashion that physiology is available to pathology. However, psychology has not sufficiently developed either the study of normal states of consciousness in everyday life or the knowledge of fluctuations over time between states of optimal and aversive experience.

The study of the daily experience of normal subjects became possible with the use of the Experience Sampling Method (ESM) (Csikszentmihalyi et al., 1977; Csikszentmihalyi & Larson, 1984, 1987; deVries, 1987; Hormuth, 1986). This method allows repeated assessment of the experience of subjects in their natural environment. At the University of Chicago it has been used to describe the phenomenon of peak experiences, also called 'flow', and as a measurement of current subjective wellbeing (Csikszentmihalyi, 1975, 1982). Through this line of research it became clear that when one's perceived challenges, that is, the intrinsic demands experienced when engaged in an activity, are greater than one's perceived skills, that is, the individual's perception of capacity to meet the demands of the activity, the person experiences worry or anxiety. In the reverse situation (skills greater than challenges), boredom and apathy are experienced (Csikszentmihalyi, 1975). Recent work at the University of Milan suggests that the ratio of challenges to skills experienced at any one time is predictive of an even wider range of human emotions (Massimini & Inghilleri, 1986).

We will examine whether varying ratios of challenge to skill can explain the

[1] Appeared in *Journal of Nervous and Mental Disease*, 1987, **175**, 9, 545–50. © Williams & Wilkins.

range of negative to positive variations in daily experience. We will also describe the activities typically associated with the different ratios of challenge to skill. Finally, we will discuss the dynamics of optimal experience in healthy adolescents and present an illustrative model to demonstrate how these insights can be applied practically in the development of personalized psychiatric rehabilitation approaches.

Methods

Subjects

Data were gathered on 47 Milanese students attending the last two years of a classic lyceum (pre-university level). Fourteen boys and 33 girls, aged 16 to 18, were included in this study.

Experience Sampling Method

The ESM was used to assess the experiences of our subjects. They were signaled repeatedly, 60 times in one week, five to eight times each day (from 8 a.m. to 10 p.m. for weekdays and between 9 a.m. and 11 p.m. during the weekend), to fill out a self-assessment form. Each of these forms contained 44 questions of the following two types:

(1) Open-ended questions about thought content, actual and preferred activities, places frequented, and companions (all coded by the researchers). Questions about the time of day at which the self-reports were filled out were also included.

(2) Seven- or 10-point scales assessed different aspects of experience and the perceived skills and challenges associated with the activity being performed. The responses to items assessing different aspects of experience were combined in four clusters of items (see Csikszentmihalyi & Larson, 1984): (a) affect: happy, cheerful, sociable, and friendly; (b) activation: alert, active, strong, and excited; (c) cognitive efficiency: concentration, ease of concentration, unselfconsciousness, and clear; (d) motivation: wish to be doing this activity, control of actions, free, and involved. On average we collected a sequence of 36 reports for each subject.

Method of analysis

The data were normalized, providing z-scores for each subject and by each item or item cluster, so that a number above zero registers experiences rated better than the subject's average for that week. Negative scores indicate experiences below the average. As a consequence of this normalization, the mean z-score for all signals, as well as any randomly selected subsets of signals, all lead to zero mean z-scores. The mean z-scores of signal subsets selected using a rule based on a discriminating variable will thus be significantly different from

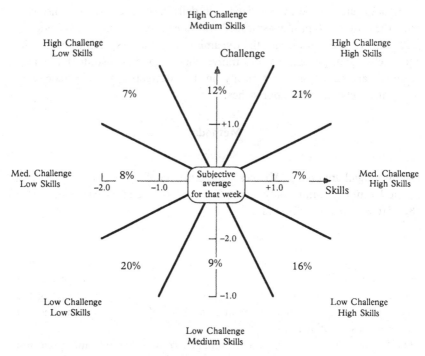

Fig. 22.1. Visual representation of the eight states of the challenge/skill ratio. Reports gathered in the different ratio states are shown as percentages ($N = 1682$).

zero. For instance, if the factor being alone captures differences in experience, the mean z-scores of the signals in that situation have to be significantly different from zero.

The discriminating variable (the ratio of experienced challenge to skill) is complex. This condition was operationalized arbitrarily as having eight different states of dimensions based on the relative z-score ratio of the challenge and skill variables (Fig. 22.1).

Results

Challenges, skills, and global experience

The percentage of observations that fell into each of the eight states, as defined by computed challenge/skill ratios, ranged from 21% (high challenge/high skill condition) to 7% (high challenge/low skill and medium challenge/high skill; see Fig. 22.1). Table 22.1 presents the mean z-score for the eight states of challenge/skill ratio, averaged over all subjects, on a number of experience items.

The means of all the experience items, including those not presented, are

Table 22.1. *Average mean Z-scores of reported experiences by challenge/skills ratios*

Challenge . . . Skills . . .	high moderate	high high	moderate high	low high	low moderate	low low	moderate low	high low	F Significance
Concentration	0.60***	0.56***	0.01	−0.36*	−0.44**	−0.46**	−0.02	.41*	23.32***
Ease of concentration	0.04	0.16	−0.13	0.23	0.15	−0.31*	−0.48**	−0.36*	7.65***
Unselfconscious	0.01	0.20	0.23*	0.25	−0.07	−0.07	−0.35*	−0.65***	9.33***
Control	0.19	0.44**	0.41	0.30*	−0.05	−0.55***	−0.71***	−0.58***	29.03***
Alert	0.15	0.28	0.09	−0.01	−0.26	−0.38*	−0.05	0.07	5.99***
Happy	0.19	0.38*	0.26	0.10	0.00	−0.37*	−0.43**	−0.16	10.37***
Cheerful	0.08	0.27	0.27	0.18	0.08	−0.24	−0.28*	−0.19	6.42***
Strong	0.15	0.35*	0.17	0.08	−0.25	−0.41**	−0.35*	−0.14	8.43***
Friendly	0.13	0.26	0.36*	0.10	−0.05	−0.23	−0.37*	−0.17	9.71***
Active	0.40**	0.45**	0.17	−0.12	−0.41**	−0.54**	−0.34*	0.21	17.04***
Sociable	0.10	0.12	0.03	0.16	−0.18	−0.18	−0.26	0.06	2.67**
Involved	0.40**	0.42**	0.00	−0.14	−0.21	−0.42**	−0.23	0.45**	13.29***
Free	0.14	0.45**	0.15	0.12	−0.11	−0.33*	−0.61***	−0.30	16.68***
Excited	0.36*	0.49**	−0.05	−0.09	−0.29	−0.47**	−0.25	0.19	14.68***
Open	0.25	0.32*	0.19	0.06	−0.28	−0.40**	−0.35*	−0.07	10.00***
Clear	0.20	0.53***	0.24	0.13	−0.15	−0.37*	−0.57***	−0.30	17.12***
Wish doing this	0.36*	0.53***	0.02	0.02	−0.27	−0.47**	−0.42**	−0.10	15.98***
Wish to be hear	0.31	0.33*	0.02	−0.02	−0.22	−0.30*	−0.23	−0.05	7.50***
N	45	47	41	45	44	46	45	42	

*P<0.05; **P<0.01; ***P<0.001.
N = frequencies.

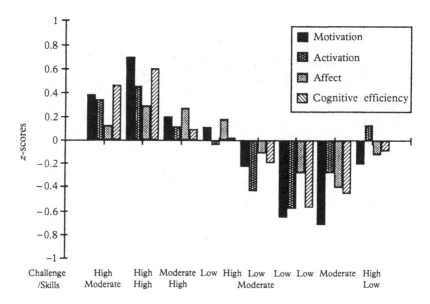

Fig. 22.2. Average mean z-scores for the four dimensions of experience by challenge and skill ratio ($N = 47$).

significantly different for the various ratios of challenge/skill (all F-tests are significant at least at a 0.01 level). As suggested by the flow model of optimal experience, the most positive values are found in the high challenge/high skill condition, whereas the opposite pole – low challenge/low skill – has only negative values. The intermediate combinations show mixed positive and negative values, while the number of significant mean z-scores is clearly smaller. In other words, depending on the ratio of perceived challenge to skill we found extremely different experiences. Therefore, the choice of the challenge/skill ratio as a discriminating variable was appropriate. From these data, optimal experience, operationalized as a congruence of positive emotions on different items, can be expected in those activities in which high challenges match high skills. A congruence of negative emotions is highly probable when activities present no challenges and skills are low.

Challenges, skills, and specific aspects of experience

The different aspects of experience were combined on an a priori basis into four clusters. As can be seen in Fig. 22.2, the optimal experience observed when a high challenge matches high skill was not restricted to good mood only. In fact, at that moment the individual also reported feeling motivated, cognitively efficient, and active.

Although the data for the different experience clusters show a comparable pattern, there are significant differences. Going from high to medium challenge in a situation with high skill, the affect cluster stays unchanged but activity, cognitive efficiency, and motivation drop dramatically. Even more interesting are the changes in the low-skill situation when going from low to medium challenge. In this situation affect and motivation are the lowest observed in any combination of the challenge and skill ratio, while activity and cognitive efficiency show slight improvement.

Challenges, skills, and activities

If optimal experience is linked to the ratio of perceived challenge and skills, it may be interesting to find out whether this ratio is an attribute of the activities themselves. Table 22.2 shows that most of the different activities were repeated at least once in each of the eight different states of the challenge/skill ratio.

In other words, the whole range of subjective experience can occur in any activity whatsoever. Nevertheless, certain activities were more probable when specific challenge/skill ratios were observed. For example, subjects involved in art had a 50/50 chance of experiencing high challenges as well as high skills. On the other hand, subjects involved in personal care perceived almost no challenge. Resting and watching television required no skills, nor did they elicit challenges. Finally, the rare combination of high challenge and low skill for these students was associated with the activities of thinking, classwork, sports, and games.

The mean z-scores for the experimental variables on a single activity, for instance, studying, matched expectations derived from the different challenge/skill ratios. Again, high challenge/high skill is associated with a congruence of positive emotions, while a congruence of negative emotions is observed when challenges as well as skills are low. The relative pattern of emotions, however, can be different. When our teenage subjects are studying, for instance, their mean z-scores on the variables 'free' and 'open' are always negative but, at moments when they experience high challenge as well as high skill in studying, they feel relatively more free and open.

Challenges, skills, and social context

The fact that one is alone or in the company of others influences experience (Larson & Csikszentmihalyi, 1983). We found that optimal experience, however, was not determined simply by being alone. The subjective perception of challenges and skills was the crucial variable determining variations in experiences. However, the frequency distribution of being with others differed for the various combinations of challenges and skills. Being with a friend of the opposite sex was reported most often when challenges and skills were high, whereas being with distant relatives was observed primarily in low-challenge-

Table 22.2. *Percentages of selected activities by challenge/skills ratios*

Challenge . . . Skills . . .	high moderate	high high	moderate high	low high	low moderate	low low	moderate low	high low	N^a
Classwork	10.88	23.85	6.69	5.02	8.37	18.83	14.23	12.13	60
Studying	19.26	23.70	9.26	6.67	6.30	16.67	10.00	8.15	270
Eating	4.40	9.89	6.59	35.16	14.29	26.37	2.20	1.10	70
Personal care	1.18	3.53	5.88	47.06	16.47	20.00	3.53	2.35	85
Transportation	5.48	19.18	4.11	20.55	16.44	21.92	6.85	5.48	73
Chore and errands	3.45	16.09	5.75	42.53	5.75	19.54	3.45	3.45	87
Rest and napping	5.26	10.53	5.26	15.79	23.68	31.58	7.89	0.00	19
Socializing	16.44	32.21	6.71	10.07	7.72	11.74	6.38	8.72	303
Sport and games	21.05	26.32	5.26	21.05	10.53	5.26	0.00	10.53	19
TV watching	5.61	2.80	6.54	24.30	14.95	39.25	2.80	3.74	105
Listening to music	23.53	11.76	0.00	11.76	5.88	17.65	17.65	11.76	17
Art and hobbies	24.53	47.17	9.43	11.32	0.00	3.77	3.77	0.00	27
Reading	14.49	24.64	5.80	21.74	7.25	15.94	4.35	5.80	69
Thinking	10.06	18.24	5.66	11.32	4.40	23.90	12.58	13.84	79
Other leisure	9.23	10.77	6.15	23.08	12.31	27.69	9.23	1.54	69

N^a = frequencies.

/high-skill situations. The company of strangers, classmates, and mixed groups was associated with high-challenge/low-skill activities.

Discussion

The data correspond well with hypotheses generated by previous research on optimal experience or flow (Graef, Csikszentmihalyi & Giffin, 1978). But can we trust conclusions based totally on self-reports? Probably, because even the most objective disciplines in the realm of behavioral science, such as ethology, now recognize the importance of self-reports (Ericsson & Simon, 1980, 1985). They may even be the only way to obtain certain kinds of important information; as Harré & Secord (1972) stated in their theoretical reconstruction of social psychology: 'In order to be able to treat people as if they were human beings it must be possible to accept their commentaries upon their actions as authentic, though revisable, reports of phenomena, subject to critical empiricism' (p. 101).

The ESM, inasmuch as it repeatedly interrogates subjects, is able to accumulate a considerable quantity of data, which permits detailed analyses and testing of the self-reports. As illustrated in this chapter, the capacity of self-reports to capture private experiences, gathered throughout the day, testifies to the utility of these approaches. These data also point out the limits of objective or behavioral observations as a means of understanding experience. For instance, the last runner to reach the finish line in a race may feel a most optimal experience whereas the winner could experience unexpected negative emotions. The only way to know is to ask. As Gergen (1982) has pointed out, the malleability of the human organism relies upon symbolization. As we hope to have demonstrated, it is what is subjectively perceived as the balance between challenges and skills that is a key factor for the understanding of changes in human emotions.

Dynamics of optimal experience

The data show that our subjects fluctuated between positive and negative states of experience. The 'ideal' positive pole, however, occurred only transitorily in everyday life, as other researchers have also observed (Csikszentmihalyi, 1975; Csikszentmihalyi & Larson, 1984; Graef, Csikszentmihalyi & Giffin, 1978). It is likely that the state of optimal experience is a state that individuals will pursue. Higher challenges and activities associated with this state will be selected (Csikszentmihalyi & Massimini, 1985). At the opposite pole, when challenges and skills are below average for the week but still in dynamic equilibrium, individuals are confronted with a situation in which, at first sight, no problems are expected. Why then is this the situation with the worst experience? According to the theory of living systems (Miller, 1970), a condition, such as balanced challenges and skills, however, leads to a regression and disorganization from a positive state of consciousness that may be characterized as apathy. The apathy of normal experiential fluctuations represents an area of risk for the individual. To avoid apathy, the search for new challenges must never end. This is akin to the parable of the oarsman on the river; if he stops rowing upstream he goes backwards (Csikszentmihalyi, 1975, 1978). States of imbalance between challenge and skill – that is, where either skill or challenge predominates – represent areas of experiential transition. Repetitive activities represent a typical everyday situation when skills are predominant. Here, negative experiences are best summarized as boredom. There is no quest for challenge and no escape from negative experiences. On the positive side, however, this state provides an opportunity to practice skills without the stress of meeting challenges. In the opposite condition, when subjects are confronted with high challenge while lacking appropriate skill, the negative experience can be summarized as anxiety.

Implications for psychiatric rehabilitation

From our observation of students, optimal experience is reported when high challenge is matched with high skill. For healthy individuals, continuing personal development is made possible only by a constant confrontation with more complex challenges weighted to the subject's self-perception of his or her own skills. Otherwise, the experience is not rewarding, because either the activity fails due to a lack of personal skills or the performance is not satisfactory because it is insufficiently challenging. This leads to atrophy in behavior. If the behavioral principle forwarded here, that optimal experience is achieved by seeking ever-growing challenges within the range of already-mastered skills, is true for psychiatric patients, such information is of use in rehabilitation programs. We believe that the process of emotional atrophy is what is experienced by chronic psychiatric patients. They are caught in an unstimulating life and are unable to achieve optimal experience on their own.

The prescription for psychiatric rehabilitation, then, is to stimulate psychiatric patients to perform activities that are challenging, while also requiring relatively high skills. These activities will probably be less complex than those performed by the subjects presented here. Because challenge/skill ratios are based on the individual subject's experience, the therapist may gather personalized information to tailor the rehabilitation programme to match the perceived challenge and skill of the patient. ESM may then serve as a supplementary rehabilitation tool by providing information about low-challenge/low-skill situations. The subject's negative pole may be identified, and a suitable program that would increase enjoyable experiences may be instituted.

In closing, we must note that although sufficiently similar to other samples (e.g., Csikszentmihalyi & Larson, 1984), the experiences of adolescents in this study may not be truly representative of a normal or, for that matter, a disordered population. We feel justified, however, in suggesting that the study of healthy subjects can offer models for the treatment of psychopathology and in urging a better collaboration between psychology and psychiatry, comparable to that of physiology and pathology in medicine. Further work is required to establish the usefulness of these data for psychiatric samples and to shed more light on psychopathology.

23

The ESM and the measurement of clinical change: a case of anxiety disorder

ANTONELLA DELLE FAVE
and FAUSTO MASSIMINI

In this chapter the Experience Sampling Method (ESM) is used to study the daily fluctuations in the mental state of an agoraphobic patient over the course of a year. This case study illustrates the relevance of the 'Flow Theory' (Csikszentmihalyi, 1975, 1985), and the key concept of 'Optimal Experience' in mental patients. Optimal experience is the state of mind that arises when high environmental challenges are balanced with high personal skills in facing them (Csikszentmihalyi & Massimini, 1985; Massimini, Csikszentmihalyi & Delle Fave, 1986, 1988). Recent studies show that this positive experiential state is recognized across cultures. The theory holds that in daily life, normal subjects tend to reproduce optimal experience selectively and to look for activities which facilitate this experience and attempt to devote as much time and psychic energy to these activities as possible (Csikszentmihalyi & Rochberg-Halton, 1981). The selected activities may include routine daily tasks, as well as leisure, but as sources of optimal experience, they are basically related to the intrinsic motivation of the subject and are performed for their own sake, regardless of material rewards.

ESM was applied to the study of daily life in a number of different samples and cultures. As deVries (1987) points out, it allows one to 'overcome the shortcomings of retrospective recall in psychiatric research'. Therefore, it is also suited to sample the experiences in the daily life of ambulatory psychiatric patients between therapeutic sessions. It allows us to understand better the moment-to-moment experience of patients in their natural settings 'with the therapeutic goal of providing context-related specific information to the patient and therapist about optimal and deviant functioning' (Delespaul & deVries, 1987).

The data discussed in this chapter concern a young woman, whose complaints corresponded to the DSM-III-R diagnostic criteria of Panic Disorder with Agoraphobia (APA, 1987). The results were gathered throughout a year of psychotherapy and were collected in nine ESM sampling weeks. A gradual disappearance of symptoms as well as an improvement in mental state was observed over the year. These changes were monitored by ESM and will be discussed in terms of the subject's interactions with her environment and treatment goals. The data presented here are meant to highlight the influences of three different levels of ESM data:

(1) Time-budgets: the distribution of the subject's activities, the places and the social contexts frequented. Time-budgets were recorded at each sampling period and systematic changes over the course of therapy are discussed.

(2) Mental state: thought content, the subject's attention and concentration in different settings, and the fluctuations in her state of mind over time were followed.

(3) The development and pursuit of optimal experience: the transformation of the subject's experience of apathy and disengagement toward a more positive and complex interaction with the challenges of daily life are described.

The subject

Caterina is a 25-year-old unmarried woman. She was born in Southern Italy, in the birth place of her parents. She was the second of three children, with a sister two years older and a brother four years younger. When she was five the family moved to near Milano, where she still lives with her mother and siblings. Her father's death after a long illness in December 1986 was a major emotional loss for Caterina.

Caterina completed high school and currently works as a clerk in an Information Services Office. She also received a traditional socialization, with typical Southern Italian cultural constraints, concerning female behavior and freedom. For example, this affected her educational decisions: 'at that time I could not go to school in Milano, because it was impossible for a girl to take a train and go to Milano. This was a taboo, since she could be raped'. Caterina's cultural education may be evidenced in her agoraphobic symptoms, such as her fear of being alone in public places, fear of falling in the street and of developing breathlessness and tachycardia in crowded places. As de Swaan (1981) and Dijkman & deVries (1987) point out, agoraphobia is influenced by culture, and by social experiences. In historical perspective, the street is a threatening place with potentially dangerous and erotic encounters for women.

Caterina started to complain about anxiety and developed agoraphobic symptoms around the age of 22. Her treatment history included group psychotherapy, interrupted after about six months, and treatment with Alprazolam, 1.5 mg per day, since 1984. In January 1987, Caterina came to us, asking for individual psychotherapy, and was followed with

281

weekly sessions until June 1988. From February 1987 until June 1988 she was tested every six- to eight-week-period with the ESM. This provided nine ESM sampling periods, each consisting of 60 random signals. Caterina completed 428 valid self-report forms, about 80% of all beeps.

The procedure

The repeated sampling was conducted with the ESM (Carli, Delle Fave & Massimini, 1988). The subject received a booklet composed of identical self-report forms and a programmed wrist-watch. She was asked to fill out a questionnaire each time she received a signal, randomly given by the wrist terminal. Five to seven signals were sent each day, ranging from 8.00 a.m. to 10 p.m. on weekdays, from 8.00 a.m. to 12.00 a.m. on Saturday, and from 10.00 a.m. to 10.00 p.m. on Sunday.

The self-report form contained 44 items, including open-ended questions concerning the activity, content of thoughts, places and companionship at the time of the beep, and 12-point Likert scales that assessed the quality of the experience: her mood, activity level, concentration and motivation, experienced challenge, physical complaints. Two additional questionnaires were filled out at the beginning of the therapy:

(1) The Flow Questionnaire (Csikszentmihalyi, 1982, 1986; Delle Fave & Massimini, 1988) that focuses on 'Optimal Experience'. It asks the subjects to describe in detail present and past activities related to optimal experience. Moreover, the Flow Questionnaire gathers general information about subjective experience in the context of daily life and about the differential use of attention in forced vs. free concentration situations (i.e. an exam versus playing a musical instrument).

(2) The Life Theme Questionnaire (Csikszentmihalyi & Beattie, 1979) which is currently used by our research group to describe positive and negative events or situations in the past, as well as present challenges and future goals. Moreover, the questionnaire asks the subjects to reflect on their lives, to describe their earliest memories, their relationships with parents and relatives, and their favorite activities. It assesses how these influence their life. Subjects' answers provide useful information about the development of their attentional processes, by eliciting on central themes which organize an individual's consciousness.

The therapy

The therapy was integrated with repeated ESM measurements. It was guided by the assumption that each individual, in order to achieve a positive state of consciousness, seeks meaningful opportunities for action in daily life (Csikszentmihalyi, 1985). The application of optimal experience theory in psychotherapy is centered on reinforcing both the patient's personal search for challenging possibilities for action in daily life, and his/her effort to develop personal skills in order to meet these challenges and not avoid them. Optimal experience is related to the subjective perception of environmental challenges: each individual in his life will selectively pursue the activities that best meet his own intrinsic motivation and his spontaneous interests. Such a therapeutic approach is therefore individualized, focusing on the personal motivation and tendencies of the subject.

To get this process under way, we ask patients at the beginning of the therapy to fill out the Flow Questionnaire, in order to register the opportunities for optimal experience they currently encounter in daily life. In February 1987, Caterina reported *no* current optimal experiences in the questionnaire, but she did refer to positive experience activities in the past, such as 'working in the White Cross', 'dancing' and 'studying English'. She described these as highly positive and challenging situations. The therapeutic approach was therefore centered on supporting Caterina's involvement in these intrinsically motivating and challenging activities. She was encouraged to pursue these activities more, thereby improving her personal skills and allowing her to meet gradually higher challenges. This was done in a number of ways. The periodic use of ESM allowed us to make a detailed analysis of Caterina's daily life experiences. ESM data were used at the level of inspection, reading the reports as pages of an inter-sessions diary. Next, these data were analyzed (after the first five samplings, and after the last one) creating a quantitative record of her experience and mental life fluctuations. This information was used in identifying goals for the therapeutic sessions. These sessions were thus centered not only around Caterina's anxiety and agoraphobia symptoms, but also on her apathy and disengagement experienced within the narrow limits of her daily routine. The session emphasized strategies for dealing with challenges and devoting time to self-rewarding activities in order to improve the quality of daily experience. Since Caterina had pursued self-rewarding activities in the past, the therapist 'could help her re-develop' these skills. For example, taking into account her interest in White Cross volunteering, books concerning first-aid practices and basic medical information, or TV programs about these topics were suggested. This approach was combined with low-key desensitization, such as accompanying her on walks on crowded Milano streets. These walking exercises, while initially experienced as an additional source of anxiety, gradually became associated with a decrease in avoidance and an increase in frequency of social events and meetings. Over that period Alprazolam was gradually reduced, until it was definitively removed in October 1987.

The ESM characterized the remarkable changes in Caterina's life. Her time-budgets shifted from a narrow routine centered on work, home and TV watching in the first samplings, to a more complex life pattern including many challenges such as volunteering in White Cross activities, meetings with friends, getting a driver's licence and beginning an English course. At the same time, Caterina reported a deep change in the quality of her subjective experiences from an apathetic to a more positive and active interaction with the environment. The results section will focus on how ESM results detect fluctuations in experiences, not just in relation to the momentary contexts of daily life, but also as a follow-up tool over a prolonged sampling period.

Results

Time-budgets

The time-budget data were analyzed separately for each of the nine sampling periods. Some remarkable changes were found in the distribution of activities, places and companionship.

(1) *Activities.* Daily routine activities, concerning her job, housework and maintenance took a constant percentage of Caterina's time through all the nine samplings. This result is remarkable in itself, in that it marks the stability of Caterina's daily life organization around basic activities. Important to note here is that the change in experience did not depend on radical modifications in routine activities or in the lifestyle of the patient. Remarkable changes occurred in the distribution of selective activities:

(a) TV watching (see Fig. 23.1) gradually decreased in frequency over the nine samplings from 45.4% of Caterina's time-budget in the first sample to 13.7% in the eighth sampling. TV watching was not reported during the ninth sampling.

(b) New activities (including White Cross volunteering, reading, studying English, attending to the driver's licence course and socializing with friends) appeared in the third sampling, consuming 3.6% of the time-budget, and remained for all subsequent samplings. The low percentage of the total time devoted to these extra-routine activities is a result of her work expenditures. She spends nine hours each day at work and four hours commuting.

(2) *Places and companionship.* The stability of daily routine, largely created by work commuting, is also demonstrated in places and companionship. Frequencies of places, such as the office, street or train and of the companionship of colleagues do not significantly fluctuate throughout the samplings. The increase of new activities, like White Cross volunteering and meetings with friends was measured in the distribution of

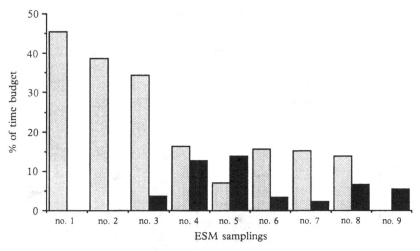

Fig. 23.1. Changes in the percentage of time devoted to TV watching (□) and to new activities (■) during the nine ESM samplings (*N* = 428).

locations: like White Cross offices or the hospital. Leisure places such as discos, friends' houses and restaurants increased in frequency from 2.5% in the first sampling to 5.4% in the ninth. Moreover, there is a remarkable increase in the time Caterina spends alone: from 19.1% in the first sampling to 43.6% in the last (Fig. 23.2). This result underlines the improving capacity of Caterina to be alone, and her diminished need for social support particularly in relation to her fear of travelling and walking alone in the street.

Mental states

(1) *Thought content.* Throughout the ESM sampling period Caterina spent a large amount of time (average 31.7%) thinking about herself, her past and future, her psychological complaints or positive moods. After sampling 4, she reported increasing thoughts about White Cross volunteering. The number of thoughts devoted to TV watching decreased from 6.1% in the first sampling to 1.7% in the ninth.

(2) *Positive congruence between thoughts and activities.* Over time Caterina began to focus her attention better and to get more involved in daily activities as demonstrated by her increase in 'positive congruence between thoughts and activity': how often, for example, Caterina's thought was more often concentrated on what she was doing. The congruence between what a subject is thinking and what he is doing is an important variable which characterizes the quality of experience. It is an indicator of the focusing of attention on the activity, which in the frame

Table 23.1. *Positive congruence (%) through the
nine samplings*

samples 1–3	samples 4–6	samples 7–9
25.1	30.7	38.1

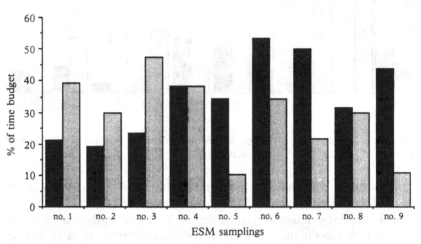

Fig. 23.2. Changes in the percentage of time spent with family (▨) and alone (■) during the nine ESM samplings ($N = 428$).

of 'Flow Theory' is one of the key dimensions for optimal experience (Csikszentmihalyi, 1975), as well as a characteristic of wellbeing in pathological samples (Delespaul & deVries, 1987). We show the percentage of 'positive congruence' through the nine samplings, grouped in three periods (samplings 1–3, 4–6, 7–9, Table 23.1). In the first batch, Caterina was rarely concentrated on her daily activities; but then there was a gradual increase in attention on situations that allowed Caterina to achieve optimal experience.

(3) *The fluctuations of the experience through the time.* Figure 23.3 shows the quality of the experience in the daily life, as Caterina described it in the 1st and 9th sampling periods. As the Figure shows, at the beginning of therapy she reported strong negative experiences and a narrow range of routine activities. Her involvement in more complex, challenging and socially valuable activities, such as White Cross volunteering, and the development of the other new activities resulted in a more positive quality of her experience. The trend began in sample no. 4, and is most clear in the last sampling.

286

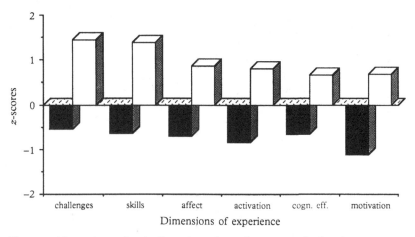

Fig. 23.3. Mean z-scores for six dimensions of experience – perceived environmental challenges, personal skills, affect, activation, cognitive efficiency, motivation – in the first (■) ESM sampling (no. of calls = 33) and in the ninth (□) (no. of calls = 55).

The role of optimal experience

The ESM data demonstrate fluctuations in Caterina's state of consciousness that can be related to the perceived environmental challenges and personal skills in a model that is based on 'Flow Theory' (Massimini, Csikszentmihalyi & Carli, 1987; Massimini & Carli, 1988; Massimini & Delle Fave, 1988).

The model is structured in the following way (see Fig. 23.4): on a Cartesian plan, perceived challenges are reported on the y-axis and skills on the x-axis; both dimensions are expressed in z-scores, and this standardization, for Caterina's data, has been calculated on the mean of the nine samples. This mean corresponds to the crossing point between the two axes. By the ratio z-challenges/z-skills the plan has been divided in eight 'Channels'. The ESM variables recording the subjective experience (also normalized) have been analyzed in their fluctuation in the channels. We theoretically expect 'Optimal Experience' in the area of Channel 2, where z-challenges and z-skills values are balanced and higher than the subjective mean. We expect an experience of 'Anxiety' around Channel 8 (z-challenges above the average, z-skills lower than the average); on the contrary, positive z-skills and negative z-challenges (Channel 4) are related to 'Boredom'. Finally, the situation characterized by z-challenges and z-skills both lower than the subjective mean (Channel 6) is theoretically associated to the state of 'Apathy', of total detachment and disengagement, very detrimental for the psychological development of the individual, in that it leads to a disruption and disorganization of consciousness (Massimini, Csikszentmihalyi & Carli, 1987).

Clinical change could be measured by means of the percentage of Caterina's

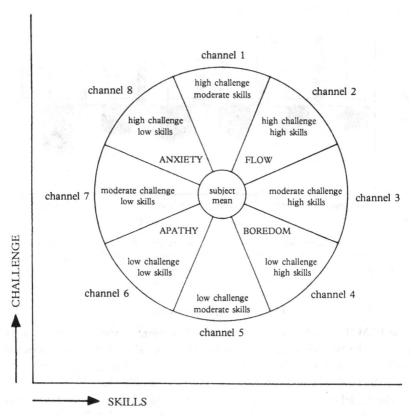

Fig. 23.4. A model for the analysis of experience. Perceived challenges are on the ordinate and perceived skills on the abscissa.

reports in each channel over the nine samplings. Here we note a clear evolution from a subjective experience dominated by the feeling of apathy in the initial samplings to a situation in which daily life frequently became a source of optimal experience.

Apathy in Channel 6 decreased from 60.6% in sampling 1 to 34.5% in sampling 9. Concomitantly, we found an increase in reports of optimal experience in Channel 2 from 15.2% to 50.9%. These results are related to the effective development of the activities quoted by Caterina herself as sources of optimal experience and the positive influence ('halo effect') of these activities on Caterina's subjective experience as she carried out her routine activities in daily life, which have been 'restructured' around the new sources of optimal experience. The increase in optimal experience provided center of order in her consciousness, which provided feelings of enjoyment and achievement in other aspects of the daily life.

Conclusions

Caterina's case study demonstrates that ESM can be used to understand better the relationship between subject and environment, and more specifically between subjective experience, time-budgets and the social context. ESM enables us to retain the personal perspective of the subject in human behavioral research. In this clinical study, it provided data about time-budgets and the situationality of pathology, clinically useful information about coping strategies of an individual patient (Dijkman & deVries, 1987).

This case study also demonstrates that ESM can be applied fruitfully in follow-up studies and in longitudinal research, since it captures relevant fluctuations in positive and negative experiences over time. ESM self-reports about the patient's interaction with her daily environment provide a quantitative evaluation of the fluctuations in her subjective experience.

Furthermore, ESM enables a new and more complex approach to the study of behavior and to the understanding of mental illness. It relates the environmental contexts of the disease to the personal coping styles. So ESM is a useful tool in psychotherapy, in that it detects both fluctuations and stability in experience over time, as well as ongoing psychotherapeutic treatment. Moreover, 'Flow Theory' and the concept of Optimal Experience provide an interpretative key to the results. The introduction of these concepts in a theory of mental health allows one to focus on the positive or potentially positive experiences of the patient. This knowledge about the subjective sources of optimal experience makes it possible to build a person-related therapy. The therapy focuses on the internal motivation and interest of the individual and his/her own strategy of reaching optimal experience by means of specific, idiosyncratic activities (Csikszentmihalyi & Csikszentmihalyi, 1988).

The case of Caterina also demonstrates the power of positive psychological processes, such as enjoyment and creativity. These issues should be central to treatment that enables the subject to find more positive experiences in daily life and develop new life styles in a positive and constructive manner.

24

The applicability of ESM in personalized rehabilitation

EGBERT G. T. VAN DER POEL
and PHILIPPE A. E. G. DELESPAUL

'The challenge of psychiatric research over the next decade seems
clear: the systematic description of mental disorders and behavior
with a high degree of situational and temporal detail.'

M.W. deVries (1987)

The de-institutionalization of mental hospitals and the movement towards a
community-integrated mental health care system is a resilient world-wide
trend in the organization of medical services. From the patients' point of view,
the central objective of this process is to optimize the functioning of individuals in their own living environment. This differs from the period prior to de-
institutionalization, when the traditional psychiatric hospital was the standard
living environment for chronic psychiatric patients. In those stable settings,
systematic treatment plans as well as relatively standard interventions were
developed and carried out. De-institutionalization, however, added complexity and re-introduced the patients' own environment into treatment planning. As a consequence mental health services had to incorporate the realities
of community life into treatment programs. Personalized rehabilitation strategies are an attempt to tailor rehabilitation to individual needs. Developing
treatment programs in such a complex context is not easy, particularly since
the data required to plan treatments, the actual interactions of the patients with
their living environments, are generally hidden from the observation of mental
health professionals. Personalized rehabilitation extends traditional treatment
approaches, that attempted to correct skill deficits through training, by
incorporating information about the patients' interactions with an active and
changing environment in the rehabilitation process. In the personal rehabilitation process as well as in de-institutionalization in general, psychiatry has
become more dependent on the existing environmental diversity of social
relationships and changing socio-cultural goals. Psychiatry by the nature of its
own development, is challenged to develop assessment strategies and interven-

tions that promote and support individual adaptive strategies (Liberman, 1988; Watts & Bennett, 1983). Leading researchers in the field of psychopathology highlight the importance of adding the dimensions of time and space to the description of mental phenomena (Zubin, 1989; Ciompi, 1989; Strauss, 1989). Research concerning the variability in illness course of depression and schizophrenia (Brown & Harris, 1978; deVries & Delespaul, 1989), has brought to our attention the host of assets and protective factors that influence the shift from health to sickness and back. The natural daily life context in which coping and adaptation occur are the target of personalized rehabilitation strategies. Today the clinical interview is the standard tool for gaining information about the quality of a person's life. We feel, however, that interview data or questionnaires for that matter do not elucidate sufficient situational detail to genuinely add to our understanding of disordered behavior. Assessment methods such as the Experience Sampling Method (ESM) go a step further and allow the collection of concurrent information on subjective experience and psychopathology with the description of the context in which they occur.

We thus propose to correct the shortcomings by supplementing the interview that is traditionally applied in the assessment of the person–environment fit with ESM. In this Chapter we will illustrate the advantage of ESM over interviewing techniques for collecting information required for implementing personal rehabilitation in a case study.

The evaluation of a year in the life of a chronic mental patient . . .

The rehabilitation process of John, a schizophrenic patient, is traced over the course of one year during which we evaluate the effect of different therapeutic interventions on the subject's mental state. We ask whether the choices made in the rehabilitation process fulfilled the goals of: (1) stabilizing his mental state; (2) enhancing his self-confidence; and (3) optimizing his quality of life?

Assessment techniques

In this case intensive interviews and the ESM were used to make personalized rehabilitation decisions.

We gathered information continually for the clinical decision-making process using a classic strategy in psychiatry: repeated intensive clinical interviews. Over the course of one year a total of 37 interviews were conducted every two weeks by the first author (EvdP) and a co-therapist (AH). The interviews focused on current mental state and experiences between interview periods. The second aim was to assess patterns in the course of the disease process, since we intended to focus rehabilitation on the experienced activities and environmental changes induced by the rehabilitation process in John's life. The interviewers and the patient developed a strong research alliance.

Although information was fed back to the treatment staff once, no direct therapeutic responsibilities were assumed.

The second method was the ESM described in more detail by Csikszentmihalyi & Larson (1987) for normals and Delespaul & deVries (1987) for schizophrenic subjects. Subjects carried a small signaling device that beeps ten times each day for six consecutive days. The signal is the well known alarmring of a digital watch which is commonplace and does not create excessive commotion in the subject's environment. At the signal, the subject is asked to fill out a small booklet containing a set of mental state Likert-type self-assessments and open-ended questions structured in subsets of items that gather information about thoughts, mood, pathology, activities, the number of people around him and relation to the persons in his environment, and the place he is at that moment. ESM is ideally suited for generating data to be used in treatment planning because such data are not distorted by retrospective recall. We attempt ecological validity further in that the data are generated in the natural context of the patients' lives, which is usually an inaccessible context for mental health professionals. In the present case study, the subject was sampled during three periods of one week each, spread over a year.

Subject

John is a 45-year-old male, the fourth of six children from a working class Dutch family that was dominated by a strict matriarch. Since childhood he has led an isolated life marked by few friends and little contact with his brothers and sisters.

John was married at the age of 20. He did not want children, but his wife insisted as soon as they were – financially and materially – prepared. After ten years of marriage, they had a daughter. John was first employed as a piper-fitter in a chemical plant, followed five years later with a job in a porcelain factory. Before his psychiatric problems began, he had been promoted to a low-level management position in this firm. He was also active in the union, being particularly concerned with health conditions at work.

After the birth of his daughter, seven years prior to the study, his mental health career began. Following an acute period of paranoia related to conflicts over his union membership and involvement, he presented to the crisis intervention team at the local mental health center. Subsequently, he lost his job, was divorced and took up residence in a caravan on a secluded lot. He felt disappointed and lived isolated from all social contact, including his family. His behavior was driven by paranoid delusions that resulted in frequent violent and aggressive outbursts toward the mayor, doctors and social workers he visited. After being threatened and robbed one night in his caravan, he refused to return. Following the advice of his priest he moved in with his mother, father, eldest brother and youngest sister. There, he was overwhelmed by his dominating brother, whom he attacked with an axe, leading to a trial conviction, and assigned to a psychiatric hospital for one year.

John remained in the hospital for three years and complied with an oral Haldol® medication regime. Since his initial period of aggressive behavior, he has today transformed into a sub-assertive behavior style, marked by paranoid delusions and persistent fears of decompensating again. He ruminates over why he has lost everything he owned: his family, his work and his health. Accordingly he developed the delusional rationale of: 'I became too important. Therefore some people (organizations) set the whole thing up to get me down and they can do it again whenever they like'. He described the goal of his sub-assertiveness as a coping strategy to keep him out of the 'limelight', to stay 'unimportant'. The role of chronic mental patient became for John a safe identity. He was thus strongly motivated to keep contact with his doctors and the psychiatric hospital. One year prior to the study he was discharged and began living on his own. John maintained regular supportive contacts with a day-treatment program, but had no social contact outside his hospital acquaintances and all contact with his family was lost. During the interviews, John presented himself as a shy, submissive person, who experienced all events in his life as if they were happening to him, events he did not understand and was not able to influence. Although most of his earlier life had been marked by a 'go getter' attitude, today he seeks the safety and security of the hospital and the industrial therapy activities. Over the last years, John had experienced all changes as frightening deviations from the daily routine. His DSM-IIIr (APA, 1987) diagnosis was schizophrenia, paranoid type, in remission.

The therapeutic process described in this case study, unfolds over the course of a year, beginning six months after his release from the hospital. We will pay particular attention to his interactions with the rehabilitation unit that formed the essential part of his life. Over the whole period John lived in a small one-person flat, and attended day care at the day-hospital. The year can be divided into three distinctive phases, related to his rehabilitation process, characterized by the type of day-care provided. During the first period, he participated in an industrial therapy program on the hospital grounds. This consisted of low-skill activities such as packing products, which were therapeutically meant to structure the day and provide social interaction opportunities. The low-skill activity was below John's abilities. Since the staff felt that the activity did not enhance his self-esteem, they experimented with tasks requiring more skill. This resulted in John's appointment as the driver of a small bus, used to transport patients to and from the day care centre. John's drivers licence rendered him qualified for the job. In addition, it provided him with the prestige of being in charge of an expensive new automobile. His promotion started six weeks before the second ESM assessment. In the six months between the first and the second phase other aspects of his life also changed: he was assigned to a new psychiatrist and regained contact with his daughter. The third assessment period was scheduled three months after his intervention as a follow-up evaluation of the long-term effects of the bus driver job and social contacts on his life situation.

Table 24.1. *Overview of major activities during the three measurement periods*

Period	Description of treatment activities	Time (months)
1	Industrial therapy on the hospital ground	0
2	Bus driver between hospital and the city	6
3	Bus driver + social contact	9

In this study we compared the relative merits of the clinical interview and ESM in providing a clear picture of John's life.

Questions and variable selection

(1) From a clinical point of view given the severity of his illness, John was stabilized at an acceptable level when he was discharged from the hospital. Our research question was therefore: was this stability preserved after the interventions that were planned to enhance his self-worth and optimize his quality of life? Measures to determine this were derived from the clinical interviews and from the pathology and mood items, that were repeatedly assessed using the ESM. The following markers of psychopathology were selected from the ESM measures: experienced suspiciousness, thought intrusion, unreal feeling, feeling out of control and mood items such as feeling happy, sad and anxious.

(2) John's primary coping strategy at discharge was to remain unimportant; regaining self-worth was reported as threatening. His reluctance to assume meaningful social roles had obstructed John's rehabilitation process. His appointment to the bus driving job for which he was skilled was meant to help with this problem. But, did bus-driving enhance his self-worth? The variables selected for this assessment were expressions of enthusiasm in the clinical interviews and the ESM mental state items

294

'relaxed', 'powerless' and 'self-assured'; activity assessments as 'being active' and feeling 'skilled'; and motivational measures such as 'concentration', 'prefer doing something else' and 'like doing' the activity.

(3) Since total symptom aleviation is usually not a realistic goal in the treatment of schizophrenia, the ultimate goal of rehabilitation should focus on the quality of life. Was John's quality of life enhanced over the year? The ESM data used in this evaluation were the frequency distributions of places, persons and activities, and the responses to Likert items of 'satisfaction' and 'loneliness'.

Results

The assessment of mental state

John's mental health history and initial clinical interviews, confirmed that he was well-adjusted, although not symptom free, throughout the first assessment period. The data in Table 24.2 from period 1 confirm this picture[1]: low scores on most of the symptom dimensions were found with the exception of suspiciousness and anxiety. Because the subject's mental state had been stable for quite some time, we assumed the bus driving intervention would not affect his symptoms. In subsequent clinical interviews, in contrast, decompensation due to overstimulation of his new work situation seemed imminent. On ESM, however, the postulated negative effect of the bus driving on his mental state was not confirmed. ESM data in fact showed no significant decrease in mental functioning and a gradual improvement of the mental health from period 1 to 3 was actually observed. One important and highly significant exception was that John gradually felt more 'unreal' between measurements 2 and 3, a finding difficult to interpret.

The assessment of self-worth

One of John's major problems was his low self-esteem and marked sub-assertiveness. These were related to the paranoid delusional thoughts that dominated his life, and his related need to remain unimportant and stay out of trouble. In the industrial therapy activities in the day-care centre during period one, John was relaxed and accepted his situation. Yet, in the interviews

---

[1] Before analysing the ESM data we have to make adjustments for the response tendencies over the 3 periods in the Likert data. The high end of the scale was almost never used. When it was used, it was used for assessing positive experiences (being active, stimulating environment, . . .). Only 15% of the scales had at least one score over 5. At the other end of the scale the score of 1 was not used for two items (ideographic complaint and suspiciousness). Both are negatively formulated and have a direct relation with pathology. 92% of the scales were answered using the most extreme low position. Accordingly we considered a range of 1 to 5 as the active range in the Likert scales and consider 1 as 'not at all' and 5 as 'very'. More information on the interpretation of ESM scores in Larson & Delespaul (this volume).

Table 24.2. *Mental state changes over time (1 = not at all; 7 = very)*

Item	Period 1 ($n=66$)	Period 2 ($n=56$)	Period 3 ($n=48$)	Test $F(2, 166)$	t-Test 1/2	t-Test 1/3	t-Test 2/3
Pathology							
suspiciousness	3.30 (0.68)	3.10 (0.37)	3.00 (0.21)	5.80 ($P<0.01$)	★	★★	—
thought intrusion	1.56 (1.07)	1.36 (0.84)	1.13 (0.64)	3.34 ($P<0.04$)	—	★★	—
feeling unreal	1.59 (0.80)	1.00 (——)	2.38 (0.70)	60.81 ($P<0.001$)	★★	(★★)	(★★)
fear of loosing control	1.33 (0.66)	1.00 (——)	1.00 (——)	($P<0.001$)	★★	★★	—
Mood (feeling . . .)							
happy	3.08 (0.27)	2.95 (1.41)	2.63 (1.02)	n.s.	—	(★)	—
sad	1.21 (0.54)	1.14 (0.65)	1.00 (——)	n.s.	—	★	—
anxious	2.80 (0.67)	2.65 (1.12)	2.88 (1.10)	n.s.	—	—	—

★$P<0.05$; ★★$P<0.01$; star values in parentheses = significant counter-expectation findings (worsening).

John continually complained that he had lost everything, that his life had lost any meaning. Therefore, the clinical decision makers decided to search for an intervention that would provide more meaning and offered him the bus-driving job. ESM data (Table 24.3) however showed a significant drop in his skill self-assessment between periods 1 and 2. The subject was a skilled driver, but he did not experience himself skilled. For example, during the second period the self-assessment of being skilled was significantly lower on weekdays when he drove the bus as compared to weekends (2.89 vs. 3.50), while the reverse relation held in the previous period (3.84 vs. 2.86).

Some mood scores such as (not being) relaxed, self-assurance and feelings of powerlessness did change in a negative direction between periods 1 and 2. In period 3, powerlessness and self-assurance did not recover. Over all measurement periods, John became less self-assured. We had expected higher scores since he would gain self-confidence by managing a highly valued and prestigious activity, for which he was skilled. Clearly, this intervention failed to reconstruct his global self-confidence. Instead of gaining strength the patient became overwhelmed with feelings of 'powerlessness'. The transition from period 1 to period 2 is the most significant one. Over all the periods the mean powerless scores on working days, compared to weekends, were the highest ($F(5,164) = 89.49$; $P < 0.001$). No systematic morning and afternoon differences were found, but an interaction effect with periods was observed. During the bus-driving periods (2 and 3), the highest experience of powerlessness was observed in the afternoon, a no-work timeblock. In period 1 no differences were found between parts of the day. Interestingly, concurrent activities showed no significant relationship to mental state. The ESM data then showed that the link between feelings of powerlessness with the activities organized by the rehabilitation staff was not direct. It could be that the effect of work is not experienced concurrent with the activity, but that the accumulated effect is experienced later when at home and alone.

The assessment of the quality of life

Enhancing the quality of life is a primary motivation for rehabilitation work. We used two criteria: (1) an objective criterion based on the level of differentiation of the frequency distributions of the places, activity and social context at time of the beep (time-budgets); and (2) a subjective criterion measured by asking someone how he feels.

Did John live a restricted life? Considering the time-budgets computed he clearly did (Table 24.4). The subject is alone and home almost all the time (see also Table 24.5). Compared to computed activity frequencies, the ranges of social context and place were more restricted. These variables are situationally linked in that the people one meets and the places one goes are often a consequence of the living situation. Activities, however, tend to be more

Table 24.3. *Activity assessment over time* ($I = not\ at\ all$; $7 = very$)

Item	Period 1 (*n* = 66)	Period 2 (*n* = 56)	Period 3 (*n* = 48)	Test $F(2, 166)$	Pairwise *t*-test 1–2	1–3	2–3
Mood (feeling . . .)							
relaxed	3.15 (0.61)	1.68 (1.05)	2.56 (0.71)	50.78 (*P*<0.001)	**	**	**
powerless	2.82 (0.68)	4.83 (0.43)	4.68 (0.77)	176.70 (*P*<0.001)	**	**	—
self-assured	2.51 (0.77)	1.15 (0.51)	1.02 (0.13)	133.41 (*P*<0.001)	**	**	—
Activity							
skilled	3.51 (0.94)	3.06 (0.73)	3.10 (0.91)	4.69 (*P*<0.02)	**	*	—
Activity motivation							
concentration	3.65 (0.84)	3.10 (0.47)	3.21 (1.48)	7.35 (*P*<0.002)	**	**	—
rather something else	1.69 (1.13)	2.46 (1.28)	1.78 (1.17)	6.34 (*P*<0.003)	**	—	**
like doing it	3.43 (0.97)	3.19 (0.82)	3.50 (1.29)	n.s.	—	—	—

P<0.05; **P*<0.01.

Table 24.4. *Time-budget changes (%) as an objective measure of quality of life*

Codes (subset)	Period 1 (n=66)	Period 2 (n=56)	Period 3 (n=48)	log-linear model M. Effect: periods	log-linear model M. Effect: codes
Where?					
home	65	70	75	d.f. = 42	d.f. = 30
network/family	0	0	2	$\chi^2 = 1108.39$	$\chi^2 = 47.70$
work/therapy	23	23	19	$P<0.001$	$P<0.02$
other	12	7	4		
What?					
nothing	2	9	13		
work/therapy	12	9	15		
socializing	5	4	6	d.f. = 63	d.f. = 44
household chores	25	18	19	$\chi^2 = 363.71$	$\chi^2 = 54.38$
leisure	37	38	40	$P<0.001$	n.s.
other	20	22	8		
Who?					
alone	75	80	88		
family	0	0	4	d.f. = 18	d.f. = 14
friends	0	0	0	$\chi^2 = 622.26$	$\chi^2 = 26.02$
colleagues	23	18	4	$P<0.001$	$P<0.03$
strangers	2	2	4		

$*P<0.05$; $**P<0.01$.

Table 24.5. *Changes in John's environment over time*

	Period 1	Period 2	Period 3	Overall 'loneliness'
alone/home	43 (65%)	39 (70%)	35 (74%)	1.57
alone/not home	7 (11%)	6 (11%)	7 (15%)	1.45
not alone/home	—	—	—	—
not alone/not home	16 (24%)	11 (19%)	5 (11%)	1.44
Total	100%	100%	100%	n.s.

personal choices less related to the living environment, especially when someone lives alone.

Over the three assessment periods the subject's living environment became even more restricted. He 'lost' 25% of his, already reduced, opportunities for social interaction between the first and the second ESM assessment periods. Alerted by these ESM data and by John's comments during the interviews, the case managers decided to adapt the daily routine and extend the opportunities for social contact. This had no effect on the time-budgets. In the three months between periods 2 and 3 John lost an additional 50% of social time, leaving only 11% for social interaction opportunities. This was statistically significant (using log linear model-fitting techniques). No significant effect of the periods was found for the activity codes. Considering this negative development we have to conclude that John's living arrangement had a deteriorating effect on the quality of his life, but John compensated for this by a differentiated activity spectrum, a differentiation that was not lost over time. How did John perceive this living situation? We restrict ourselves to 'satisfaction' and 'loneliness' variable. Table 24.6 shows a progressive deterioration of satisfaction from period 1 to 2 and, also significant, from period 2 to 3. Interestingly, the subject complained of loneliness in the repeated clinical interviews. This complaint is understandable considering the global assessment of his living situation. However, the experience of loneliness was almost totally unreported in the ESM reports in period 1 to 2 and remained at this low level in period 3. Broken down by environmental situation (as in Table 24.5), no differences were found in the loneliness scores.

Discussion

Summarizing the clinical information we conclude the following: we have investigated by interview and ESM a paranoid schizophrenic patient living alone in a small flat after discharge from the hospital. The working hypothesis of the clinical staff was that the patient attempted to limit drawing attention to himself, assuming that this would lead to self-destruction. The rehabilitation

Table 24.6. *Changes in satisfaction and loneliness (1 = not at all; 7 = very)*

Items	Period 1 (n=66)	Period 2 (n=56)	Period 3 (n=48)	Test $F(2, 166)$	t-Test 1–2	1–3	2–3
Mood (feeling . . .)							
satisfied	4.50 (1.07)	3.55 (1.52)	3.15 (0.36)	22.78 ($P<0.001$)	**	**	*
lonely	2.26 (0.88)	1.02 (0.14)	1.11 (0.45)	76.12 ($P<0.001$)	**	**	—

$*P<0.05$; $**P<0.01$.

effort was, therefore, not focused on psychopathology but on recovering self-worth and developing new activities. The medium was meaningful 'work'. Following Gruenberg's Social Breakdown Theory (1967) and considering the intrapsychic dynamics of the patient, the clinical staff anticipated the possibility that this task would overstimulate him. They were, therefore, prepared for negative consequences after their initial intervention. The uneasiness reported by the patient at the second measurement was interpreted promptly as an imminent decompensation, requiring admission to the hospital. However, in response to John's loss of social meeting opportunities, a simpler intervention was chosen: a day-program providing additional social hours with other patients over lunch.

A closer look at the subjective experience reflected in the ESM showed that contrary to interview information a decompensation was not imminent at period 2. Moreover, his repeat measures of psychopathology showed that the subject gained in health over the different assessment periods after his discharge. Nevertheless, a negative appraisal of his life situation was also observed in that the subject became less satisfied and happy. These negative feelings were not associated with the bus-driving intervention, nor could the loss of self-confidence and the dramatic rise in feelings of powerlessness be related to it. It is of course possible that the feelings of powerlessness are not concurrent with activities but are delayed to a time when the subject gets the chance to evaluate his activities, when at home or alone. Moreover, the feelings of powerlessness were higher during working days but not during the bus-driving activity per se, nor were they present in the morning when the bus driving took place. We do, however, think the influence of the driving job did cause part of the negative observations at period 2, but that this influence was temporary and recovered in period 3. This is supported by the motivational data of 'rather doing something else' and being 'relaxed'.

To describe further the negative changes reported at moment 2 we investigated the feelings of loneliness. In contrast, between periods 1 and 2 the assessment on loneliness improved significantly, even though a rather dramatic change in time-budgets took place, resulting in more time spent alone. The subsequent intervention made by the treating staff, aimed at broadening his social opportunities, had no effect at time 3. Considering that the subject was only provided with opportunities for interaction with patients and former patients, our interpretation is that a 'normal' extinction curve of interactions with his former colleagues after discharge is observed. No compensation for this loss was created within the patient's life. John's ambulatory life in a small one-person flat became a lonely life and the small changes in the daily routine initiated by the staff had only marginal effects. The intervention did not go far enough, since it did not create additional opportunities for broadening his network of acquaintances.

Clinically, it is interesting to note that when comparing the answers on the Likert type scales, improvement over time could be observed primarily on those items measuring positive symptoms of schizophrenia (suspiciousness, thought intrusion, . . .) while negative symptoms assessments (tension, feeling unreal, . . .) deteriorated, but this was probably less related to the rehabilitation interventions than to the living situation (alone in a flat). In terms of setting effects the data are similar to those of Hamilton et al. (1989) who found correlations between negative symptoms and smaller social networks. The question remains whether inherent psychopathology, or the difficult-to-cope-with living situation, is responsible for this trend.

What advantage has the ESM offered over the interview in this particular case? While ESM did not always generate straightforward answers, it did provide a closer look at John's actual experience which is especially important when one aims at tailoring the rehabilitational process to the subject's individual needs. Neither the clinical working hypothesis, that the patient would decompensate as a consequence of the rehabilitation intervention, nor the predictions based on the overstimulation of 'new activities' proved correct. The self-perception of skills, as compared to objective skills, proved most important for the rehabilitation process. The patient's narrative seemed confounded by the distortions resulting from the problems with accurate retrospective recall of experience, John's communication of dependency needs and personal goals for therapy as protection. Those may have mislead the staff. Rehabilitation interventions therefore tended to be based on projections of the therapist institutional goals and the patient's unconscious needs, clearly another world from the patient's actual living environment. ESM helps us to break out of this mold by visualising the patient's world better in a more cost-effective way. This in turn, provides better treatment opportunities such as increasing his 'out of the hospital' social network that in turn may be evaluated. We do not argue that the intensive involvement of personal counseling contacts should be diminished and substituted by the ESM assessment technique but it points out the importance of supplemental information about real-life experience for adequately assessing and tailoring individual rehabilitation interventions.

25

Everyday self-awareness: implications for self-esteem, depression, and resistance to therapy
THOMAS J. FIGURSKI

The significance of self-awareness to the therapeutic process has long been recognized by psychiatrists and clinical psychologists. Freudian psychoanalysis encourages the conscious exploration of one's emotional and behavioral responses to facilitate the resolution of an emotional conflict. In Kohut's (1971) self-psychology, the focus is even more specifically on the individual's inner experience of relations between self and others (Wolf, 1987). Client-centered therapists (Rogers, 1961; Gendlin, 1973), although espousing a very different theoretical orientation, also encourage their clients to focus directly on and explore their personal experience in order to actualize their full potential as human beings. Similarly, cognitive therapies (Beck, 1976; Ellis, 1973) direct clients' attention to their maladaptive ways of thinking about themselves and their interpersonal interactions. Even behaviorists, dissatisfied with the focus on mental and emotional content (Skinner, 1953; Wolpe, 1958; 1969), will direct their clients' attention to observable behavioral symptoms and the development of more functional and desirable behavior.

Whatever the clinician's particular bias, the nature of psychotherapy is such that the person is required to attend to the self, whether the focus is on one's emotional experience, cognitive processes, or behavioral patterns. It would be ludicrous to suggest that the client could participate effectively in the therapeutic process without paying attention to the self. Yet while self-awareness is generally understood to be a fundamental element of psychotherapy, relatively little consideration has been given by clinicians to the direct effects of this basic cognitive operation.

Experimental social psychology has, over the last two decades, given considerable attention to the relationship between self-awareness and emotional experience. In particular, Duval & Wicklund (1972) have argued that self-awareness is generally an aversive experience, because when people become self-aware, they tend to evaluate themselves against an ideal, and thus usually focus on their shortcomings as compared to that ideal.

This pattern of response certainly has implications for psychotherapy, which relies on the client's ability to process information about the self. Such a pattern would help to explain why people are resistant to therapy. If the necessary self-awareness is going to produce the emotional discomfort associated with a negative self-evaluation, then resisting therapy represents an attractive alternative. Indeed, experimental research (Ickes, Wicklund & Ferris, 1973; Duval & Wicklund, 1973) has found that avoiding self-awareness is a typical response under conditions of negative self-evaluation. Accordingly, under the conditions that generally draw people to therapy, i.e. experiencing a particular emotional or functional difficulty, one would expect the aversiveness of self-awareness to be manifest.

To the extent that this cognitive-emotional process leads the individual to resist therapy, the Rogerian position that one of the therapist's primary functions is to encourage the client's self-esteem by creating an atmosphere of unconditional positive regard is supported. If the client can become self-aware without evaluating himself negatively, then the resistance to therapy breaks down.

Other clinical implications of the relationship between self-awareness, negative self-evaluation, and aversive emotional experience are developed by recent research on depression. Following Beck (1976), Pyszczynski & Greenberg (1987) have noted that depressives have a tendency to perseverate their negative self-evaluation, whereas non-depressives do not. They suggest that the depressive's style of perseverated self-awareness under conditions of low self-evaluation serves to exacerbate the low self-esteem and negative affect that are symptomatic of depression.

Experimental studies of self-awareness have relied primarily on inducing self-awareness in a laboratory or measuring general tendencies toward self-consciousness by self-report questionnaires. In contrast, the Experience Sampling Method (ESM) allows us to collect information on one's awareness and emotional experience across a range of specific everyday-life situations. This makes it possible to examine situational differences in the relationship between self-awareness and emotional experience as it occurs in the natural context of everyday life.

Early studies (Csikszentmihalyi & Figurski, 1982; Franzoi & Brewer, 1984) of this issue indicated that naturally-occurring self-awareness was *not* generally associated with a negative affect. To the extent that ESM research can identify the conditions under which self-awareness is or is not aversive, it can suggest approaches for clinically addressing the related problems of low self-esteem, depression, and resistance. Knowing under what conditions self-awareness is aversive can be very helpful to the clinician whose task is to create a therapeutic context within which the client can attend to the self without automatically generating a negative self-evaluation. A clinical process that does not threaten the client's self-esteem is less likely to exacerbate depression or produce resistance.

The present paper will discuss how ESM research on the conditional relationship between self-awareness and emotional experience can aid the therapist's efforts to create the most therapeutically effective context. Relevant to this general consideration is the more specific question of how emotional experience is related to the particular type of self-awareness that is encouraged.

Private and public self-awareness

Research in social psychology has distinguished between 'private' and 'public' self-awareness, according to whether one is attending to internal or external aspects of the self. Whereas private self-awareness focuses on content not directly observable to others, such as emotional experience, physical sensations, thoughts, and attitudes, public self-awareness focuses on externally-observable aspects of the self, such as appearance, behavior, and expressions (Fenigstein, Scheier & Buss, 1975).

While the difference between private and public self-awareness was originally defined as a difference in content, it essentially depends on the differential use of perspective (see Figurski, 1987a). The publicly observable aspects of one's own external presentation (e.g. appearance) are accessed by considering the perspective of the other. In contrast, the more private, internal aspects of one's own personal experience (e.g. emotions, bodily sensations) are directly accessible only to the 'privileged' point of reference one has by virtue of *being* the object of attention. Thus, internal or experiential self-content is addressed from the 'egocentric' perspective, which relies on a point of reference anchored in one's physical self. External self-content is addressed from the 'allocentric' perspective, which uses a point of reference outside the self.

The ability to take the perspective of the other was emphasized as critical to the development of the self by early theorists interested in identity formation. Cooley (1902) and Mead (1934), in particular, articulated how the child develops an understanding of the self by interpreting the responses of significant other people (see also Flavell, 1968).

Effective communication and healthy relationships with others require an accurate understanding of how one is perceived by others. Consideration of these different perspectives can thus be helpful for purposes of self-understanding and interpersonal relationship. If there are different emotional responses to the different kinds of self-awareness, then this is important to the therapeutic process.

A study of everyday self-awareness

In light of self-awareness theory and the difference between private and public self-awareness, a study (Figurski, 1985) was specifically designed to address the question of how the everyday occurrence of these two forms of self-awareness is related to self-evaluation and the quality of affective experience. Using the ESM, 31 subjects provided repeated reports of their self-awareness, self-evaluation, and affect across a variety of situational contexts over the course of one week. Consistent with the standard procedure for this method (Csikszentmihalyi & Larson, this volume), subjects were signalled via an electronic paging device on eight occasions each day according to a schedule randomized within two-hour segments. Subjects were instructed to fill out a short report form each time they were signalled.

Information regarding the subjects' self-awareness was provided by their responses to a series of four-point rating scales (0 = 'not aware' to 3 = 'very aware') on the Experience Sampling Form (ESF) that addressed the content of their awareness. Two of these items provided separate summary ratings of their public and private self-awareness. Public self-awareness was indicated by a rating of the extent to which one was 'aware of how you looked, sounded, or appeared'. Private self-awareness was operationalized by a rating of the extent to which one was 'aware of how you were personally experiencing something'. Intercorrelations with more specific awareness items (e.g. 'your physical appearance', 'your words and expressions', 'your feelings and emotions', and 'your plans and intentions') were consistent with the definition of public and private self-awareness as focusing on external and internal self-aspects, respectively, indicating construct validity.

The quality of one's self-evaluation in each reported experience was designated by the mean score of four items, which specifically addressed the subjects' feelings of evaluation toward themselves. These included the semantic differentials 'self-critical–self-approving', 'embarrassed–proud', 'inadequate–competent', and 'weak–strong', each rated on a seven-point scale. The four ratings were found to correlate with each other 0.50 or more (Pearson's r, $P < 0.001$).

The general affective quality of a reported experience was designated by the mean of the ratings on three other semantic differentials: 'irritable–cheerful', 'sad–happy', and 'hostile–friendly'. Earlier ESM research (Csikszentmihalyi & Graef, 1980; Csikszentmihalyi & Larson, 1984) had found these scales to intercorrelate highly. This study was consistent with that, producing correlations greater than 0.70 (Pearson's r, $P < 0.001$).

The everyday use of self-awareness

Both the frequency with which subjects indicated they were privately or publicly self-aware and the mean intensity for each form of self-awareness are informative (Figurski, 1987a). Subjects indicated they were at least 'somewhat aware' of their personal experience on 88% of the 1298 reports. They indicated at least some public self-awareness on 77% of their reports. Previous estimates of the frequency with which attention is focused primarily on private self-aspects (37%) or public self-aspects (23%) were considerably lower (see Hormuth, 1986, p. 285). The difference is probably attributable to the earlier research indicating the primary focus of attention and thereby not including low levels of self-awareness. Whereas use of the four-point rating scale still allows for the identification of high self-awareness situations, it also indicates that at least some degree of private and public self-awareness is the rule, not the exception.

This points to the need for examining variations in the degree of self-awareness. A more precise indication of the relative use of the two forms of self-awareness is provided by the mean intensity, which refers to the full range of the four-point rating scale. Mean ratings of intensity were 1.84 for private self-awareness and 1.39 for public self-awareness ($t = 5.90$, $P < 0.001$). Thus, private self-awareness is more prevalent than public self-awareness, whether the indicator is frequency or mean intensity. This finding is expecially important because it indicates that, while people may use both perspectives to attend to the self, the tendency to consider the perspective of another is not as great as the tendency to use one's own egocentric perspective. Thus theories that emphasize public self-aspects as critical to self-definition and the formation of a self-concept fail to acknowledge appropriately those internal/experiential aspects that are the primary focus of self-awareness.

Furthermore, personal self-awareness tendencies were found to be related to the way the individual attended to other people as well, although perhaps not as might be expected. Subjects who were more aware of their own public aspects were found to be more attentive to the internal experience of others. That public self-consciousness is related to a more empathic awareness of others' experience demonstrates how taking the perspective of the other addresses different content for self and others. The implication of these data is that public self-consciousness and empathy, both grounded in the ability to use the allocentric perspective, may develop and even function together. Theoretically, perhaps people (including therapists) can develop their empathic skills by first directing their attention to their own public aspects and thus facilitating their use of the allocentric perspective. For clients who have difficulty with interpersonal relationships, perhaps public self-awareness can develop their perspective-taking skill, which will improve the quality of their interpersonal interaction by making them more sensitive to the experience of others (see Figurski, 1987a).

The relationship among self-awareness, self-evaluation, and affect

Such discussion illustrates how ESM data can be used to examine both group patterns and individual differences in everyday interpersonal attention. Further analysis, addressing the relationship that self-awareness has with emotional experience, demonstrates the utility of the ESM for investigating situational differences and patterns within individuals. Results from this set of analyses produced three general conclusions (Figurski, 1987b):

(1) Self-awareness was not negatively related to self-evaluation, as suggested by original self-awareness theory.
(2) However, self-evaluation and affect were positively related, as expected by self-awareness theory.
(3) Self-awareness interacted with self-evaluation in its relationship to affect, but differently for private and public self-awareness. Specifically:
(a) private self-awareness was associated with a more negative affect, but only if self-evaluation was negative; and
(b) public self-awareness was associated with a more positive affect, but only if self-evaluation was positive. (See Fig. 25.1.)

The significance of self-evaluation to these relationships between self-awareness and affect is partially consistent with self-awareness theory. Certainly, the prediction that self-awareness is aversive is based on a hypothesized increase in negative self-evaluation. Furthermore, Wicklund (1975) acknowledged that if self-evaluation is positive, then self-awareness would be expected to produce a correspondingly positive affect. However, he maintained that such positive self-evaluation when self-aware was relatively rare, arguing that as people come to match or exceed their standards they continue to adjust them upwards and subsequent self-evaluation is generally negative.

To the contrary, the ESM data indicated that, in everyday life, neither private self-awareness nor public self-awareness correlated strongly with self-evaluation (Pearson's $r = -0.04$ and 0.13, respectively). Similarly, self-evaluation was not more negative for conditions specifically identified as either high private or high public self-awareness (using each subject's personal median to create split-halves). Self-evaluation even tended to rise slightly if public self-awareness was high.

Allowing that self-evaluation varies independently of self-awareness, its role as a variable important to the relationship between self-awareness and affect was nonetheless supported. What is especially important about the results of this study is that private and public self-awareness related differently to affect and that these relationships existed under different conditions of self-evaluation.

These data suggest that the aversiveness of self-awareness as it occurs in everyday life is limited to particular conditions, specifically those in which self-evaluation is low and the self-awareness is focused on experiential aspects of the self. It also suggests that self-awareness can be a positive, reinforcing experience under other conditions: when self-evaluation is high and attention

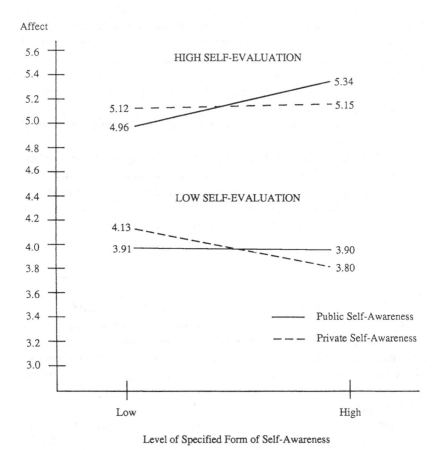

Fig. 25.1. The relationship between self-awareness and affect for conditions of high and low self-evaluation.

is focused on external aspects of the self. These findings may be related to a combination of methodological factors that differentiate ESM from experimental approaches as discussed elsewhere in this volume (Csikszentmihalyi & Larson).

The finding, however, that the relationships between self-awareness and affect occur only under particular conditions of experience suggests that the two forms of self-awareness serve different functions. Specifically, that private self-awareness is related to a more negative affect only under conditions of negative self-evaluation suggests it performs some function specific to feeling bad. Conversely, that public self-awareness is related to a more positive affect only under conditions of positive self-evaluation suggests it performs some function specific to feeling good. One plausible interpretation of this pattern is that private self-awareness serves to troubleshoot negative experience, with the function of determining what adjustments are necessary, while public self-awareness operates primarily under conditions of positive experience, with the function of reinforcing one's positive image (Figurski, 1987b).

Clinical implications

While these findings have implications for the applicability of self-awareness theory to everyday life, they also have implications for clinical practice, particularly with regard to the depressive self-focusing style, the significance of the client's self-evaluation, and resistance to therapy.

As indicated, Pyszczynski & Greenberg (1987) have suggested that depression is characterized by a perseveration of self-awareness that serves to maintain a negative evaluation of oneself. The ESM study discussed here suggests that private self-awareness (and not public self-awareness) is especially instrumental in this process. Thus, a heightened attentiveness to one's internal, experiential aspects under the miserable affective conditions of depression could easily facilitate an unending depressive loop of the kind Pyszczynski and Greenberg describe. If public self-awareness is unrelated to affect under these conditions, it has no function in maintaining depression and is thus less likely to characterize this pathology. Such a high private, low public self-awareness is consistent with the inner-directedness and social withdrawal that typifies the classic depressive symptomology.

Similarly, the interaction of negative self-evaluation and private self-awareness may explain client resistance to therapy. The ESM data suggest that the self-awareness that accompanies psychotherapy will not in and of itself produce a negative self-evaluation. However, under conditions of negative self-evaluation, an increase in private self-awareness has been indicated to be associated with a more negative affective experience. Whereas (1) negative self-evaluation is more likely to occur among individuals forced to acknowledge a dysfunction, and (2) private self-awareness is required by those clinical approaches that seek to process one's emotional and cognitive functioning, most psychotherapy represents just the kind of condition that would be expected to precipitate aversion. The negative affect found to accompany such conditions may explain the tendency of clients to resist. Furthermore, the two conditions specify two forms of resistance. The client can either (1) avoid negative self-evaluation by denying the problem, or (2) avoid private self-awareness by refusing to attend to internal emotional or cognitive processes.

Likewise, this pattern of relationship among self-awareness, self-evaluation, and affect identifies how the therapist may intervene. That resistance is in part a response to felt or threatened negative self-evaluation illustrates the utility of the Rogerian emphasis on establishing a context of unconditional positive regard for the client. To the extent that the client can become less critical of the self, attending to one's private emotional and cognitive processes will not be so aversive, and the likelihood of resistance will be reduced.

Whereas decreasing the negative self-evaluation is one therapeutic intervention suggested by this pattern of relationship, another would be the deliberate manipulation of private and public self-awareness. Specifically, the options would be to reduce private self-awareness or increase public self-awareness, the effectiveness of which would depend in part on the level of self-evaluation. Behaviorists attempt both, rejecting what they see as an unproductive focus on private aspects of the self and directing attention to behavioral functioning.

Often, it may not be possible to reduce private self-awareness, either because it is part of the pathology, as in the depressive's perseverated self-focusing style, or because it is necessary to address a particular emotional difficulty or inappropriate cognitive response. Under such circumstances, however, it may be possible to raise the client's public self-awareness. If, under conditions of low self-evaluation, private self-awareness is especially aversive and responsible for resistance, then perhaps directing the client's attention to public aspects of the self will be more tolerated and – at least initially – allow the client to be more responsive to the therapeutic process. Similarly, if private self-awareness is perseverated and thereby responsible for exacerbating depression, then perhaps a heightened public self-awareness will help to disrupt this pattern.

As suggested earlier, directing clients' attention to their own public aspects forces them to consider the allocentric perspective. Developing this perspective-taking skill will not only allow them to become more responsive to the experience of others. It may also enable them to emerge from an overwhelming focus on their own personal misery. In either case, focusing on external self-aspects may operate in conjunction with the therapist's unconditional positive regard until the client becomes comfortable enough within the therapeutic relationship to pursue more private issues productively.

Conclusions

These clinical implications of the ESM research on self-awareness need to be addressed more directly with continued investigation. Yet, this discussion demonstrates how the ESM can be used to elucidate the relationship among cognitive, emotional, and situational variables as they occur in the naturalistic context of human functioning. With regard to this particular research on the emotional experience of everyday self-awareness, the role of self-evaluation and the different patterns found for private and public self-awareness serve to inform earlier work on self-awareness theory and the depressive self-focusing style.

It is only by exploring the implications of this research that we can identify the issues that need to be addressed. Toward that end, consider the following:

private self-awareness and public self-awareness are related differently to affective experience, such that private self-awareness is more likely to be associated with aversive experience than public self-awareness. This is conditional on a negative self-evaluation, which is determined by factors other than the level of self-awareness. This suggests that (1) resistance to therapy may be due in part to the aversiveness of attending to the private aspects of the self under conditions of negative self-evaluation; (2) the perseverated self-focusing style associated with depression may be specific to private self-awareness; (3) the raising of self-esteem, whether by unconditional positive regard or other measures, is an important element to the therapeutic process; and (4) public self-awareness may serve as a useful means of (a) increasing client responsiveness without increasing negative affect and (b) exercising the client's perspective-taking ability and empathic skills.

PART V

Psychiatric research applications: practical
issues and attention points

26

Practical issues in psychiatric applications of ESM

MARTEN W. deVRIES

In spite of the success of ESM in describing mental disorders in context, there are limitations. ESM asks more of the subject than a survey instrument, questionnaire or interview. It demands a look into the private world and experience of the individual over an often prolonged period of time. Creating an environment of trust, required for compliance and accurate reporting, is a crucial and practical part of the Experience Sample process that may not be casually passed over. In this Section, the article discussing compliance in elderly depressed patients is a good example of the care that is required in sampling certain groups. Heroin addicts, studied by Kaplan, serve as a good example of research methods tailored to the life style of the population under investigation. Special care must be taken in creating a research alliance and in selecting appropriate questions that speak to and access the experiental world of a specific group, while remaining true to the diagnostic requirements of the mental disorder under study. In addition, careful attention needs to be paid to planning the timing and intensity of the time-sampling procedure. The ability of patients to comply with the signaling schedule and a 'good fit' with temporal nature of the phenomena under study such as stress, panic or 'getting high', are crucial considerations. Although smaller than expected initially there are specific limits to the use of the ESM. Difficulties have been encountered in sampling elderly subjects with dementia, individuals with severe melancholia and the acutely psychotic. Limitations in sampling have further been experienced in specific social contexts. Families with disordered relations, for instance, have proved problematic in that a conspiracy against reporting accurately can influence the data. Such family and communication dynamics also play a role in the sampling of dependent individuals like the elderly. When these problems present, the active involvement and engagement of the mental health worker and the family in the research process is recommended for the establishment of a research alliance.

Practical problems and attention points not covered in previous sections in this volume are discussed here. The first chapter addresses question selection for the self-report. The process of determining the psychometric validity of the items chosen for a study on depression is described. The chapter is followed by a discussion of the limits of compliance in a sample of depressed elderly. In the other chapters practical attention points are highlighted within the context of ongoing studies. Analytic strategies, such as the importance of calculating base rates for understanding behavior and the utility of analyzing infrequently occurring events in time-use data, are presented. The last article discusses the practical consequences of the time-sampling schedule for the quality of the data gathered and the analyses performed. In the remainder of this introductory chapter, to round out the practical considerations, issues of subject recruitment, research alliance and informing the subject about the goals of the study, i.e. briefing and debriefing, as well as a coding strategy for the 'open-ended' questions, are presented.

Sample recruitment

When using a method that spends so much time and energy on accumulating detailed information about the person, it is easy to overlook requirements for sampling individuals at the group level. ESM studies to date have been primarily concerned with demonstrating the use and feasibility of the method in psychiatry. While diagnosis was stringent and subjects were carefully chosen, the studies were not rigorously designed to control for demographic and individual influences. Since ESM seeks the high resolution of experiential variables, subjects should be grouped as homogeneously as possible. One sampling strategy that achieves this is Snowball Sampling (Kaplan et al., 1987), a technique that requests individuals to name others like them, who in turn again name others like them. This creates a sample saturated for a particular characteristic such as heroin use. Careful diagnoses and comparability in demographic characteristics, age, sex, chronicity etc., are also important. Severity and duration of illness are also important factors, if we wish to determine whether the findings that discriminate groups, are, indeed, attributable to a particularly psychopathological type, and not due to other factors. For example, the idiosyncratic experience of the individual and the pervasive effect of being ill must be controled for. Control groups should be matched and selected with care. Chronic mental patients, for example, should be compared not to normals from whom they differ greatly, but to other individuals with a chronic disorder, medical or not. Such a procedure could discriminate the psychopathological effects from the long-term effects of illness represented in both groups. In short, the confounding effects of illness, sex, age and employment are important elements to consider in setting up an ESM study, particularly if time-use, activities and setting effects are of interest.

Future studies will require intensive attention to subject selection and sample size. As ESM data accumulate and provide insight into psychiatrically valid and meaningful measures of mental state and situations, larger samples may be required to clarify their impact. In larger samples, the effects of individual characteristics may thus be ascertained and sufficient data on the relatively low frequency of important situations and states may be gathered. Another solution to the problem of sampling low frequency but important instances has been to sample only the event under study, such as panic attacks (Margraf et al., 1987). While event-sampling introduces confounding reactivity factors into the description of situations, for some problems and syndromes it may be ideally suited. A quasi-experiential, multimethods approach that includes the oversampling of certain periods of the day or sampling in situations where an event is likely to occur, such as at work, is perhaps a better approach that preserves the ecological validity of the report as well as providing baseline data.

Research alliance

Obtaining ESM data requires care and concern. The method is a means for communicating with people about their daily lives; this requires an alliance and mutual understanding about the research procedure and aims of the study. Most participants find the procedure both taxing and rewarding. Cooperation and compliance depend on their trust, and their belief that the research is worthwhile, as well as on standardized instructions. Before beginning, during the briefing, the purpose of the research is explained to the subjects, an interest in learning about their daily experience, as well as the occurrence of their symptoms is communicated. The participants are given control of the signaling device in that they can turn it off, if they do not want to be disturbed. It is stressed, however, that as complete a set of reports of the week as possible, needs to be obtained in order to carry out a proper analysis of the data. At the conclusion, during the debriefing, the sampling period is reviewed and the self-report forms are checked. Some weeks later the data obtained may be shared with the subject. This standard procedure may need to be adapted to the specific disorders under study. A group may require more or less incentive to participate. For example, heroin addicts required additional contact and support during the week to retain participation, while subjects in a myocardial infarct study could be left alone for up to three weeks without a decrease in response rate.

Subject recruitment

Subjects participating in ESM research are asked to carry a programed terminal watch or other signaling device over a period of time ranging from roughly three to 30 days. Each time they hear a signal – usually ten times a day, at randomized moments – they fill in a questionnaire concerning their physical and mental status at the moment of the beep. Compliance is often highest when a person is in active treatment. In health care settings, the researcher together with the therapist may decide whether a subject meets the criteria for a particular study. The subject is approached by the therapist who remains an important ingredient in the research compliance. When the subject's informed consent is gathered, a brief explanation of the research is given and an appointment for the 'briefing' is made. Alternative recruitment approaches to that sketched here are discussed in other chapters in this volume. One potentially useful and often clinically helpful strategy is the testing of individuals who are temporarily on waiting lists for clinical care. ESM information is thus available to both client and therapist when treatment ensues. It may further help the patient to clarify his problem to himself.

The briefing

During the briefing, instructions are given about the use of the beeper and how to fill out answers to the questions in the booklets. Subjects are asked to go through the self-report form and each item is discussed with them. Additional, cross-selectional data, diagnosis, etc. are gathered at this time. At the end of this session the patient is asked to fill in the questionnaire after a simulated beep, to check whether the instructions have been well understood. As a reminder, the instructions are also printed on the inside cover of the booklet. The name of the responsible researcher is provided, who may be contacted if there are any questions or difficulties. Next, the signaling device is described; how it works, how to turn it on and off and how to turn the beep off after a signal has been received. Subjects are instructed to fill out self-reports as soon as possible after a signal. Situations in which this will be difficult (e.g. driving a car, etc.) are discussed. They are asked whether there are any circumstances when they would not want the beeper to disturb them (e.g. in church) or when it might be difficult to carry it on their person (e.g. during sports). Strategies for how they could still be signaled (e.g. by having someone on the sidelines carrying the watch) are discussed. The random schedule of signals is described. Patients are told that the beeper may be turned off if they go to bed or nap during the sampling period. Next, the organizational form of the self-report may be discussed in greater detail. Since thoughts at the time of a signal are the most difficult to catch, they are asked about first. Response difficulties such as these are shared with the subject. They are asked to do their best in providing as much detail as possible. The intent of questions is fully described, for example, 'Where were you?' should be answered as specifically as possible, i.e. room in the house, etc. They are also asked to be specific about their activities and social contact, without overly compromising their privacy.

Likert-scale items, (semantic differentials or other question types) are rehearsed to ensure the subject has a feel for the concept of grading his internal state. The entire list is run through to make sure the subject understands the meaning of each question. Likert scales have proven most efficient for ill populations since other types of self-report scales (semantic differentials, etc.) often proved too difficult to interpret for people under stress. Further, the subjects are discouraged from showing their completed booklets to others and asked not to look back through previously completed forms. At the end, the need for privacy is again supported, but response to as many of the signals as possible is encouraged.

The debriefing

The actual sampling period usually starts the morning after the briefing. At the end of the sampling period, a new appointment is made for the debriefing. Here, the subject is given an opportunity to describe his experiences during the week. The researcher checks the following items:

> The influence of the ESM on mood, activities, social contacts during the period.
> If the sampling was disturbing to the individual's normal routine.
> If the subject had been able to give a representative picture of his experiences.
> If there had been any difficulty in answering the questions.
> Special events that occurred during the sampling period.
> If the subject is willing to participate in the research again.

The researcher checks the booklet at this time for legibility, ambiguities, etc. to minimize coding and analytic mistakes during the next phase of the research.

Data transformation and coding example

The ESM booklet structures the data in the form of Likert scales and open-ended questions. Only responses to a beep signal given within 15 min after the beep are considered valid and used in the analysis. A subject must have given 20 valid responses to be included.

The Likert scale scores from 1–7 or semantic differentials are punched directly into the computer for analyses. Open-ended questions: what are you doing (activity), where are you (place), who are you with (social environment), and thought content are coded according to the schemes shown in Table 26.1. The coded categories are examples of reduced categories partly based on the international time-budget study, for use in group level analyses (Robinson, 1987; Szalai et al., 1972). Consistent inter-rater reliability for these reduced codes as well as more specific categories (not discussed here) have been good to excellent with a range of Kappa values from 0.83 to 0.97. The detailed responses to open-ended questions are also available for more detailed analyses at the individual level.

Table 26.1. *Reduced coding categories*

Activity	Place
Inactivity	At home
Work and study	Network (family friends)
Maintenance activities	Work/study
Introspection	Health care setting
Leisure	Public places outdoors (street, park)
Socialization	Public places indoors (shop, pub)
Meals	Transport
Organizational activities	
Other activities	
Social environment	**Thought content**
Alone	Nothing
Alone with pets	Self-physical
Household members (relatives at home)	Self-psychic
Non-resident 'family' members	Other persons
Friends	Environment, context
Colleagues, neighbours, health care	Activities
Professional, other acquaintances	Experience Sampling
Strangers	Cannot score
	Empty

The following dimensions of thought are given special attention and coded separately:

(1) The *content* of the thought: what were you thinking about?
(2) The *evaluation* of the type of thought: such as planning, anticipating, neutral evaluation? etc.
(3) The *orientation* of the thought in *time* (prospective, retrospective, here and now)?
(4) The *congruency* of the thought with the activity (thinking about what you are doing)?
(5) The *experience* of the thought content (positive/negative)?
(6) The *pathology* of the thought (ruminating, delusional, etc.).

Further, what is written on the report form may be coded. The coding of handwriting style, the number of words used, neologisms, spelling, etc. have all been tried with success. For example, with this method, changes in handwriting style have been a good indicator of both anxiety and the extrapyramidal side-effects of neuroleptic medication, such as micrographia. A variant of this approach using more open-ended reporting schemes was developed by Hurlburt (1987, 1989). A narrative description of thoughts at a signal is requested followed by an intensive interview at the end of the day or sampling period. This allows a more detailed analysis of individual thoughts and experience than is typically carried out. In the chapters that follow the authors discuss practical aspects of ESM in the context of ongoing studies. The Section is meant to provide a practical guide for those interested in research applications as well as for the interested clinician.

27

Selecting measures, diagnostic validity and scaling in the study of depression

HERRO KRAAN, HELENA MEERTENS, MARCEL HILWIG, LEX VOLOVICS, CHANTAL I. M. DIJKMAN-CAES and PIET PORTEGIJS

Over the last decades research on depression has expanded considerably. Improved classification (DSM-III-R) and psychometric testing (Hamilton rating scale, Zung scale, etc.) resulted in an increase in reliable epidemiological data. The latter confirm the importance of depression as a health problem: the prevalence of major depression is 6–10%, mounting to 25% when 'minor syndromes' are taken into account (a.o. Goldberg et al., 1980).

In addition to improved classification and psychometric evaluation of depressive phenomena, psychosocial determinants have also been studied from broad theoretical viewpoints. Distortions in cognition (Beck et al., 1979), negative attributional styles (Peterson & Seligman, 1984; Tennen et al., 1987), lack of social skills (Coyne, 1976, 1985) and inadequate stress appraisal and coping (Lazarus & Folkman, 1984) have been conceptualized as causal intrapsychic mechanisms in depression. From a social psychiatric viewpoint the interaction between life events and long-standing difficulties on the one and and vulnerability factors (e.g. lack of intimacy, young children at home) and protective factors ('buffering social support') on the other hand have strengthened the theoretical base for preventive and curative interventions (Brown et al., 1986, 1987; Lin et al., 1985; Holahan & Moos, 1987).

In spite of the many theoretical approaches research on depression suffers from methodological one-sidedness. In an overview of the broad field of depression research, some salient features can be observed. The designs are generally experimental or quasi-experimental with a paucity of naturalistic studies that take the influence of psychosocial contexts of daily life into account. Furthermore, the studies tend to test one theoretical hypothesis at a time, attending primarily to precipitating and causal factors and not those factors that maintain depression. Finally, the concept of 'depression' leans heavily on the 'objectivistic', expert-based DSM-III criteria, neglecting the subjective experience by patients.

The Experience Sampling Method (ESM) challenges this one-sidedness by creating a data set, which is qualitatively different from those obtained with the retrospective approaches cited above. The ESM uses repeated self-assessments to study the variability in cognitions, emotions, symptoms, motivation and activities of depressive patients prospectively in their natural settings. To these self-assessments of depressive states, we link assessments of daily microstressors (Zautra et al., 1986; Folkman et al., 1986) and perceived social support (Lin et al., 1985; Holahan & Moos, 1987). Moreover, ESM collects systematic data about the ongoing experience of physical and social contexts to which the ever-changing clinical picture of depression is related. Finally, ESM prevents retrospective bias, because subjects are requested to report about a moment immediately after a signal. In this sense, ESM data might be called 'spective', because subjects only use their immediate memory functions as opposed to more traditional psychometric and epidemiological instruments whose primarily short- and long-term memory functions are used. This is particularly important in depression, since the retrospective memory bias of the depressive patients (Blaney, 1986) can be circumvented. ESM thus creates fundamentally new data on depression.

The ESM has the potential to offer clinicians and researchers a supplement to the objectivistic and expert-based DSM-III by providing a systematic and standardized assessment of the subjective experience of depressive state characteristics and intensity. Using this subjective approach it may become evident that the symptoms from which the patient suffers the most, may differ from current diagnostic criteria. For instance, a patient with a major depressive episode may be suffering from fatigue (not a core symptom, like dysphoric mood or loss of interest or pleasure) or from loneliness (not a diagnostic criterium at all). In a standardized way ESM may shed light on the subjective dimensions of depressive states, that allow new ways to dimensional classification of depression. Furthermore, the ESM provides a possibility of assessing concomitantly important contextual variables such as experienced daily stress and perceived social support in order to investigate possible factors that maintain depression.

In this chapter we describe the results of a pilot study in which we adapted the ESM for research in depression, and ask the following questions:

Which of the items, derived from expert-based criteria are selected by depressive patients to describe their subjective, psychological states?
Are the selected items suitable for repeated self-reports and do they show variability?
Do the selected items cluster into internal consistent and scalable dimensions?
What is the reliability (individual consistency of self-assessment over six days; intercoder reliability of the open ESM categories) and the validity

(convergency and divergency patterns; distinction of levels of intensity) of the ESM in depression?

Assembling the item domain

First we created a panel of clinical and research experts on depression who selected items and questions from a range of psychometric and clinical sources. Items were selected from the DSM-III-R (APA, 1987) and Research Diagnostic Criteria (Spitzer et al., 1978) concerning major depressive episode, dysthymia and the depressive period of cyclothymic disorders. The panel also studied depression questionnaires like the Zung Depression Scale (Zung & Durhan, 1965), the Beck Depression Inventory (Beck et al., 1961), the Hamilton Depression Rating Scale (Hamilton, 1960), the PVP (Plutchik & van Praag, 1987) and the Carroll scale (Carroll et al., 1981) for items and scaling possibilities.

The Likert-type items and open-ended questions were included using the following criteria:

The ESM item-domain should define depression in terms of disturbances of mood, affect, thinking, activity/initiative, social behavior and somatic functioning.
Items should describe state-like properties (instead of traits).
Item content and number should be suitable for rapidly repeated measurement: within four to five minutes.

The items were organized in modules starting with a module about depressive thinking. The open question:'What did you think at the moment of the beep?' raises important theoretical issues. According to Beck (Beck et al., 1979) negative thoughts about the self, the future and the world are determinants of a depressive mood. Further, depression may be characterized by particular modes of thought like brooding, worrying, obsessing and by loss of concentration. These thoughts may be coded according to content of the thinking. Next, Likert items allowing a cognitive self-appraisal on a seven-point scale are offered (e.g. concentration, speed of thinking, brooding, pleasant thought). The next module deals with mood and affect and starts with the question 'How did you feel at the moment of the beep: . . .', after which Likert items like sad, cheerful, guilty, anxious, self-assured are filled in. Next, a module about somatic functioning assesses states such as energetic, hungry, tired, main and other complaints. The question 'What were you doing at the moment of the beep?' starts the activity/motivation module. In depression, psychomotor disturbances are often involved; these are reflected in a decrease of motivation and activity. The coding system of the open question encompasses activities like work, household, self-care, doing nothing, etc. Next, Likert

326

items about the motivation for the specific activity are rated. The physical context module opens with the question 'Where were you at the moment of the beep?'. The answers to this open question are coded with categories like at home, work, public places, transport, etc. Finally, open questions about the social context ('with whom?') are asked. Coding categories pertinent to this question are alone, partner, children, friends, strangers, etc.

Especially for the research in depression, theoretically important concepts like perceived social support and experienced microstressors have been included. Perceived social support and its underlying dimensions (emotional support, practical and material help, cognitive guidance) derive their import-ance from the buffering theory of stress. According to this theory social sup-port may protect individuals from developing depressive symptoms in case of stress (Alloway et al., 1987). From the underlying dimensions of social support Likert-type items are derived, like feeling appreciated, secure, rejected, disap-pointed, etc., which are included in the ESM form. Microstressors as an operationalization of daily stress are assessed with the question 'Did something (un)pleasant occur to you between the present and the previous beep?'. Microstressors are defined as observable events, experienced by the individual as salient, dangerous, threatening ('a hassle') or meaningful and favorable to his/her wellbeing ('an uplift'). These daily events should be discernible from the severe, drastic, sporadically occurring 'major life events'. Microstressors are considered as aetiological and maintaining factors in depression (Kanner et al., 1981; Monroe, 1983). At the beep the subject is asked to recall whether a hassle or uplift occurred during the period starting from the previous beep. In this way characteristics of a microstressor prior to a present beep (to a maxi-mum of 90 min) are measured during this present beep. Because of this time interval such a daily event cannot directly be connected with the mental states measured at the beep-level. In contrast with the other modules the assessment of microstressors has a more retrospective character and relies upon short-term memory.

Theoretically, important aspects in microstressors are their predictability, (un)desirability and meaning (e.g. the event being a social entrance or exit). Further the impact of daily events depends on the degree to which it can be prevented, initiated and controlled by the subject (Dohrenwend & Shrout, 1985; Zautra et al., 1986; Zautra et al., 1988; Lazarus, 1984). These theoreti-cal aspects are reflected in several Likert-type items and coding categories. Coding takes place only when the daily event passes the criteria derived from the aforementioned definition of 'microstressor'. If so, the event is coded, according to its content, e.g. work, education, household, social network, health, children, etc.

Finally, socalled contextual assessment (Brown & Harris, 1978) is carried out during the coding. This is an estimation of the impact of an event on the individual by a well-informed interviewer. The latter is told during the brief-ing interview about the history and biography of the subject, and has addi-tional, standardized information about chronic life difficulties and their subjective severity. The latter are obtained with the socalled Groningen List of Long-standing Difficulties (GLLM; a Dutch adaptation of a comparable instrument used by Brown et al., 1988). Armed with this information a rater attributes an impact weight to the microstressor based on his/her knowledge of the subject's chronic difficulties.

The pilot study

The pilot study was carried out in an ambulatory mental health centre with a catchment area of 200,000 people. About 60% of the new patients from this catchment area with mental health problems are admitted to this centre (2000–2100 yearly). The remaining new patients are admitted to the out-patient departments of the general or the psychiatric hospital. More severe depressives slightly prevail in the psychiatric hospital. The ambulatory mental health center provides a variety of short- and long-term psychotherapy, psychopharmacological treatments and offers programs for chronic mental patients. The center has a strong primary care orientation to mental health.

Subjects

Over a two-month period we recruited subjects from newly referred patients to the ambulatory mental health centre. To obtain a broad spectrum of depres-sives we started with the DSM-III-R criteria for major depressive episode, but attenuated the obligatory number of symptoms from five to four to include a group with a less-severe clinical picture. Excluded were subjects with psycho-organic, substance-abuse and psychotic disorders. Next, from other depart-ments of the ambulatory mental health center depressive patients in remission have been recruited. Non-depressive subjects from the community were asked to participate as controls. The following subjects were selected:
- −16 newly admitted patients (with minimally four DSM-III-R criteria for major depression). 8 male; 8 female; age, 22–50.
- −6 patients with a depression in remission: 2 male; 4 female; age, 34–67.
- −4 normals: 1 male; 3 female; age, 19–43.

Instruments/procedure

The composition of this group of subjects does not mirror the prevalence of depressive disorders in the general or referred population. To describe our pilot group better we collected demographic data (age, sex, social class) and measured the subject's severity of depression with the SCL-90.

The subjects followed the ESM-procedure for six consecutive days. Each day 10 beeps with a semi-random interval of 90 min were given. In the debriefing interview following the ESM procedure the subjects were asked to comment on the comprehensibility of the items and were asked about their problems filling out the ESM forms.

Analysis

Frequencies, variances, score distributions (skewness) of the ESM and the cross-sectional data were analyzed. The open categories of the ESM were coded. Finally, the scalability, reliability and validity studies were carried out.

Results

Which of the items derived from expert-based criteria are selected by depressive patients to describe their subjective psychological state?

Are the selected items suitable for repeated self-reports and do they show variability?

The Likert type items and the open-ended questions were tested using two criteria: comprehensibility and a 'not-skewed' score distribution over the spectrum from normal to severely depressed. Items that performed poorly were removed. This decreased the burden on the subject, diminishing the number of items. Next, based on data from the debriefing interviews, incomprehensible items have been removed, especially when they correlated highly (r >0.80) with more understandable ones. Further, it was examined whether the score distribution had a normal shape without pronounced skewness over the spectrum of normals, remitted depressives, depressives and depressives who dropped out of the study. In the Appendix the selected items are presented.

During this selection process some theoretically important items have been removed. Some examples: an item about the speed of the thinking process was removed because of its skewness; this item might be important for differentiating depressive from manic states in bipolar depression and might throw some light on the variability of the cognitive impairment in depression. Further, the item 'did you feel hopeless' did not survive the item selection because of its skewness. This item is important to the theories of 'hopelessness' in depression (Tennen et al., 1987; Abramson et al., 1989). Also psychodynamically interesting items like 'did you feel guilty?' and 'did you feel ashamed?' showed, in contrast with our expectations, a score pattern with strong skewness and low variance. All these items were removed with regret.

How do depressive patients undergo the ESM procedure?

Of the 236 people who were referred to the ambulatory centre during the two month study period, 40 (17%) were eligible for the study. Twenty-two (55%)

329

agreed to participate. At this level, refusal appeared to be selective. More women, married people, more subjects aged between 35 and 55, and subjects of lower education refused. The group that consented had a dropout rate of 50%. All dropouts stopped their participation after one to three days. They had the following characteristics:

– High severity of depression (SCL-90).
– Age above 35.
– Lower level of education: the dropout rate of people with only elementary school education was greater compared to these with secondary or higher education.

From the debriefing interviews some additional characteristics were inferred:
– For some subjects the repeated confrontation with the items, requesting continuous introspection, was unbearable.
– Subjects experiencing strong social control or expressed emotion by important others.

Moreover, we noticed that for the more depressed patients the time to fill out the sheet sometimes increased to 15 to 20 min instead of the usual five minutes. The subjects who completed the study responded on the average to 6.6 beeps each day. There was only a slight response decrease in filling out the ES forms, over the week (see Fig. 27.1). Apart from the relatively high dropout rate and the selection bias in consenting to participate, the compliance in the group that completed the study is satisfactory.

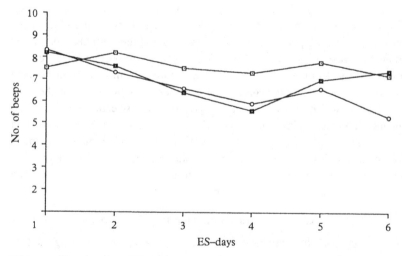

Fig. 27.1. Mean number of beeps filled in per ES-day for the onset depressives (o), depressives in remission (▢), and the normals (■).

Do selected items cluster into internal consistent and scalable dimensions? When depressive patients assess their own psychological states, which dimensions can be discerned in their self-ratings on the selected Likert items? Do the items pertaining to each of such dimensions or latent variable constitute a homogeneous, unidimensional scale?

In this respect a factor analysis has been carried out on the raw scores of the Likert-type items of the pilot group. Two factors appeared after principal component analysis with varimax rotation: a positive and a negative mood (or depression) factor. After dichotomizing the highest loading items (>0.50) both factors have been submitted to a Mokken scale analysis, which is a probabilistic version of Guttman scale analysis (Stokman et al., 1980). After dichotomizing the items the probability of a positive response on each item concerned has to increase monotonically over the subject's value. Items have different difficulties and the value of an item on the latent variable is equal to that of a subject giving a positive response with a probability of 0.50. When a subject gives a positive response to a more difficult item, the answer to all easier items should be positive too. The 'goodness of fit' of a Mokken model can further be tested by calculating the Loevingers coefficient of homogeneity (*H*). A high homogeneity coefficient means that a scale has been identified with only a few deviations from a perfect scale. When this Loevingers coefficient of homogeneity is >0.50, then a good scale has been identified. Furthermore, in the Mokken analysis a measure of internal consistency, the reliability ϱ, is produced. (See Table 27.1.)

Table 27.1. *Negative and positive Mokken scales, underlying the ESM items and their coefficients alpha*

Negative mood factor		Positive mood factor	
Items	Mean item score	Items	Mean item score
empty	0.19	energetic	0.40
lonely	0.22	cheerful	0.48
down	0.28	satisfied	0.52
brooding	0.33	self-assured	0.54
main complaint	0.33		
Loevingers coefficient of homogeneity	0.67	Loevingers coefficient of homogeneity	0.67
Reliability, ϱ	0.87	Reliability, ϱ	0.85
Coefficient α	0.89	Coefficient α	0.89

The Mokken scale analysis yielded two scales (with Loevingers coefficients of homogeneity of respectively 0.67 and 0.65, indicating robustness), but one methodological restriction should be made. Although the analysis has been carried out on 960 beeps the pilot group contains only 26 subjects. The repeated measurement of such a restricted number of subjects might have inflated the robustness of these scales. However, the results suggest that self-assessment of a depressive psychological state has a two-dimensional structure, instead of one single, bipolar dimension (negative mood being the counterpart of positive mood). Self-assessment of mood is likely to proceed according to two dimensions: high to low positive mood; and high to low negative mood. The depressive factor with the main complaint (most: down, loss of interest, fatigue) as lowest intensity and emptiness in severe levels of depression. The positive mood factor shows that feeling energetic is affected early whereas the level of self-assuredness is relatively less easily disturbed. The data suggest that both factors that have a negative correlation of 0.51 to 0.70 are used as rather independent measures by the patient. These results are in accordance with recent findings of other investigators (see for an overview Watson & Tellegen, 1985).

In future when a larger and representative data set will be available, advanced techniques like LISREL-analysis or more strict probabalistic scale analyses like Rasch-analysis will be applied in order to replicate these preliminary findings.

What is the reliability and validity of the ESM in depression?

Individual consistency of self-assessment over six days   The ESM is based on the assumption that responses of individuals are not constant during the day and over the days of the week. Life situations are considered to exert effects on psychological states. Therefore, perfect consistency or stability would defeat the purpose of ESM. However, relative stability of means and variances within individuals is expected to persist over time. With respect to the positive and negative mood factors it can be expected that their means and standard deviations (as measures of mood variability) have a trait-like stability (Csikszentmihalyi & Larson, 1987; Larsen, 1987). Therefore, we correlated the subjects' mean scores on the negative and the positive mood factors on two work days in the ES-week, one in the first half and the other in the second of the ES-week. These (Pearson) autocorrelations are $r=0.86$, $P <0.001$ for the negative mood factor and $r=0.81$, $P <0.001$ for the positive mood factor, witnessing a fair stability. In variance terms the proportion of stable trait variance is 65%, leaving 35% for variability. In the same way autocorrelations between the standard deviations of the negative and positive mood factors have been calculated. They are respectively $r=0.91$, $P <0.001$ and $r=0.45$, $P = 0.04$. It is noteworthy that the variability in positive mood swings is greater

332

than the variability in negative mood swings; the latter shows more trait-like stability in its variability.

Intercoder reliability of the categories used in the open-ended questions For the categories in the open-ended questions intercoder reliabilities, by means of unweighted Cohen's Kappa, have been assessed: thought content, 0.51; place, 0.92; social context, 0.77; and activities, 0.69. The intercoder reliability for the microstressors was not computable in this way, because the computer program is restricted to a maximum of 10 categories. The reliability of most categories is satisfactory, except for thought content.

Validity issues of the momentary experience (beep-level) Inspecting the cross-correlations between variables of depressive states we can discern patterns of convergence and divergence. It may be hypothesized that moments of low mood, emptiness and brooding are not compatible with moments of cheerfulness, self-assurance and vitality. The data confirm these expectations by showing for instance a correlation coefficient of -0.70 between cheerful and down; a coefficient of -0.51 between empty and energetic and a coefficient of -0.55 between brooding and self-assured.

ESM data compared with individual scores on cross-sectional instruments Convergent and divergent validity has been assessed by comparing individual scores on the depression dimension in the Symptom Complaint List (SCL-90) (Derogatis et al., 1973) with the mean negative mood (depressive) factor of subjects derived from the ESM data. For reasons of comparison also the correlations with the anxiety and somatization dimensions of the SCL-90 are given in Table 27.2.

Table 27.2. *Correlations between subjects mean positive and negative mood factors with the anxiety, somatization and depression dimensions on the SCL-90* (n = 26)

	Positive mood		Negative mood	
	r	P	r	P
SCL-90 total score	−0.42	0.03	0.71	0.000
anxiety	−0.37	0.06	0.68	0.000
somatization	−0.17	0.49	0.62	0.001
depression	−0.51	0.008	0.68	0.000

The convergent and divergent validity of the positive mood factor is very satisfactory and better than the validity of the negative mood factor. The high correlation between the depressive factor and the anxiety and somatization dimensions of the SCL-90 indicate a lack in divergent validity. The good validity figures of the positive mood factor should be placed in the light of the well-known fact that in the SCL-90, the discrimination between the depression, anxiety and somatization dimensions is not great (Brophy et al., 1988).

Differences between groups with distinctive levels of depression The ESM should also differentiate well between groups with distinctive levels of depression. Therefore, we compared the scores on the depression factor of our four small groups from the pilot study (normals, moderate to severe (onset) depressives, depressives in remission and depressives dropped out of the study). First, we calculated the scores of these groups on the SCL-90.

Table 27.3. *Mean scores of the pilot study groups on the SCL-90 compared with scores in a psychiatric out-patient population*

	Depression	Anxiety	Somatization	Total score
normals	21.5 L	12.3 L	16.3 L	115.8 L
onset depressives	55.8 M	29.8 M	31.5 M	234.5 M
remitted depressives	34.6 M	17.3 L	19.7 L	155.9 M
depressive drop-outs	56.8 M	30.6 M	31.4 M	395.1 H

L = low, M = medium, H = high in comparison with a psychiatric out-patient population.

In Table 27.3 the mean scores on the SCL-90 subscales (depression, somatization, anxiety) are given, compared with the standards of out-patient psychiatric populations and normals. According to scores on the SCL-90 the four groups are well-defined: normals and remitted depressives have low to intermediate scores, whereas onset depressives, and depressives who dropped out of the study have intermediate to high scores according to the standards of psychiatric out-patient populations. In Table 27.4 we present the mean scores of the positive and negative mood factors (on beep level) for these four groups. A one-way analysis of variance showed significant differences among the scores of the groups for both mood factors.

These findings demonstrate that the four groups are clearly distinguished by the positive mood factor, whereas the negative mood factor is not able to discriminate between the remitted and the onset depressives. An explanation might be that remitted depressives have a residual negative response set in a repeated self-assessment. This group may be discriminated better by a retrospective, cross-sectional method, like the SCL-90.

Table 27.4. *ANOVA means and standard deviations of the negative mood factor in the normals, onset depressives, remitted depressives, and the depressive drop-outs*

	Negative mood			Positive mood		
	mean	SD	n of beeps	mean	SD	n of beeps
normals	1.37	0.65	315	4.22	1.11	315
onset depressives	2.77	1.55	394	2.89	1.44	387
remitted depressives	2.86	1.81	260	3.20	1.84	260
depressive drop-outs	3.80	2.20	79	2.34	1.28	79
ANOVA	$F = 90.2$ ($P<0.000$)			$F = 64.4$ ($P<0.000$)		

Concluding remarks

The use of ESM in depression research has the promise to create a rich, prospective, phenomenological data set, mirroring the daily depressive experience and its variability. Contextual factors like daily stress and perceived social support can also be taken into account. A pilot study showed that reliability figures are generally satisfactory. The intercoder reliability of the open categories is encouraging. Factor analysis and subsequent Mokken scale analysis suggest a two-dimensional structure in the self-assessment of the depressive psychological state. Two probabilistic Guttman scales appear: one for negative mood with the following items ranging from 'difficult' to 'easy': empty, lonely, down, brooding and the individual main complaint, and one scale for positive mood with the following items ranging from 'difficult' to 'easy': energetic, cheerful, satisfied and self-assured. When individual mean scores on both mood factors during a day in the beginning and one at the end of the week are correlated, the means show a good stability. Also the stability in the degree of the variability, measured by the correlation between the standard deviations, is satisfactory for the negative mood factor, but moderate for the positive mood factor. In terms of test-retest reliability these results are promising, whereas they also leave sufficient room for the subjects' daily variability of mood.

The validity on the 'state' (beep-) level shows a divergency and convergency pattern between items like down, energetic, cheerful, empty, self-assured and brooding, according to the expectations. Further, the ESM, especially the positive mood factor, is able to discriminate between levels of severity of depression. Finally, both mood factors reveal a pattern of convergency with the SCL-90 depression dimension. The negative mood factor shows no divergent validity with the SCL-90 somatization and anxiety dimensions in contrast to the positive mood factor. Therefore, the positive mood factor surprisingly has better validity properties than the negative mood factor. The empirical finding that self-assessment of depression has a two-dimensional pattern with a negative and a positive mood factor, replicates studies by Watson & Tellegen (1985). Depressive patients are probably characterized best by a decrement in positive mood, than by an increase in negative mood. This two-dimensionality contrasts with the expert-based 'objectivistic' DSM-III approach to depression, that focuses on negative mood phenomena and supports the notion of Leff (1978) that depression is more a caretaker than a patient concept.

In this respect the procedure of the scale construction should once more be stressed. The ES items have originally been taken from sources with high expert validity (RCD; DSM-III). Next, they have been extensively commented on by a 'panel' of depressive patients. Consequently, the items were adapted and selected according to their views, enhancing 'member validity'. This procedure illustrates the 'middle ground' item selection of experts and patients. The two probabilistic Guttman scales arising from the score patterns of these depressive patients are a result of this 'negotiated validity'.

These promising findings are clouded by the high and selective dropout of more severe, older (>35) and lower-educated depressives. Furthermore, from the debriefing interviews this seemed to be due to the burden of introspection demanded by the ESM. The selection caused by this dropout hampers the generalizability of results for severe depressives.

The counter-intuitive finding of better validity of the positive mood factor inspires, however, to further theoretical and empirical study. When a larger data set is available these preliminary findings may provide more insight into the clinical picture of depression.

Appendix to Chapter 27: Experience Sampling Form for depression

---

what did you think at the moment of the beep?

....

	not		a little		rather		very
was this a pleasant thought?	1	2	3	4	5	6	7
could you concentrate?	1	2	3	4	5	6	7
were you brooding?	1	2	3	4	5	6	7

---

at the moment of the beep, did you feel:	not		a little		rather		very
– cheerful?	1	2	3	4	5	6	7
– down?	1	2	3	4	5	6	7
– angry?	1	2	3	4	5	6	7
– self-assured?	1	2	3	4	5	6	7
– empty?	1	2	3	4	5	6	7
– anxious?	1	2	3	4	5	6	7
– satisfied?	1	2	3	4	5	6	7
– lonely?	1	2	3	4	5	6	7

---

at the moment of the beep, did you feel:	not		a little		rather		very
– energetic?	1	2	3	4	5	6	7
– tired?	1	2	3	4	5	6	7
– agitated?	1	2	3	4	5	6	7
were you hungry?	1	2	3	4	5	6	7
did your main complaint bother you?	1	2	3	4	5	6	7
did you have other complaints?	none /						

---

what did you do at the moment of the beep?

....

	not		a little		rather		very
did you do it with pleasure?	1	2	3	4	5	6	7
was it an effort to do this?	1	2	3	4	5	6	7
did you prefer to do something else?	1	2	3	4	5	6	7

---

where were you at the moment of the beep? ....

were you with others? yes/no, if so – with how many people?...........

name	with whom?	did you do something together? what?	were you talking?
....	....	....	yes/no
....	....	....	yes/no

please answer the following questions if you were not alone:

In this company, did you feel:	not		a little		rather		very
– secure?	1	2	3	4	5	6	7
– appreciated?	1	2	3	4	5	6	7
– rejected?	1	2	3	4	5	6	7
did you get help/assistance?	1	2	3	4	5	6	7

---

	not		a little		rather		very
did you need support?	I	2	3	4	5	6	7
did you prefer to be alone?	I	2	3	4	5	6	7
did you receive what you needed?	I	2	3	4	5	6	7

---

did you use something between this and the previous beep?
      o nothing   o drugs, viz. ....
      o alcohol   o other substances, viz. ....

Did something pleasant or unpleasant occur to you between the present and the previous beep?
If yes, what is it?
....

Was this event:

O	O	O	O	O	O
very	rather	a little	a little	rather	very
pleasant	pleasant	pleasant	unpleasant	unpleasant	unpleasant

In case if an unpleasant event:	not		a little		rather		very
did you expect it?	I	2	3	4	5	6	7
could you have prevented it?	I	2	3	4	5	6	7
how much influence could you exert on the situation?	I	2	3	4	5	6	7

In case if a pleasant event:	not		a little		rather		very
did you expect it?	I	2	3	4	5	6	7
did you owe it to yourself?	I	2	3	4	5	6	7

| did this beep bother you? | I | 2 | 3 | 4 | 5 | 6 | 7 |
| what time is it now? | ....hrs ....min | | | | | | |

28

Research alliance and the limit of compliance: Experience Sampling with the depressed elderly

KENNETH C. M. WILSON,
RICHARD HOPKINS, MARTEN W. deVRIES
and JOHN R. M. COPELAND

Introduction

After a one-year follow-up period Murphy was able to show that only one third of elderly depressed patients had a satisfactory outcome (Murphy, 1983). Baldwin & Jolley (1986) found that 60% of subjects in their patient series either remained well or had further episodes followed by full recovery, when observed for a variable time of up to two years. In both studies, concomitant physical illness was associated with poor outcome. Copeland et al. (in press) in their community study of subjects aged 65 and over reported that more than 30% of those diagnosed as depressed at initial interview were depressed three years later. These studies demonstrate that depression in the elderly can present considerable therapeutic problems and that only a minority of patients seem to make a full recovery without suffering relapse or chronicity. Moreover, the onset of depression in the elderly has been shown to be associated with severe life events, major social difficulties and poor physical health, while those elderly people without a confiding relationship appear to have increased vulnerability to depression (Murphy, 1982). Such studies suggest that the elderly individual's perception of their environment, physical illness and social relationships clearly influence both the genesis and prognosis of depression.

Most clinical or psychological assessments have been limited to a single interview or to periodic, daily observer or self-report ratings. Recent research has employed a repeat measure, longitudinal design which emphasises the relationships between the individual's external environment and his or her cognitions and mood (Lader, Lang & Wilson, 1987). Using a related single case method, Blackburn et al. (1988) studied the order of change in mood, cognition and cortisol concentration in a group of eight subjects recovering from depression. The subjects completed the rating procedures at a fixed time on consecutive days but serial cortisol levels were measured daily.

Randomized sampling of an individual's mood, cognition and environment, using the technique of Experience Sampling (ESM) has already been attempted in a number of psychiatric settings (Johnson & Larson, 1982; deVries et al., 1983–9). The advantage of this technique is that it captures the well-recognized diurnal variation in mood and other within-day fluctuations so commonly experienced by elderly subjects suffering from depression. The technique is also suitable for longitudinal case studies (Hurlburt & Melancon, 1987a,b).

This pilot project examined the practicality of ESM techniques in elderly subjects suffering from physical illness and depression in order to prepare for a more detailed investigation of the relationships between mood, physical illness, cognition and external environment.

First study

The first part of the study examines the practical difficulties of the technique when used in an elderly population having common physical illnesses.

Subjects

A consecutive series of eight non-psychiatrically ill patients, over the age of 65, admitted to a Geriatric Day Hospital were interviewed using the Geriatric Mental State interview (Copeland et al., 1976) in order to exclude those subjects suffering from a psychiatric illness.

Of the eight subjects, two were recovering from cerebral infarction and were unable to write as a consequence. Of the remaining six, one had Parkinson's disease, one a hemi-paresis and one peripheral neuropathy, two were suffering from multiple sclerosis and diabetes mellitus and one was attending for social reasons.

The two subjects who could not write were asked to mark the questionnaire to the best of their ability.

Procedure

The period of study was limited to each subject's single day of attendance at the day hospital.

The subjects received extensive briefing and debriefing interviews during which they were given a booklet of questionnaires, one to be completed at each time signal. At the end of the sample period the investigator gave the subject a semi-structured interview and completed a questionnaire designed to identify difficulties experienced by the individual in carrying out the procedure.

Questionnaires

Each booklet consisted of 10 questionnaires, printed in bold black type on A4 paper. The forms incorporated questions and scales used in previous studies of younger psychiatric subjects (deVries, 1985). Each questionnaire provided data on two problem areas identified in discussion with the subject during the introductory interview. It also included questions concerning the subject's thoughts, feelings and immediate environment. Ratings were made using Likert scales.

Random signal generators

Two RC-1000 Seiko wrist terminals were used in both projects. The terminals were programmed to signal nine times on a semi-randomized basis within each 12-h period.

Results

Response to the signalling

Of the eight subjects with physical illness, one failed to complete any of the booklets, saying that the signal was not heard, and two (both with associated stroke) were unable to indicate clearly which scale number they intended to ring. One subject failed to hear three out of the total of five signals. More specific problems experienced by some of those subjects who nevertheless completed all the booklet questionnaires, included difficulty in understanding the numerical nature of the Likert scale, and the meaning of some of the items such as 'agitated thought' and 'feeling uncertain'.

Second study

The object of the second study was to identify additional problems which might arise when the method was applied to depressed elderly subjects over a period of several days.

Subjects

Four subjects over the age of 65 participated in the second study. Each had a different clinical presentation of the illness according to the descriptions of DSM-III, namely, early dementia of the Alzheimer type and depression, major depressive illness with psychotic features, major depressive disorder with melancholia, and dysthymic disorder.

Procedure

Each subject had a series of interviews aimed at establishing a research alliance, introducing the nature of the project and teaching the technique of ESM.

Questionnaires

The design of the booklets for the second study was similar to that used in the first except that semantic scales were substituted for Likert scales. The questionnaires incorporated randomly selected questions from the Cognitive Style Test. This test has been used in longitudinal case studies to measure the degree of those negative interpretations of pleasant and unpleasant events which relate to self, the world and the future (Wilkinson & Blackburn, 1981).

Random signal generators

Each subject was supplied with an RC-1000 Seiko wrist terminal, programmed to generate five random signals within a 10-h period.

Results

The subject with early Alzheimer's disease succeeded in completing only two interviews, because he was unable to understand either the design or the purpose of the study. He refused to complete the self-rating scales even with supervision despite having agreed to participate in the project.

The subject suffering from major depressive disorder with psychotic features was interviewed on an in-patient ward, as soon as it was judged that she was capable to giving informed consent. Following an introductory interview she said that the questionnaire looked too complex. During the following interviews she was encouraged to complete the questionnaires with the help of the investigator. However, after four interviews the patient withdrew her consent, having found the required concentration too difficult to sustain.

Mrs F. presented with major depressive illness and melancholia. She was an articulate lady who lived at home in the care of her husband and sister. For this subject the questionnaires had now been modified by substituting semantic scales for the Likert scales. After five interviews she withdrew consent. At the initial interview it was decided to encourage the subject's husband to support his wife and help her complete the questionnaires and to comply with the protocol. At first, the subject was keen to participate. She was able to complete the initial questions with little difficulty under supervision. By the time of the fourth interview the subject was able to complete the questionnaire on her own without supervision. However, it became apparent that other members of the family were suspicious about the purpose and design of the study. At the next interview the wrist terminal was introduced. This provoked the family's concern and opposition to continuation of the study. After the next interview the patient stopped completing the questionnaires and withdrew consent. It was apparent that the subject's family played a key role in influencing her decision.

Mrs T., who had recently moved to a new house, developed dysthymic disorder. Since moving house she had suffered from loss of confidence and lowered self-esteem and had become increasingly reliant on her husband for decision making and for carrying out daily chores. She cried most days and had a pessimistic view of the future with the feeling that her illness would never recover. Both she and her husband accepted the idea of diary keeping and agreed to participate in the project.

During the introductory period the subject showed some initial difficulty over interpretation of the severity points on the emotional scales. During the fourth interview the wrist terminal was demonstrated to the subject. At the fifth interview the subject had had the watch for 24 h although she was experiencing some anxiety concerning both the protocol and the loudness of the signal which she found embarrassing in company. Nevertheless, she completed all the questionnaires. She continued with the study for a total of six weeks, engaging in ESM for four days in each week. During this time it was apparent that both her ratings of mood and her ability to 'catch' thoughts when the wrist terminal signalled, were improving. During the first days of the study she had tended to record what she was doing at the time of the signal rather than what she was thinking.

Discussion

During the first study the authors were surprised at the perseverance of the subjects in completing the protocol while at the same time suffering from considerable physical illness. In each case, the subject was helpful to the investigator and keen to participate, but liable to become worried about the possibilities of failing to complete the recordings. The investigator had to take particular care to reassure the individuals about their performance, despite the preliminary interview in which the nature of the project had been explained in detail.

Most of the subjects were able to complete the questionnaires successfully, but the Likert scale proved confusing to some of the participants who were unable to appreciate the relevance of a numerical scale. A semantic scale proved more acceptable. One subject failed to hear the signal from the wrist terminal and four others had difficulty in understanding the descriptive terms used to evaluate 'thought content'. This latter problem could have been reduced by undertaking more extensive rehearsal.

Subjects suffering from depression had difficulty following the protocol due to cognitive impairment, poor volition and poor concentration. However, the patient suffering from dysthymic disorder completed a series of recordings clearly showing an improvement in mood and a change in thought content. In the one case suffering from a mixed dementia and depression the patient appeared threatened by the questionniare and refused to participate. Interference by close relatives also proved a problem.

343

As a result of this study a format has been devised for the introduction of ESM techniques with depressed elderly subjects.

It was apparent early in the project that one interview was insufficient to familiarise the subject with the aims and procedure of the study and that this was best undertaken in the context of an established rapport with the subject. A relationship of trust and confidence between the investigator and the subject proved crucial for establishing compliance. This usually developed after a number of interviews of relatively short duration during which the investigator did not pressurise the subject into complying with the protocol but on the contrary offered support and encouragement. The investigator may have to collude in the examination of the patient's experiences. It may be necessary for the introduction, during which the technique is explained to the subject, to be carried out in an unhurried manner over a number of days. This may take up to five or six short semi-structured interviews. The authors found that elderly depressed subjects seemed unable to tolerate more than one interview per day.

Simple teaching strategies, including modelling, rehearsal and appropriate reinforcement proved to be successful. The investigator must be aware of the subject's domestic circumstances, including the personal role of relatives and carers, and be prepared to recruit their help and support where necessary. The authors identified three sources of poor compliance caused by the subject's relatives. They included distrust of the investigation with consequent break-down of the research alliance, distraction of the subject at the time when the wrist terminal operated (e.g. conversation of visitors, family, television or other concurrent sounds) and interference from a close family member or other person in the way the subject completes the questionniare.

As expected, structured interviews proved useful. Each interview commenced with a review of the content of the previous interview and the details of the procedure already learned. The middle part of the interview consisted of the introduction and learning of a new component of the protocol with appropriate rehearsal and modelling. The interview finished after the subject had summarised the information learnt.

The authors concluded that the first interview should concentrate on establishing a research alliance and consist of diary keeping during which a collaborative relationship is cultivated. At the second interview, the booklet should be introduced and demonstrated using role play and modelling techniques. The third interview can be used to rehearse the filling in of the questionnaires under supervision but without interference from other persons, recording the thoughts and moods that the subject is currently experiencing. The need to complete the questionnaire a number of times in the day should be introduced at this stage and the use of an alarm clock for timing the recording of information discussed. At the fourth interview, the random signalling can be introduced, taking care to familiarise the subject with the device. The authors found it helpful to supplement this interview with written instructions. The working and fitting of the unit should be explained to the subject in detail and where necessary modified. A rehearsal of the subject's response to the signal should also be arranged. Finally, the subject should be provided with sufficient questionnaire booklets for a 24-h period and a follow-up interview arranged for the following day.

The final introductory interview was used to identify areas of difficulty experienced by the subject over the preceding test period. Considerable reassurance is often necessary at this stage, in order to ensure further compliance.

The elderly person undertaking ESM requires regular and relatively frequent meetings with the investigator, for support. Use of the telephone for support may appropriately be combined with personal interviews, thus reducing some of the burden on the investigator. The authors have also found that randomized 'break periods' from ESM may encourage the patient to remain in the study for a longer overall period.

Wrist terminal and modifications

Six signals in a 24-h period provided the best compliance and data quality for this type of sample. Reassurance had to be given to the subject that the wrist terminal signal would not interfere with sleep. Most of the subjects found that the liquid crystal display was of poor visual quality and difficult to view comfortably. The elderly people studied were also unaccustomed to digital displays.

The particular terminal used by the investigator had no facility for cancelling the everyday alarm system which sounded independently of the study signals, causing confusion and upsetting the order of the questionnaire completion.

Questionnaires

The form of the questionnaires had to balance simplicity of layout and clarity with practical size. The print had to be a little larger than normal and the number of items on each page had to be restricted, as subjects tended to refuse to complete questionnaires which to them looked too complex.

Likert scales seemed too complicated for subjects in this study to complete, so where appropriate, either a visual analogue or semantic scale was substituted. This resulted in better compliance.

The ability to think in the hypothetical or abstract terms necessary for the completion of questions was limited in both the severely depressed and in the subject with co-morbid dementia. Severe depression caused obvious problems in decision making and volition which made it difficult for the subject to complete all but brief questionnaires. Some subjects tended to perseverate when answering the questions.

This pilot study has examined the problems inherent in applying ESM techniques to elderly subjects suffering from both physical illness and depression. From those subjects with physical illnesses it is clear that despite considerable disability, elderly subjects are receptive and generally enthusiastic about participating in this form of data collection. The authors were surprised and encouraged by the ability of the subjects to complete the protocol. The authors found that severe degrees of depression often present cognitive and volitional difficulties for the subject attempting to complete complex questionnaires. In those cases of milder depression, characterised by a less-endogenous clinical picture, extensive data can be collected over longer periods of time. The authors suggest that this technique is likely to prove of considerable research value in longitudinal studies of milder depression in the elderly, and could be used as a vehicle for data collection in elderly subjects undergoing cognitive behavioral psychotherapies. Further research is being undertaken in the validation of the technique in this population using random community samples to assess the diagnostic and prognostic value of ESM in other forms of depression and early dementia and for studying normal subjects.

29

The importance of assessing base rates for clinical studies: an example of stimulus control of smoking

JEAN PATY, JON KASSEL
and SAUL SHIFFMAN

Cigarette smoking poses serious health risks, including cancer (US DHHS, 1982), cardiovascular disease (US DHHS, 1983) and chronic obstructive lung disease (USD DHHS, 1984); it is the leading cause of premature death and disease in the Western World. Despite these dangers, one quarter to one half of adults smoke in North America and Europe. Several theoretical models have attempted to explain – with limited success – why people continue to smoke in the face of such severe consequences.

Most current theories emphasize the role of nicotine and nicotine dependence in smoking. These models assert that, once smokers become addicted, their smoking is driven by the need to avoid the nicotine withdrawal symptoms they experience when they go without tobacco (e.g. Jarvik, 1979; Schachter, 1978). This implies that smokers smoke in order to keep nicotine from dropping below a certain level in their bloodstreams. Additionally, it has been suggested that smokers may also strive to achieve acute peaks or surges of blood nicotine that produce direct and immediate pharmacological effects (Russell & Feyerabend, 1978). Some of these effects seem to include: enhancement of pleasure, stimulation, improvement of learning and performance on cognitive tasks, and anxiety reduction (see Pomerleau & Pomerleau, 1984, and Russell, 1976, for reviews).

A simple pharmacological dependence model predicts that smoking will occur at regular intervals, as nicotine is depleted from the bloodstream. However, studies indicate that smoking is cued by a variety of environmental and proprioceptive stimuli. Laboratory studies have demonstrated that the social context can influence smoking (Glad & Adesso, 1976; Miller, Frederiksen & Hosford, 1979). Smoking can also be cued by alcohol and coffee consumption (see Lichtenstein & Brown, 1982). Among the most important cues for smoking are affective states; negative affect is posited to be a major cue for smoking (Ikard, Green & Horn, 1969; Rose, Ananda & Jarvik, 1983; Pomerleau, Turk & Fertig, 1984). Smoking can thus be elicited by both interoceptive (e.g., affective states) and exteroceptive (e.g. coffee or food) stimuli. In order to account for environmental cueing of smoking, pharmacological theories are forced to acknowledge the role of learning in smoking behavior (Pomerleau & Pomerleau, 1984).

Learning models of smoking emphasize the role of environmental stimuli as conditioned cues or discriminative stimuli for smoking. Environmental stimuli may become conditioned to smoking through repeated contiguity, or may come to signal that smoking will be reinforced. Under these models, smoking is considered to be under stimulus control; smoking and craving are said to be elicited by stimuli that have become linked to smoking through association and conditioning (e.g., drinking coffee) or by conditions that make smoking more reinforcing (e.g., stressors motivate smoking to reduce negative affect).

According to these stimulus control models, the stimuli that cue smoking should vary across smokers, based on their unique learning histories. Individual differences in smoking patterns have been a cornerstone of theory and clinical treatment (Niaura, Rohsenow, Binkoff, Monti, Pedraza & Abrams, 1988). Ideally, treatment approaches should be tailored to the individual smoker based upon the cues which elicit his/her smoking. For example, the links between these cues and smoking might be extinguished through repeated exposure (i.e., 'cue exposure'; Niaura et al., 1988); or smokers can be taught to anticipate and cope with urges to smoke which may arise when they are faced with a smoking cue (Shiffman, Read, Maltese, Rapkin & Jarvik, 1985). Unfortunately, treatment programs which follow these procedures do not seem to succeed better than treatment programs based upon other models of smoking. Failure to adequately assess individual differences in smoking patterns may be part of the problem.

Individual differences in smoking patterns have been most commonly assessed by self-report. Several questionnaires purport to measure smoking occasions or smoking motives (Ikard, Green & Horn, 1969; McKennell, 1970). These measures are quite reliable and have very stable factor structures (Leventhal & Avis, 1976). Their validity is less well-established. Smoking 'typology' measures do not correlate well with data from self-monitoring, a more direct method of assessing smoking patterns (Shiffman & Prange, 1988; Joffe, Lowe & Fisher, 1981). Self-monitoring methods have a distinct advantage over self-report questionnaires because they rely on subjects' real-time observations, rather than on retrospective recall.

Computerized self-monitoring of smoking antecedents

Recently, we used self-monitoring methods to study the role of various stimuli in smoking. Typically, subjects in self-monitoring studies record data on a piece of paper which is folded and carried in their cigarette package. However, this method has two important limitations: (1) poor compliance, due to subject

burden, and (2) doubtful validity, because subjects have been known to complete a week's worth of data on their way in to the laboratory. To overcome
these limitations, we developed a computerized method of self-monitoring.
Using hand-held computers, subjects in our study monitored their mood,
activity, and social situation just prior to smoking. Subjects carried the computer for two weeks; when they indicated they were about to smoke, the
computer administered an assessment of the antecedent situation. To reduce
subject burden, the computer randomly sampled these occasions so that
smokers completed the assessment only about five times per day. The computer also recorded the time and date of each entry.

Our assessments focused on stimuli thought to be relevant to smoking.
Besides activity and mood, we asked whether subjects had been eating or
drinking in the five minutes before smoking. Eating food and drinking coffee
or alcohol are important antecedents of smoking and relapse (Shiffman, 1982;
Istvan & Matarrazo, 1984). Subjects first indicated if they had eaten at all;
those who had were then asked specifically about food, coffee, and alcohol.

As a basis for discussion of stimulus control, we present data from two
subjects. Figure 29.1 contrasts data from these subjects: male smoker of 30
cigarettes per day; female smoker of 40 cigarettes per day. The figure shows
the proportion of cigarettes that were preceded by alimentary consumption,
and specifically by food or coffee consumption. (The drinking of alcohol was
not included because of its low frequency.)

On the assumption that the proportion of smoking under each of these
conditions reflects stimulus control, the figure suggests that nutrient consumption plays a very different role in each subject's smoking. Compared with the
female subject, the man's smoking is more likely to be accompanied by eating
or drinking. Turning to specific types of consumption, we find that both
subjects were equally likely to have eaten food just before smoking, but that
the man was much more likely to have been drinking coffee. Thus, we might
conclude that the male subject's smoking is cued specifically by drinking
coffee (though not by eating food).

If these two smokers presented themselves for treatment, we might use these
data to design individual treatment strategies. We might prescribe that the
man avoid coffee in order to avoid being cued to smoke. We might perhaps
warn both subjects equally to take care lest they be tempted to smoke after
eating. Thus, data from self-monitoring seem useful in designing individual
programs for smoking cessation.

The importance of base-rate data: use of ESM

Unfortunately, the above conclusions are faulty. For example, we concluded
from the fact that the male subject often smokes after drinking coffee that he is
prompted to smoke when he drinks coffee. However, without knowing how

349

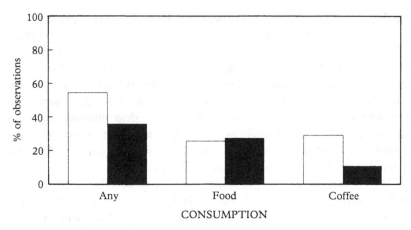

Fig. 29.1. Consumption: subject comparisons. □, male smoker; ■, female smoker.

often he drinks coffee (with or without smoking), we cannot possibly know whether there is an association between coffee drinking and smoking. That is, we need data on the *base rate* of the behavior. Only if it can be shown that the proportion of 'coffee-drinking when smoking' is significantly higher than the proportion of 'coffee-drinking when not smoking' would it be reasonable to conclude that smoking is *associated* with coffee drinking. Thus, the above conclusions may be erroneous because they have not accounted for base rates.

To collect base-rate data, we borrowed a technique from the ESM. We programmed the computer to 'beep' subjects at random when they were *not* smoking. At these times, subjects again entered data on their consumption of food and coffee (as well as mood, activity, etc.). (To avoid beeping subjects while they were smoking, the computers were programmed not to beep or prompt subjects within 10 min of smoking. We also excluded data from signals that fell five minutes before a cigarette.)

Figure 29.2 contrasts data from smoking entries with data from randomly-prompted 'base-rate' entries. Considering base-rate data alters our perception of these two subjects' smoking patterns. We have concluded that the male was more likely to smoke when he had eaten or drunk. In fact, his consumption is not associated with smoking; there is little difference in the proportion of time that he is eating or drinking when he is smoking compared to when he is not smoking (phi=0.03, n.s.; phi is a correlation coefficient for 2×2 tables). His high rate of smoking while eating or drinking simply reflects frequent consumption. (The subject was a store clerk who 'nibbled' throughout the day.)

Conversely, there *is* a link between consumption and smoking for the woman. She was much more likely to have been eating or drinking when she was about to smoke than when she was prompted at random (phi=−0.20,

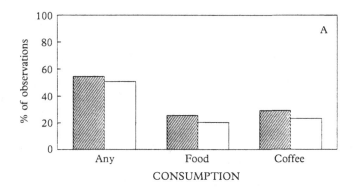

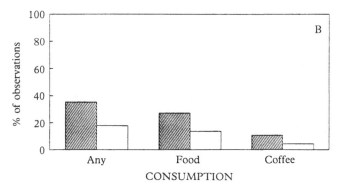

Fig. 29.2. Consumption: smoking vs. base rate. (A), male subject; (B), female subject. ▨, smoking; □, not smoking.

$P < 0.007$). In short, considering base-rate data causes us to reverse our initial conclusions.

The same reversal occurs when we consider the base rate of coffee-drinking. The man's smoking is preceded by coffee drinking three times as often as the woman's smoking. Both subjects seem more likely to smoke after drinking coffee, but this association is (marginally) significant only for the woman (phi=0.12, P=0.10); there is no relationship between coffee-drinking and smoking for the male. Again, our initial conclusions were dreadfully wrong.

We had concluded initially that food was not associated with smoking for either subject; both subjects had eaten before smoking about a quarter of their cigarettes. Examination of Fig. 29.2 shows, however, that the man had also eaten before a quarter of the random prompts; i.e., there is no association between smoking and eating. In contrast, the woman had been eating twice as often when smoking as when prompted at random, resulting in a significant association between eating and smoking (phi=0.17, P <0.03). Although eating food originally appeared to be a stimulus eliciting smoking for both subjects, taking into account base rates shows that it is a smoking-contingent cue for only one of the subjects.

Conclusions

These comparisons demonstrate the importance of taking base rates into account when determining whether a cue is associated with smoking. Some stimuli that at first glance appeared to cue smoking were shown to be irrelevant; other stimuli that originally seemed irrelevant proved to be important. Clinical approaches based on assessments of individual smoking patterns and stimulus-control principles may yet prove effective when they are based on adequate assessment. These issues are also important to theoretical accounts of smoking, many of which posit that smoking is associated with stimuli such as affect (e.g., Tomkins, 1966). These theories have been based on and supported by inadequate data. Properly constituted data on *when* people smoke may yet help us understand *why* people smoke.

These issues go beyond smoking to the assessment of any behavior in relation to antecedent conditions. Self-monitoring is a powerful naturalistic approach to assessment, but may also prove misleading if not sufficiently fine-grained. When supplemented with data on base rates by methods such as ESM, it can help us understand many aspects of psychopathology.

30

Infrequently occurring activities and contexts in time-use data[1]

PHILIP J. STONE and NANCY A. NICOLSON

During 1965 and 1966, social scientists from 12 countries collected 24-h time-use diaries and interviews from over 25,000 people. Efforts to ensure uniformity of data-gathering and coding methods paid off, resulting in one of the richest data bases in the history of cross-cultural research. A full description of the Multinational Comparative Time-Budget Research Project, including several applications of the results and a bibliography of publications derived from these data, can be found in *The Use of Time* (Szalai et al., 1972). Since this definitive work appeared, developments in the use of computers in the social sciences (for example, more flexible software for data management and statistical treatment) have made possible more detailed analyses of this massive data set. We completed a major reformatting and reordering of data from the Multinational Time-Budget Study to undertake studies of particular activities. In this paper we provide some examples of the kinds of insights that can be gained from focusing on infrequently occurring behaviors and behavioral settings and suggest how this approach might be applied in studies of mental disorder.

To put into perspective the applications for which data organization at the level of activities are most suitable, it is useful to contrast them with more traditional time-budget applications. The more conventional researches include the categories detailed below.

(1) Social accounting trade-offs

This approach, whether based upon the time-budget of the individual or of the entire household (As, 1978), focuses on trade-offs between activities as a form of social accounting (Harvey, 1978; Juster, 1975; Juster et al., 1979; Minge-Kalman, 1980). For example, an earlier paper (Stone, 1978) reported that in all countries studied, women who had both a family and an outside job got significantly less sleep than either employed husbands or women who had only a family. Such analyses of trade-offs generally aggregate the data to make

[1] This work appeared in *Journal of Nervous and Mental Disease*, 1987, **175**, 9, 519–25.

comparisons between major activity allocations, such as work, sleep, house-work, and so on. Indeed, almost all analyses based on the Multinational Time-Budget Project have used a collapsed activity code of 37 categories (or even a further reduction to nine categories), rather than the 96 separate categories into which the activities were originally classified. In the large statistical appendix to *The Use of Time* (Szalai et al., 1972), only the first few tables are based upon the full set of activity categories.

(2) Characterization of particular populations

As part of a more general ethnographic approach, some researchers have used time-budgets to characterize time allocations of a subculture or a group such as English or French urban workers (Chombart de Lauwe, 1956; Cullen & Godson, 1975) or women villagers in Upper Volta (McSweeney, 1979). In some cases, family time-budget diaries have been part of a larger descriptive data-gathering endeavor, often including family financial budgets for comparisons. Again, this approach usually aggregates activities into more general categories.

(3) Focus on particular, high-frequency activities

Many investigators have been interested in studying a particular activity. The time-budget may be a useful tool if enough instances of the activity under consideration are likely to occur in the time period sampled. Time-budget data have been used, for example, by Robinson (1977) to study television watching and by Vanek (1974) and Walker (1982) to study household work. The study of a much less frequent kind of activity will often require a specially designed survey targeted to that activity. One common example is the targeted survey of travel behavior, in which travelers over a particular route are stopped and asked about the trip they are making.

In contrast, the approach presented in this paper focuses on medium- to low-frequency activities in everyday life. An anthropologist gains insight into a culture through studying special events such as rituals; relatively infrequent activities in time-budgets may, similarly, characterize particular cultures or groups of individuals, perhaps even better than common everyday events. In addition, activities that are rather rare in the time-budgets of the population – playing a musical instrument or sleeping during daytime, for example – can clearly represent significant aspects of individual lifestyles. Borrowing from the work of R. Barker (1968; Barker & Schoggen, 1973) and others who have studied 'behavior settings', we can explore not only infrequent kinds of events but also less-frequent settings for more ordinary events, such as when there are children present at work, or people have work associates home for dinner, or some of the other examples we present below.

The Multinational Time-Budget Study, in which diaries from over 25,000 respondents resulted in more than 640,000 recorded events, provides a unique opportunity to examine the nature of uncommon events. What sorts of people engage in such activities and in what contexts? To explore this question, we first reorganized the original data (see Stone, 1972) so that each event is a separate record, labeled according to its respondent number. For each event, we have the following information: (a) the time of day the event started; (b) the duration of the event; (c) the serial position of the event (i.e., its place on the list of events reported in the 24-h period); (d) the original primary activity code, retaining also any auxillary activity codes used by any survey for further categorization; (e) the secondary activity, if any; (f) where the activity took place; (g) with whom the activity took place. For any event record, the investigator can also directly access the 'module card' of background information about the person doing the act. A total of 29 background variables were coded, including demographic information about the respondent and the head of the household, number of adults and children in the household, location and characteristics of the dwelling, work schedules, transportation used to commute between house and work, and specific details about the diary day (see Szalai et al., 1972, Statistical Appendix, Section I).

The event records were then sorted by the primary activity two-digit code to produce 96 separate files, one for each kind of activity. The number of event records in each of these files is shown in Table 30.1. By thus combining persons and countries, we can begin to obtain enough occurrences to study infrequent kinds of behavior (such as the 70 cases of museum going or 60 instances of participating in a factory council). In short, we can now begin to study those events that are between one in 200 and one in 10,000 in occurrence frequency. Behavior settings can be studied by breaking down the event categories further, according to when, where, with whom, or by whom the activity was performed.

To illustrate some insights and some cautions to be drawn from frequency data, we have graphed in Fig. 30.1 the frequencies of married men doing the laundry, adjusted for the sample size of each survey.

Perusing the graph, one might conclude initially that if a woman were to expect help from her husband with the laundry, she would do well to go to a socialist country, especially the German Democratic Republic, Czechoslovakia, or Poland. Inasmuch as the Federal Republic of Germany surveys show quite low rates (separate studies of the town of Osnabruck and a German national sample) compared with the German Democratic Republic survey, these results evidently reflect more the economic system than a culture. To pursue the question of why married men were more than twice as likely to do the laundry in socialist (0.015 events per respondent) than in non-socialist (0.007 events per respondent) countries, we would want to adjust the frequencies for the percentage of married men in each survey and to compare

Table 30.1. *Frequency of each event in the multinational time-budget study*

Event	Frequency	Event	Frequency
00 Regular work	36,240	50 Attend school	764
01 Work at home	4,075	51 Other classes	466
02 Overtime	312	52 Special lecture	84
03 Travel for job	2,078	53 Political courses	42
04 Waiting, delays	442	54 Homework	1,587
05 Second job	965	55 Read to learn	673
06 Meals at work	8,531	56 Other study	364
07 At work, other	13,306	57 Blank	
08 Work breaks	4,742	58 Blank	
09 Travel to job	39,979	59 Travel, study	1,913
10 Prepare food	41,042	60 Union, politics	253
11 Meals cleanup	21,618	61 Work as officer	161
12 Clean house	22,608	62 Other participation	252
13 Outdoor chores	1,428	63 Civic activities	195
14 Laundry, ironing	10,152	64 Religious organization	121
15 Clothes upkeep	4,025	65 Religious practice	1,282
16 Other upkeep	3,298	66 Factory council	60
17 Garden, animal care	7,036	67 Miscellaneous organization	245
18 Heat, water	7,354	68 Other organization	284
19 Other duties	4,546	69 Travel, organization	2,909
20 Baby care	5,281	70 Sport event	228
21 Child care	13,732	71 Mass culture	539
22 Help on homework	3,158	72 Movies	949
23 Talk to children	979	73 Theatre	150
24 Indoor playing	1,544	74 Museums	70
25 Outdoor playing	753	75 Visiting with friends	8,344
26 Child health	308	76 Party, meals	1,596
27 Other, babysit	813	77 Cafe, pubs	1,945
28 Blank		78 Other social	235
29 Travel with child	3,388	79 Travel, social	13,578
30 Marketing	14,448	80 Active sports	927
31 Shopping	888	81 Fishing, hiking	413
32 Personal care	626	82 Taking a walk	4,754
33 Medical care	853	83 Hobbies	595
34 Administrative service	768	84 Ladies' hobbies	3,760
35 Repair service	697	85 Art work	109
36 Waiting in line	1,436	86 Making music	240
37 Other service	1,091	87 Parlor games	973
38 Blank		88 Other pastime	476
39 Travel, service	25,198	89 Travel, pastime	2,631

Table 30.1. *Contd.*

Event	Frequency	Event	Frequency
40 Personal hygiene	73,443	90 Radio	5,439
41 Personal medical	628	91 TV	18,150
42 Care to adults	1,268	92 Play records	270
43 Meals, snacks	63,996	93 Read book	4,703
44 Restaurant meals	7,502	94 Read magazine	1,866
45 Night sleep	52,018	95 Read paper	10,719
46 Daytime sleep	2,561	96 Conversation	12,926
47 Resting	7,742	97 Letters, private	1,910
48 Private, other	3,463	98 Relax, think	4,872
49 Travel, personal	4,122	99 Travel, leisure	262

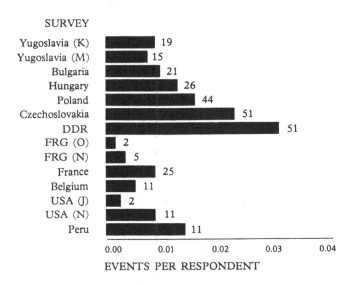

Fig. 30.1. Frequency of doing the laundry by married men, adjusted for the total number of respondents in each survey: Yugoslavia (K) = 2125 respondents; Yugoslavia (M) = 1995; Bulgaria = 2096; Hungary = 1994; Poland = 2759; Czechoslovakia = 2193; German Democratic Republic (DDR) = 1650; Federal Republic of Germany (FRG) (O) = 978; FRG (N) = 1500; France = 2805; Belgium = 2077; USA (J) = 778; USA (N) = 1243; Peru = 782. The raw event frequencies are shown to the right of each bar. Descriptions of survey sites and methods can be found in Szalai et al., 1972. In three countries, two separate surveys were conducted as follows: Yugoslavia: (K) = Kragujevac, (M) = Maribor; FRG: (O) = Osnabruck, (N) = national; USA (J) = Jackson, Michigan, (N) = national.

357

surveys as well as individual launderers on a number of coded background variables, such as size of household, number of children, plumbing conveniences, or schedule of paid work on the diary day.

An earlier publication (Stone, 1978) used the Multinational Time-Budget data to conclude that family women in socialist countries were not particularly better off than women in Western countries, based on a study of trade-offs against free time and time for sleep. Does the laundry illustration contradict this conclusion? Note that there were in all 10,152 occurrences of doing laundry (Table 30.1, event 14), while Fig. 30.1 shows that married men (when combined from all the survey sites) did the laundry only 294 times. Thus, although a woman was indeed likely to do relatively better in a socialist country, she still was not likely to do very well in any absolute sense in achieving a major trade-off with her husband. In this example low-frequency statistics are clearly more relevant to understanding cultural or situational dynamics than to making personal plans.

The laundry illustration demonstrates the frequency with which an activity occurs rather than the amount of time spent at the activity. In many cases these two kinds of indexes will lead to somewhat different pictures. In Fig. 30.2A, we have compared the frequencies of trips (3388 occurrences in all) made to transport children.

Three surveys stand out: one from France and two from the United States. If, however, one considers the large suburban distances to be covered in the United States, it stands to reason that the total time parents spent transporting children in the United States was probably more than in France. A new graph is produced simply by weighting each event by its duration. The resulting Fig. 30.2B, using total daily durations rather than frequencies, shows our expectation to be confirmed, for now the United States stands out by itself. This graph also shows that, in every survey, transporting children was done primarily by women.

In carrying out secondary analyses using such detailed activity categories, it should be carefully noted how a category has been defined. 'Travel with child' (Table 30.1, event 29), for example, refers to travel with regard to achieving some objective for the children. From other analyses not shown here, it is clear that this was mainly recorded on weekdays. In contrast, weekend family travel was likely to show the presence of children only in the 'with whom' category. Given that 'transporting children' was coded mainly with respect to child-related errands, it may be that a country like West Germany scored low because children there transported themselves at a younger age, using good transportation facilities in relatively safe urban environments.

With the primary data organization at the level of the event record, it is much easier to focus on characteristics of a behavior, such as the people typically present or the location where it is typically carried out. For example,

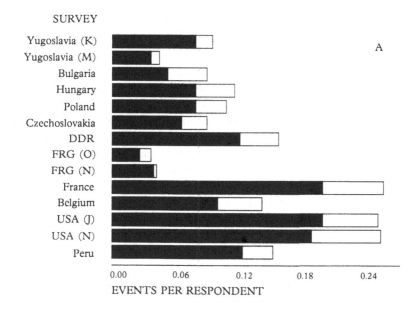

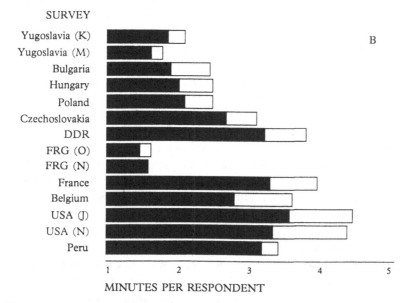

Fig. 30.2. Transporting children performed by adult men (□) and women(■). Number of respondents per survey as in Fig. 30.1. A, frequency (mean number of events per respondent); B, time spent (mean number of minutes per 24 h per respondent).

what are the characteristics of taking a walk? Is it primarily a meditative activity that is done alone, or is it a time to share with one's spouse, or is it a family occasion with the children? This can be analyzed by examining the 'with whom' information in the 4754 occurrences of 'taking a walk'. In terms of overall frequencies we expected that countries with more established traditions (such as French 'promenade') would show higher frequencies of taking a walk than, for example, America, where, at least back in the 1960s, there were not even many footpaths. As shown in Fig. 30.3, Americans did indeed take the fewest walks and, when they did walk, they tended to do so alone. Contrary to expectation, the French were outdone by most other Europeans surveyed, especially the West Germans, who often took walks with their spouses.

Looking toward the future, it seems likely that time-budget analyses will be able to handle more geographic information, such as the location data included in the Halifax time-budget study (Elliot & Clark, 1978) and that these will be analyzed with innovative spatial displays such as those proposed by the Lund group of geographers (e.g., Carlstein, 1978). General time-budget studies may also be more frequently linked to targeted surveys of specific activities. One example of this is Robinson's (1978) comparisons of television viewing indexes from time-budget surveys with the data from media surveys. Future surveys that combine such targeted time-allocation information with time-budget overview diaries from the same household would provide a better context for analyzing more specialized behaviors. Finally, the study of time use and the flow of daily events will gain an important dimension when methods of assessing the respondent's subjective experience of activities can be coupled to the diary approach (see Robinson, 1987).

We have used the Multinational Time-Budget data to demonstrate a method for analyzing relatively infrequently occurring behaviors and behavioral settings. It was not the purpose of the Multinational Study to collect data relevant to mental health issues; nevertheless, how time is allocated is arguably an important aspect of the quality of life. Bearing in mind that the data were collected 20 years ago, we could still derive useful information on patterns of time use through secondary analysis. For example, the overall time-budgets or specific activities of disabled, unemployed, or retired respondents could be compared with those of employed respondents.

In future research, time-use studies could also be carried out with specific diagnostic groups. From diary data we could ask how the time-budgets of particular diagnostic or risk groups differ from those of normal controls in amount and patterning of sleep, time spent alone, participation in social activities, and so on. Clinical experience, as well as recent Experience Sampling (ES) research (see Dijkman & deVries, 1987; Margraf et al., 1987), suggests that particular activities and contexts are related to symptomatology in some disorders. In these cases, the approach we have outlined in this paper would be

SURVEY

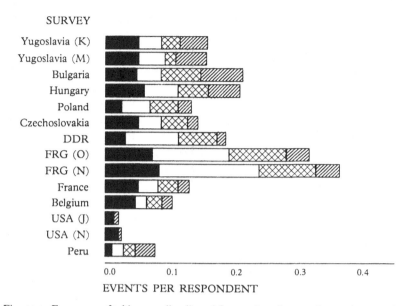

Fig. 30.3. Frequency of taking a walk adjusted for number of respondents per survey (see Fig. 30.1.). The graph also indicates with whom walks were taken: alone (■); with spouse only (□); with children only or with children and spouse (▨); or with a friend (▧).

particularly appropriate. Shopping, for example, although not a very pleasant activity for normal people (Robinson, 1987), has been reported to be highly aversive for individuals with certain anxiety or panic disorders (Wender & Klein, 1981). From diary data, we could examine shopping (or other activities outside the home) performed by anxiety patients to find out how frequently this activity typically occurs, at what time of day, how long it lasts, with whom it occurs, which other activities precede or follow it, etc.

There are several problems inherent in this sort of analysis that should be mentioned. First, the activity we wish to study may not occur frequently enough to appear in an individual's 24-h diary. Second, we may not know in advance which activities and contexts are relevant to a given disorder. Finally, because the diary can only provide limited information about cognitive and affective states associated with activities, the interpretation of differences between normal and disturbed individuals is difficult. The solution to these problems will probably lie in some combination of diary and repeated, sampling approaches, as described elsewhere in this volume.

If we wanted an unbiased estimate of frequencies and durations of activities for individuals or small groups, for example, it would be necessary to collect data over extended periods of time. A 24-h diary is too taxing, however, to fill in for much longer than a day. An alternative is to signal the subject with a paging device once or twice a day over a period of two weeks or longer, at times

361

scheduled to give a representative sample of the person's waking hours. The 'beep' initiates a fixed period (e.g., one or two hours) of continuous, detailed, activity recording, terminated by a second signal. This method is equivalent to 'focal sampling' in ethological research (Altmann, 1974), except that subjects observe themselves. It would not be applicable, of course, when trade-offs within a person's daily time-budget are of interest, but it might prove especially useful in longitudinal or intervention studies. It is not yet clear what clinical significance such activities might have to the associated disorders; continuous recording methods such as the diary can suggest what role the target activity plays in the subject's daily routine.

Finally, the method we have described for examining infrequently occurring daily activities in 24-h diaries has a direct parallel in the analysis of ESM data. Certain clinically relevant behaviors or situations may be recorded only infrequently under standard ESM protocols (e.g., panic attacks, psychotic symptoms). By focusing then at the level of the event ('beep') record, rather than at the subject level, enough cases can be aggregated that we can begin talking about the situational characteristics of panic attacks, hallucinations, and so forth, to the extent to which these phenomena are similarly experienced by different individuals. Johnson & Larson (1982) used this sort of analysis to describe binge-purge sequences in an ESM study of bulimia.

In conclusion, the systematic and quantitative study of daily activities can be expected to yield new insights into mental disorders. Because many of the most clinically relevant behaviors and behavioral settings are likely to occur only infrequently in the diaries or periodic self-reports of individuals, novel strategies will have to be used at both the data collection and analysis stages to obtain unbiased results from small samples or individual subjects. One such strategy, as illustrated in this paper, is to organize data at the level of the event or setting, which allows the researcher to explore differences between normal and disordered individuals in the nature of specific activities as well as in the overall use of time.

31

Technical note: devices and time-sampling procedures

PHILIPPE A. E. G. DELESPAUL

(1) Choice of the sampling device

A device that meets all the needs of researchers does not exist. The researcher who plans to buy or hire signaling devices faces a difficult decision. The starting point of the decision-making process should be a commonsense analysis of the purpose of the study and the nature of the target population. A pilot run with different devices before making hardware investments is recommended.

(a) General choice considerations

The shape, size and use of the ESM device should create minimal disturbance for the subject and his environment. It should have flexible applicability and allow full control over the sampling process by the researcher.

Non-reactivity: The goal of many ESM studies is to gather an ecologically valid dataset. The ideal device should lend itself to the feeling that nothing strange is happening in daily life, for both subjects and their environment. Reactivity can best be minimized by using small, reliable and inexpensive devices that emit unpredictable signals and can be fully employed within a range of environmental constraints.

Size: Small devices usually create less reactivity. Large devices may be forgotten because they are not easily carried by the subject and require extra attention. This further increases the chances of unwanted reactions from the environment. A large device is no real problem if the sampling environment is relatively small or when the technological intrusiveness of the device is exploited to enhance compliance or reporting accuracy (Nelson, 1977). Considerations are many, e.g.: even a men's wrist-watch may attract the attention of others when carried by a woman, while women, on the other hand, may hide larger devices in their handbags.
Reliability: The researcher should be convinced that the device will signal the subject in the way intended by the research protocol. The

device should not be an encumbrance or be fragile. If the subject has to keep the unit operational this will have an untoward effect upon the subject's daily life. Many high-tech beepers available on the market are not reliable for use in ESM studies, because the conditions of daily life, like extremes of humidity and temperature, may compromise the equipment.

Expense: Inexpensive devices or 'cheap'-looking ones are best. An expensive device tends to create over-concern in the subject. Cheaper devices also relax the researcher.

Unpredictability: The random or unpredictable nature of the beep can avoid anticipation effects on behavior and thoughts and therefore minimize reactivity. Random signal generation also has repercussions for analysis (see next paragraph on time series).

Subject controlability: For example, a beeper may be too loud for people working in a library while presenting no problem in the market place. Accordingly, a volume control for the beeping signal is useful. On the other hand, with pre-programmed devices there should be a limit to adjustments the subjects might make, particularly they should not be able to inspect or change the beeping times.

Flexibility: Because you cannot anticipate all conditions of future research you should use flexible devices. Avoid devices that are overly restrictive or provide just one sampling scheme. Programmable devices are best suited for this.

Verifiability: Researchers should generally have access to: (1) the time the beep was emitted; and (2) the time the subject answered the beep. When analyzing experience patterns over time we need to know when the subject actually received the signal (not when he should have received it). If only reported frequency and experiential description are the object of the study, knowledge of signal time is less crucial. Furthermore, the beep moment should be known because it is important to check the delay between beep and response. Delay may distort the quality of the reports (Ericsson & Simon, 1984). Therefore 'real-time' devices with pre-programmed (or stored) sampling schedules are best.

(b) Sampling devices

Early devices: Early mechanical devices, primarily used in observation studies, signaled at quasi-random intervals. The first generation computerized pocket instruments were usually developed specifically for research of this type, but usually did not link the beeps to a real time clock. The random timer used by Hurlburt (1990) is a good example. A creative alternative is the use of a standard digital watch (Brandstädter, 1983). These methods, however, do not meet ESM requirements.

Real time devices: Most current ESM devices use the signal-generating techniques of the modern computer. They can be summarized in three groups: radiotransmission-based systems; pre-programmed systems; and small-scale computer systems.

Csikszentmihalyi & Larson (1984) and deVries et al. (1984) have used 'doctor pagers' linked to a telephone network. A host computer with a modem generates the beeps and phones the pagers. This provides a flexible time series, restricted only by the options available on the host computer.

A diversity of paging devices are currently offered by telephone and electronic companies, but most of these devices give overloud signals, that disturb the environment. One interesting exception is a vibrating buzzer. This signal method is probably the best option for the non-intrusiveness intentions of ESM, because only the subject and not his environment will feel the signal. However, pagers are costly, usually have to be rented, and their operation requires a computer as well as repeated telephone connections which can increase research costs. Furthermore, signals may be lost because of the restricted working radius of the transmitter, while the presence of buildings and hills in the environment may obstruct the radio signals. Another important handicap is that one cannot be sure if the telephone connection was made at a specified time. Telephone lines may be overcrowded and the numbers may need to be repeatedly dialed, leading to significant delay or signal loss. We have found that when sampling subjects simultaneously, technical limits may be quickly reached. Radio-transmitted systems have an advantage over other devices, in that additional signals may be sent simultaneously by an external observer who monitors target events.

Delespaul & deVries (1987) and de Vries et al. (1988) use SEIKO RC-1000 and RC-4000 wrist terminals. These watches do not generate a time-series themselves but execute schedules prepared by PCs. When the current time matches a pre-programmed moment, the watch will beep and, if necessary, provide information on display. Because the SEIKO watches are commercial products targeted for managers they are relatively inexpensive. The fact that the device is also a watch, solves the problem of synchronization between the researcher's clock that generates the beeps and the subject's clock. A variety of sampling schedules can be executed, limited only by the program options on the time-series-generating PC. The device is a men's wrist watch (normal size), therefore the portability is optimal, while the minor aesthetic inconveniences for women can be dealt with using a 'clip-on' version of the RC-4000 (the

RC-4400). The sound, a digital beeping signal, is often heard in modern society and causes little extra commotion in the environment. For people living or working in noisy places or for the elderly, the beep may be insufficiently loud. The watch is also sensitive to humidity which may affect reliability, but this did not create a problem in over 200 subjects.

Recently, pocket or laptop computers have become available commercially and can be used for sampling and data recording. They allow a new way of data gathering (Van Egeren & Madarasmi, 1988) and the total control of the data-insertion process. An interesting development is the combination of the ESM and the sampling of biophysiological data (e.g. Thakor et al., 1989; Meldrum, 1988a, b) for which new hardware developments are planned. The *Journal of Ambulatory Monitoring* is devoted to following these developments. The portability, price and standardization of those devices are still a problem but the future medical applications of time-sampling techniques will follow this trend.

(2) Choice of the sampling process

The sampling process depends upon the purpose of the study. If the intention is to compute stable assessments of the frequency and duration of events it is essential that all moments within the target period have an equal chance of being selected at a beep. Representativeness may only be realized with *random* sampling schemes. If the assessment of an underlying time dimension for, say, cortisol (Nicolson, this volume) is the object of study, it is important to sample with *fixed* interval lengths. Once the distance between beeps is selected, randomization around those moments is possible, thus still meeting the criterion of unpredictability for the subject.

(a) The sampling frequency

Sampling frequency, signal density and the between-beep-time-interval are interchangeable notions. Theoretical and pragmatic considerations will be discussed.

(i) Theoretical approach to sampling frequency For an appropriate choice of the sampling frequency two questions are important:
  (1) How many observations are needed? This depends upon the frequency and duration of an event. Fewer beeps are required for the assessment of highly frequent, long-duration events than for rarely occurring, short events. Precision in estimating event duration is limited by the sampling interval, e.g. sampling every 90 min gives assessments of duration in multiples of 90 min.

(2) What is the minimal between-event interval of interest? Interval length depends on the answer to the following two questions:

(a) What periodicity is expected in the phenomenon under study? Ideal, theory-based sampling intervals must be half the period-length of the sampled process, e.g. when we expect a one-hour cycle we should sample every 30 min.

(b) What is the expected time frame of an event effect? When we intend to describe how the subject recovers after a target event, say a panic attack, we have to sample in a frequency corresponding to that expected duration. Here intervals should be chosen which are half of the recovery time of anxiety.

(ii) Practical factors in selecting sampling frequency ESM is a very demanding assessment method. It is therefore currently impossible to sample subjects in the ideal frequency range because it would exhaust them or have a drastic impact on the sampling environment. A standard procedure should seek a compromise between compliance and sampling requirements. In Maastricht, we use beep intervals of 90 min producing 10 beeps per day between 7.30 (a.m.) and 22.30 (p.m.). This 90-min period was initially selected based on the basic activation/rest cycle of human behavior (Minors & Waterhouse, 1981; Daan & Gwinner, 1989), but pragmatic sampling considerations weigh more heavily.

Our 'rule of thumb' for the sampling density is based on 10 years of experience with a large number of populations. Assessing subjects for one week makes 10 beeps each day an acceptable rate, giving at least 60 observations for each subject. When sampling is carried out for shorter periods of time, higher sampling frequencies may be possible. When sampling over longer periods (e.g. three weeks) we advise not to cross a six beeps/day threshold. Of course, compliance may be influenced by using other factors such as shorter or longer questionnaires, additional recording of physiological parameters, and the introduction of incentives.

(b) Parameters for the sampling process

An unlimited number of sampling schedules is possible. Because of the influence of the sampling procedure upon the nature of the data and for the purpose of replicability we strongly recommend conformity with schedules that have been used in earlier ESM studies. Sampling schemes should be described using the following parameters:

The *interval:* This is the average period between two beeps. When using random schedules it is appropriate to provide the standard deviation of the intervals, e.g., intervals of 90 min ± 30 min; three hours; . . .

The *type*: Fixed or random generation of the sampling series, e.g., a fixed schedule could start at 7.30 with 90-min intervals; . . .

The *sampling period:* This is the period over which the sampling took place, e.g., a day; a week; a month. If the period is shorter than one week mention should be made of the starting weekday. When sampling over longer periods, the starting day, season, and relation to the therapeutic or other process should be included.

Period restrictions: Sampling of experience is necessarily restricted to waking hours: between 7.30–22.30 (weekdays) and 9.00–23.30 (weekends) for adolescents or between 12.00 p.m.–3.00 a.m. for heroin addicts and prostitutes, for example (Kaplan, this volume). Alternating day periods with frequent, infrequent or no sampling such as intensive 'saturated sampling' of late afternoon, social time for morning affective style and concentration; or sampling mental patients with 30-min intervals during industrial therapy activities while using two-hour intervals for the rest of the day are examples of approaches that have worked with good result.

The researcher should be aware that changes in the basic time-series structure may lead to complication in analysis of the data and the interpretation of the results. ESM data are very complex and we strongly recommend the use of standardized sampling series. With the availability of user-friendly software in programming devices, or when 'smart' devices are developed that can generate their own sampling schemes, it will be increasingly tempting to use a different sampling series for each subject. This can be defended from a methodological point of view, but in the short run it is best to restrict the number of sampling schemes used, until improved statistical capacities for time-series analysis are available.

(c) Variation in types of sampling series[1]

We differentiate two types of sampling series: fixed and random schedules.

(i) Fixed schedules In fixed schedules beep-moments have a regular periodicity. As a consequence, each possible moment of the target period has a different probability of being selected. Probabilities may range from 0 to 100%. Fixed schemes are advisable whenever the use of a time-related statistical analysis is planned, such as time-series analysis, Markov processes, etc.. Fixed schedules, however, compute time-budgets of activities poorly. Infor-

---

[1] All the time series presented can be generated for RC-1000 and RC-4000 Seiko watches by custom developed software for ESM. For information about purchase of hard and software: IPSER, P.O. Box 214, 6200 AE Maastricht, The Netherlands.

mation about smaller intervals is also lost. As a consequence, modeling of experiental processes is restricted to periods of two intervals. This may be too slow in most instances. Most importantly, with fixed schedules the periodicity is easily recognized by the subjects (and their environment) and this generates anticipatory behaviors, thoughts and emotions. Although reactivity cannot be avoided in this type of sampling series, small random variations around a fixed point can minimize this reactivity.

Figure 31.1 shows standard fixed schedules. Reactivity may be minimized by disguising the fixed time-series, starting each day with different (random) starting time and using unexpected but fixed intervals (A). For example, periods of 52 min starting on Monday at 8.23, Tuesday at 9.07, . . .

B and C (Fig. 31.1) are modifications of the basic fixed-series. Here, the actual beep will occur at a random moment within a period around the fixed-scheduled-beep-time. The algorithm used for the randomization in Fig. 31.1B is based on random numbers drawn from the standard normal distribution. When using this kind of series the probability that a beep will occur at a certain moment will be highest when the moment is near to the fixed-scheme-beep-time. In Fig. 31.1C, however, the probability for the selection of a moment is equal within the sampling range. Outside this range the probability is zero.

When a schedule contains periods in which, due to the algorithm used, some moments can never be selected, or are selected using different probabilities, the computation of time-budgets becomes very difficult and perhaps impossible. The fixed periodicity, however, allows the use of the more sophisticated statistical analysis techniques.

(ii) Random   Random schemes are sampling schedules in which each possible moment of the target period has the same probability of being selected at a beep. This is a prerequisite for computing time-budgets. Randomization techniques further reduce the likelihood of anticipation. Figure 31.2 presents two schedules. In the truly random schedule (A), a random number of beeps will be selected each day. The intervals between beeps may vary. We do not advise this schedule because the possible long between-beep interval may demotivate the subjects. The stratified random scheme (B) generates one or more beeps within each time block of the target sample period. Each beep has the same probability of being selected. Each time block will also have the same number of beeps. Thanks to the stratification, shorter sampling periods can be sufficient to represent the whole period.

When sampling experience, particularly thought content, it is necessary to use schedules which signal the subject with a range of uncertainty about the beep of approximately 20 min. In our experience, this can be achieved by introducing randomization in fixed schedules. Stratified random series are best if the sampling period is rather short (e.g. one week, 10 times per day) and true

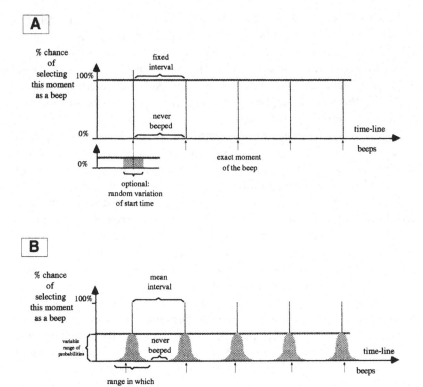

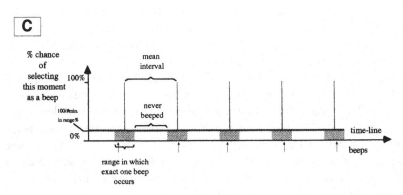

Fig. 31.1. Fixed interval time-sampling schedules. (A) Standard fixed interval time-series; (B) Fixed internal time-series with variations of random normal deviates; (C) Fixed interval time-series with variations of fixed probabilities.

370

Table 31.1. *Summary table for making device choices*

Device	Non-reactive	Flexible	Controllable	Description of elements to be weighted
a. *no 'real time' devices* egg-timers; random beepers; . . .	+	–	–	cheap reactivity; beep time can be checked (exc. external observer) timing control weak (no time-linked modelling possible)
b. *'real time' devices* radio transmission devices	+/– (noise)	+	–	expensive in acquisition and use: only for small samples restricted mobility (acti-radius): e.g. on hospital grounds allows sampling (time budgets) but not time-linked modelling allows event triggering by external observation
Pre-programmed devices	+	+	+	cheap; can be used for large samples allows sampling (time-budgets) and time-linked modelling allows real time control (e.g. interactions in families) allows total free mobility (long distances , . . .)
Laptop computer devices	– (size[1])	+	+	expensive; only for small number of subjects allows branched questioning (e.g. on computed events) allows concurrent signal monitoring (e.g. EEG, heart rate, . . .) allows direct data-input allows total control of the data-collecting process

[1] Hand-held computers are becoming available that overcome the size problem.

Table 31.2. *Pros and cons of fixed and random ESM sampling*

Purpose	Fixed series	Random series
Reduce reactivity (no anticipating behavior or thoughts of subject and/or the environment)	only in mixed series	+
Stable interval length (requirement of high-tech statistical model-building)	+	only in long series
Assessment of time-budgets	−	+
Assessment of event duration	only for long events (> interval)	only for the most frequent events
Assessment of time patterns (e.g. response decay)	only for long time patterns (> 2 × interval)	only in long series

+ controlled; − not controlled.

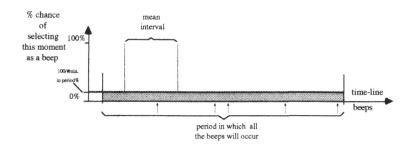

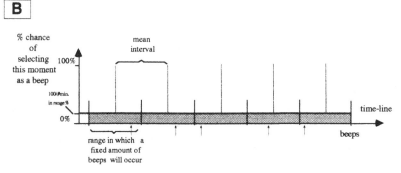

Fig. 31.2. Random interval time-sampling schedules. (A) Standard random interval time-series; (B) Stratified random interval time-series.

random schemes for longer (one or two months with six beeps per day) or high density, very short sampling periods (one day 40 times).

Summary

Selecting a sampling device is not easy. It will depend on the focus of the study, the available hardware at a specific time, and on the research budget. Table 31.1 summarizes the elements that can be weighted.

Selecting the sampling procedure is independent of hardware availability and cost issues and depends entirely on the research goals. A number of options have been discussed. The pros and cons of the basic sampling schedules are summarized in Table 31.2.
Good luck!

CLOSING

Looking to the future

MARTEN W. deVRIES

Initially, the idea of introducing Experience Sampling in psychiatric research aimed at incorporating ethnographically and ecologically relevant variables into clinical care. More provocatively, we sought to challenge psychiatric thinking with a new data set anchored more solidly in the experience of the person. We wanted to investigate if variables such as daily time-budgets, variations in mental state, situational reactivity and temporal patterning of symptoms would better describe and predict course and outcome. We wished to manufacture more valid psychiatric diagnostic profiles that would be able to specify treatment requirements more concretely. Quantitative descriptions of daily life patterns of ill and normal individuals would provide these data. Theoretically, the day and its behavioral components would open the window from which the history of the person, and the dynamics of his relationships, could be viewed. We wished to place the person more central than he currently stands in diagnostic formulations by emphasizing individual variation in experience and treatment tailored to individual needs. We thought that by confronting directly the often-ignored reality of individual differences, a powerful and persuasive argument for expanding the scope of treatment strategies could be made, ultimately resulting in a better fit between the person and the medical system.

Most of these challenges are as yet premature. The studies in this volume do take a first step; they are the beginning of systematic evaluation in this area. The data thus far demonstrate that detailed ESM information describes the patient well and can guide treatment successfully. The studies stand on the shoulder of psychiatric giants such as Adolf Meyer and Henry Stack Sullivan, who had previously formulated similar social, behavioral and clinical ideas and programs. Since then many men and women have theorized about the 'adaptive' person in relation to the environment. The authors in this book have added a methodological advance to this historical quest. Moreover, they are beginning to develop models for understanding psychopathology as well as optimal experience and wellbeing. From a research point of view, statistical packages and computer software are now available to manage these larger data sets. New instruments for ambulatory monitoring, including improvements in the ease with which data may be logged in, downloaded and analyzed, are being developed. The *Journal of Ambulatory Monitoring* is a focal point for technical and theoretical developments in this area. Theoretical, technical and critical advances testify to the growth in this field.

ESM studies describing psychopathology will continue into the 1990s producing a data base that may be archived for secondary analyses and comparison across a range of mental disorders. Such a data base will include descriptions of the experience as well as the situational aspects of psychopathology. Whether ESM will be able to clarify psychiatric issues in the future hinges on its capacity to elucidate systematically the power of daily life variables for psychiatric classification, treatment and research. ESM researchers will have to formulate testable hypotheses that will demand experimental refutation or support. Clinically, one useful contribution to care and classification would be the use of ESM data to flesh out the hitherto underdeveloped axes IV and V of the DSM-III classification system. Here, ESM descriptions of stressors, adaptive style and coping capacity of the individual may bring these diagnostic qualifications into quantitative perspective. Further, development of biopsychosocial research approaches by means of simultaneously collecting physiological measures such as cortisol and blood pressure along with the moment-to-moment measures of mental state, remain promising. Such naturalistic studies that measure physiological parameters accurately and repeatedly outside the laboratory can facilitate the exchange of information between more rigid, designed experimental studies within the laboratory. Community-based field studies, such as the study of heroin addicts in Amsterdam and Rotterdam, exploit the 'natural laboratory' created by the less-restrictive Dutch drug scene which provides an environment in which a research alliance with drug addicts can be developed. These studies thus gain access to hidden populations, which are often out of reach for clinicians and researchers. In the future, ESM may be used opportunistically in such field sites for clarifying epidemiologically significant health and behavioral problems related to AIDS, sexual behavior and addiction. Non-clinical studies pioneered by M. Csikszentmihalyi, R. Larson and F. Massimini are developing models for normative adolescences and adult experience; such models will provide the framework for comparing psychopathological behavior. Therapeutic applications of ESM could then be formulated and find many creative adherents.

The future seems bright for time-sampling and Experience Sampling approaches in psychiatry and medicine. In the early 1990s, the sister fields of biological psychiatry and psychopharmacology require information about the nature of setting effects as well as diurnal patterns of social behavior in order to understand their findings. Converging interests of social and biological oriented researchers can only be beneficial for scientific understanding and the treatment of patients. Researchers and clinicians active with ESM will continue to develop models and technology that will increase our capacity to collect data in the natural environment more easily, perhaps resulting in a decade of increased understanding of the person and his or her context of pain and joy.

References

Ablanalp, J.M., Livingston, L., Rose, R.M. & Sandwich, D. (1977). Cortisol and growth hormone responses to psychological stress during the menstrual cycle. *Psychosomatic Medicine*, **39**, 158–77.

Abraham, S.F. & Beumont, P.J.V. (1982). How patients describe bulimia or binge eating. *Psychological Medicine*, **12**, 625–35.

Abramsom, L.J., Metalsky, G.I. & Alloy, L.B. (1989). Hopelessness depression: A theory-based subtype of depression. *Psychological Review*, **96**, 2, 358–72.

Agar, M. (1973). *Ripping and Running: A Formal Ethnography of Urban Heroin Addicts*. Seminar Press: New York.

Alexander, B.K. & Hadaway, P.F. (1982). Opiate addiction: The case for an adaptive orientation. *Psychological Bulletin*, **92**, 367–81.

Alexander, B.K. (1990). The empirical and theoretical bases for an adaptive model of addiction. *Journal of Drug Issues*, **20**, 1, 37–65.

Allen, P., Batty, K., Dodd, C., Herbert, J., Hugh, C., Moore, G., Seymour, M., Shiers, H., Stacey, P. & Young, S. (1985). Dissociation between emotional and endocrine responses preceding an academic examination in male medical students. *Journal of Endocrinology*, 107, 163–70.

Allison, P.D. (1984). *Event-history Analysis*. Paper series on quantitative applications in the social sciences. Sage, Beverly Hills.

Alloway, R. & Bebbington, P. (1987). The buffer theory of social support: A review of the literature. *Psychological Medicine*, **17**, 91–108.

Alloy, L.B., Abramson, L.Y. *et al.* (1988). The hopelessness theory of depression: Attributional aspects. *British Journal of Clinical Psychology*, **27**, 5–21.

Allport, G.W. (1937). *Personality: A Psychological Interpretation*. New York: Holt.

Altmann, J. (1974). Observational Study of Behaviour: Sampling methods. *Behaviour*, **49**, 227–67.

Altschuller, M.I. (1923). *Byudzhet Vremeni (Time Budgets)*. USSR: Perm.

American Psychiatric Association. (1980). *Diagnostic and Statistical Manual of Mental Disorders*, 3rd edn (DSM III). Washington DC: APA.

American Psychiatric Association. (1987). *Diagnostic and Statistical Manual of Mental Disorders*, 3rd edn, revised (DSM-III-R). Washington DC: APA.

Anderson, C.M. (1983). A psychoeducational program for families of patients with schizophrenia. In: W.R. McFarlane (ed.), *Family Therapy in Schizophrenia*, pp. 99–116. London: Guilford.

Andreasen, N.C. (1982). Negative symptoms in schizophrenia: definition and reliability. *Archives of General Psychiatry*, **39**, 784–94.

Anisman, H. & Zacharcko, R.M. (1982). Depression: the predisposing influence of stress. *The Behavioral and Brain Sciences*, **5**, 89–137.

Ansseau, M., Sulon, J., Doumont, A., Cerfontaine, J.L., Legros, J.J., Sodoyez, J.C. & Demey-Ponsart, E. (1984). The use of saliva cortisol in the Dexamethasone Suppression Test. *Psychiatry Research*, **13**, 201–11.

APA *see* American Psychiatric Association (p. 381).

Appels, A. (1989). Loss of control, vital exhaustion and coronary heart disease. In: *Stress, Personal Control and Health*, eds. E. Steptoe & A. Appels, pp. 215–35. Brussels: Wiley and Sons.

Appels, A., Höppener, P. & Mulder, P. (1987). A questionnaire to assess premonitory symptoms of myocardial infarction. *International Journal of Cardiology*, **17**, 15–24.

Appels, A. & Mulder, P. (1988). Excess fatigue as a precursor of myocardial infarction. *European Heart Journal*, **9**, 758–64.

Appels, A. & Mendes de Leon, C.F. (1989). The association between vital exhaustion, unstable angina and future myocardial infarction. In: *Predisposing Conditions for Acute Ischemic Syndromes*, eds. T. von Arnim & A. Maseri, pp. 51–8. Darmstadt: Steinkopf Verlag.

Appleby, I.L., Klein, D.F., Sachon, E.J. & Morton, L. (1981). Biochemical indices of lactate induced panic: A preliminary report. In: D.F. Klein & Y. Rabkin (eds.), *Anxiety: New Research and Changing Concepts*. New York: Raven Press.

Aronson, T.A. & Craig, T.J. (1986). Cocaine precipitation of panic disorder. *American Journal of Psychiatry*, **143**, 643–5.

Arrindell, W.A. (1980). Dimensional structure and psychopathology correlates of the Fear Survey Schedule (FSS III) in a population: A factorial definition of agoraphobia. *Behavior Research & Therapy*, **18**, 229–42.

As, D. (1978). Household and dwellings: New techniques for recording and analyzing data on time-use. In: W. Michelson (ed.), *Public Policy in Temporal Perspective*. The Hague: Mouton.

Babor, T., Cooney, H., Hubbard, R., Jaffe, J., Kosten, T., Lauerman, R., McLellan, T., Rankin, H., Rounsaville, B. & Skinner, H. (1988). The syndrome concept of alcohol and drug dependence: Results of the secondary analysis project. In: L.S. Harris (ed.), *Problems of Drug Dependence 1987* (NIDA Research Monograph 81). Rockville, MD: NIDA. pp. 33–9.

Baldwin, R.C. & Jolley, D.J. (1986). The prognosis of depression in old age. *British Journal of Psychiatry*, **149**, 574–83.

Bannister, D. (1977). The logical requirements of research into schizophrenia. *Schizophrenia Bulletin*, **4**, 72–77.

Barker, R.G. (1963). *The Stream of Behavior*. New York: Appleton-Century Crofts.

Barker, R.G. (1968). *Ecological Psychology*. Stanford, CA: Stanford University Press.

Barker, R.G. (1978). *Habitats, Environments and Human Behavior: Studies in the Ecological Psychology and Eco-Behavioral Science of the Midwest Psychological Field Station: 1947–1972*. San Francisco: Jossey-Bass.

Barker, R.G. & Wright, H.F. (1951). *One Boy's Day*. New York: Harper & Row.

Barker, R.G. & Wright, H.F. (1955). *Midwest and Its Children*. Evanston, Il: Row, Peterson.

Barker, R.G., Wright, H.F., Barker, L.S. & Schoggen, M.F. (1961). In. K.S. Lawrence (ed.), *Specimen records of American and English Children*. University of Kansas Press.

Barker, R. & Schoggen, P. (1973). *Quality of Community Life*. Jossey Bass.

Bebbington, P. (1980). Causal models and logical inference in epidemiological psychiatry. *British Journal of Psychiatry*, **36**, 317–25.

Bechtel, R., Achepohl, C. & Akers, R. (1972). Correlates between observed behavior and questionnaire responses on television viewing. In: E.A. Rubenstein, G.A. Comstock & J.P. Murray (eds.), *Television and Social Behavior*, vol. 4, *Television in Day-to-day Life: Patterns and Use*. Washington DC: U.S. Government Printing Office.

Beck, A.T. (1976) *Cognitive Therapy and the Emotional Disorders*. New York: International Universities Press.

Beck. A.T. (1979). *Cognitive Therapy and the Emotional Disorders*. New York: Meridian.

Beck, A.T. (1987). Cognitive models of depression. *Journal of Cognitive Psychotherapy*, **1**, 1, 5–57.

Beck, A.T., Ward, C.H., Mendelsohn, M. *et al.* (1961). An inventory for measuring depression. *Archives of General Psychiatry*, **4**, 561–71.

Beck, A.T. & Beamesderfer, A. (1974). Assessment of depression: The depression inventory. In: *Psychological Measurements in Psychopharmacology, Modern Problems in Pharmacopsychiatry*, ed. P. Pichot, vol. 7, pp. 151–69. Basel: Karger.

Beck, A.T., Rush, A.J., Shaw, B.F. *et al.* (1979). *Cognitive Therapy of Depression*. New York: Guilford.

Becker, H. (1963). *The Outsiders: Studies in the Sociology of Deviance*. New York: Free Press.

Beers, C. (1986). *A Mind that Found Itself*, Revised Edn. New York: Doubleday.

Bellak, L. (ed.) (1979). *Disorders of the Schizophrenic Syndrome*. New York: Basic Books.

Benner, D.G. & Joscelyne, B. (1984). Multiple personality as a borderline disorder. *Journal of Nervous and Mental Disease*, **172**, 98–104.

Berger, M., Bossert, S., Krieg, J.-C., Dirlich, G., Ettmeier, W., Schreiber, W. & von Zerssen, D. (1987). Interindividual differences in the susceptibility of the cortisol system: an important factor for the degree of hypercortisolism in stress situations? *Biological Psychiatry*, **22**, 1327–39.

Bernard, H.R., Killworth, P., Kronenfeld, D. & Sailer, L. (1984). On the validity of retrospective data: The problem of informant accuracy. *Annual Review of Anthropology*, **13**, 495–517.

Bernheim, K.F. & Lehman, A.F. (1985). *Working with Families of the Mentally Ill*. New York: Norton.

Bevans, G.E. (1913). *How Workingmen Spend Their Spare Time*. New York: Columbia University Press.

Biernacki, P. (1986). *Pathways from Heroin Addiction. Recovery Without Treatment*. Philadelphia: Temple University Press.

Blackburn, I.M., Whalley, L.J. & Christie, J.E. (1987). Mood, cognition and cortisol; their temporal relationships during recovery from depressive illness. *Journal of Affective Disorders*, **13**, 31–43.

Blaney, P.H. (1986). Affect and memory: a review. *Psychological Bulletin*, **99**, 229–46.

Bleuler, E. (1911). *Dementia Praecox and the Group of Schizophrenias*. New Haven: International University Press.

Bleuler, M. (1978). *The Schizophrenic Disorders: Long Term Patient and Family studies*. New Haven CT: Yale University Press.

Bliss, E.L. (1980). Multiple personalities: A report of 14 cases with implications for schizophrenia and hysteria. *Archives of General Psychiatry*, **37**, 1388–97.

Bliss, E.L. (1984). Spontaneous self-hypnosis in multiple personality disorder. *Psychiatric Clinics of North America*, **7**, 135–49.

Blum, R. (1969). *Drugs*. San Francisco: Jossey-Bass.

Bohannan, P. (1963). *Social Anthropology*. New York: Holt, Rinehart & Winston.

Booth-Kewley, S. & Friedman, H. (1987). Psychological predictors of heart-disease: a quantitative review. *Psychological Bulletin*, **101**, 343–62.

Borkovec, T.D. (1985). Worry: a potentially valuable concept. *Behavior Research & Therapy*, **23**, 481–2.

Boskind-Lodahl, M. (1976). Cinderella's stepsisters: A feminist perspective on anorexia nervosa and bulimia. *Signs: Journal of Women in Culture and Society*, **2**, 2, 342–56.

Boskind-White, M. (1985). Bulimarexia: A sociocultural perspective. In: S.W. Emmett (ed.), *Theory and Treatment of Anorexia Nervosa and Bulimia: Biomedical Sociocultural and Psychological Perspectives*, pp. 113–26. New York: Brunner/Mazel.

Bossert, S., Berger, M., Krieg, J.-C. Schrieber, W., Junker, M. & von Zerssen, D. (1988). Cortisol response to various stressful situations: relationship to personality variables and coping. *Neuropsychobiology*, **20**, 36–42.

Bouman, T.K. (1987). *The Measurement of Depression with Questionnaires*. PhD Thesis, Groningen, The Netherlands.

Bowers, K.S. (1973). Situationism in psychology: An analysis and critique. *Psychological Review*, **80**, 307–36.

Bracht, G., Brakarsh, D. & Fellingstad, D. (1973). Deviant drug use in adolescence. *Psychological Bulletin*, **79**, 92–106.

Bradburn, N. (1969). *The Structure of Psychological Well-being*. Chicago: Aldine.

Brandstätter, H. (1983). Emotional responses to other persons in everyday life situations. *Journal of Personality and Social Psychology*, **45**, 871–83.

Breier, A., Charney, D.S. & Henninger, G.R. (1986). Agoraphobia with panic attacks: Development, diagnostic stability, and course of illness. *Archives of General Psychiatry*, **43**, 1029–36.

Bronfenbrenner, U. (1979). *The Ecology of Human Development*. Cambridge, USA: Harvard University Press.

Brophy, C.J., Norvell, N.K. & Kiluk, D.J. (1988). An examination of the factor structure and convergent and discriminant validity of the SCL-90 R in an outpatient clinic population. *Journal of Personality Assessment*, **52**, 2, 334–40.

Broughton, J. (1981). The divided self in adolescence. *Human Development*, **24**, 13–32.

Brown, G.W. (1974). Meaning, measurement and stress of life event. In: D.P. Dohrenwend (ed.) *Stressful Life Events: Their Nature and Effects*. New York: Wiley.

Brown, G.W. & Harris, T. (1978). *Social Origin of Depression. A Study of Psychiatric Disorder in Women*. London: Tavistock.

Brown, G.W., Andrews, B., Harris, T. *et al.* (1986). Social support, self-esteem and depression. *Psychological Medicine*, **16**, 813–31.

Brown, G.W., Bifulco, A. & Harris, T. (1987). Life events, vulnerability and onset of depression: some refinements. *British Journal of Psychiatry*, **150**, 30–42.

Brown, G.W., Adler, Z. & Bifulco, A. (1988). Life events, difficulties and recovery from chronic depression. *British Journal of Psychiatry*, **152**, 487–98.

Brunswick, E. (1949). *Systematic and Representative Design of Psychological Experiments*. Berkeley and Los Angeles: University of California Press.

Brunswick, E. (ed.). (1952). The conceptual framework of psychology. *International Encyclopedia of Unified Science*, vol. 1, no. 10. Chicago: University of Chicago Press.

Buck, O.D. (1983). Multiple personality disorder as a borderline state. *Journal of Nervous and Mental Disease*, **171**, 62–5.

Bukstein, O.G., Brent, D.A. & Kaminer, Y. (1989). Comorbidity of substance abuse and other psychiatric disorders in adolescents. *American Journal of Psychiatry*, **146**, 1131–41.

Buse, L. & Pawlik, K. (1984). Inter-Setting-Korrelationen und Setting-Persönlichkeits-Wechselwirkungen: Ergebnisse einer Felduntersuchung zur Konsistenz von Verhalten und Erleben. *Zeitschrift für Sozialpsychologie*, **15**, 44–59.

Cameron, O.G. & Nesse, R.M. (1988). Systemic hormonal and physiological abnormalities in anxiety disorders. *Psychoneuroendocrinology*, **13**, 287–307.

Carli, M., Delle Fave, A. & Massimini, F. (1988). The quality of experience in the flow channels: Comparison of Italian and U.S. students. In: M. Csikszentmihalyi & I. Csikszentmihalyi (eds.), *Optimal Experience. Psychological Studies of Flow in Consciousness*. New York: Cambridge University Press.

Carlstein, T. (1978). A time-geographic approach to time allocation and socioecological systems. In: W. Michelson (ed.), *Public Policy in Temporal Perspective*. The Hague: Mouton.

Carney, M.W.P., Roth, M. & Garside, R.F. (1965). The diagnosis of depressive syndromes and the prediction of E.C.T. response. *British Journal of Psychiatry*, **111**, 659–74.

Carroll, B.J., Feinberg, M., Smouse, P.E. *et al.* (1981). The Caroll rating scale for depression. 1. Development, reliability and validation. *British Journal of Psychiatry*, **138**, 194–200.

Casper, R.C., Eckert, E.D., Halmi, K.A., Goldberg, S.C. & Davis, J.M. (1980). Bulimia: Its incidence and clinical importance in patients with anorexia nervosa. *Archives of General Psychiatry*, **37**, 1030–5.

Chabon, B. & Robins, C.J. (1986). Cognitive distortions among depressed and suicidal drug abusers. *International Journal of the Addictions*, **21**, 12, 1313–39.

Chambless, D.L. & Goldstein, A.J. (eds.) (1982). *Agoraphobia: Multiple Perspectives on Theory and Treatment.* New York: Wiley.

Chapin, S. (1974). *Human Activity Patterns: Things People Do in Time and Space.* New York: Wiley.

Chapman, L.J. & Chapman, J.P. (1980). Scales for rating psychotic and psychotic-like experiences as continua. *Schizophrenia Bulletin,* **6,** 3, 476–89.

Chapple, E.D. (1970). *Culture and the Biological Man: Explanations in Behavioral Anthropology.* New York: Holt, Rinehart & Wilson.

Cherek, D.R., Smith, J.E., Lane, J.D. & Brauchi, J.T. (1982). Effects of cigarettes on saliva cortisol levels. *Clinical Pharmacology & Therapeutics,* **32,** 765–8.

Chesney, M.A. & Ironson, G.H. (1989). Diaries in ambulatory monitoring. In: N. Schneiderman, S. Weiss & P. Kaufmann (eds.), *Handbook of Research Methods in Cardiovascular Medicine.* New York: Plenum.

Chombart de Lauwe, P.H. (1956). *La Vie quotidienne des Familles ouvrières.* Paris: CNRS.

Ciompi, L. (1989). The dynamics of complex biological-psychosocial systems. Four fundamental psycho-biological mediators in the long-term evolution of schizophrenia. *British Journal of Psychiatry,* **155,** 15–21.

Ciompi, L. & Müller, C. (1976). *Lebensweg und Alter der Schizophrenen. Eine Katamnestische Langzeitstudie bis ins Senium.* Berlin: Springer-Verlag.

Cloninger, C.R., Martin, R.L., Guze, S.B. & Clayton, P.J. (1985). Diagnosis and prognosis in schizophrenia. *Archives of General Psychiatry,* **42,** 15–25.

Cochran, W. (1953). *Sampling Techniques.* New York: Wiley.

Collins, A., Eneroth, P. & Landgren, B.-M. (1985). Psychoneuroendocrine stress responses and mood as related to the menstrual cycle. *Psychosomatic Medicine,* **47,** 512–27.

Combessie, J.-C. (1985). Oubli et paradoxes. *Bulletin de Méthodologie Sociologique,* **6,** 29–38.

Combessie, J.-C. (1986). A propos de méthodes: effets d'optique, heuristiques et objectivation. *Bulletin de Méthodologie Sociologique,* **10,** 4–24.

Cook, N.J., Ng, A., Read, G.F., Harris, B. & Riad-Fahmy, D. (1987). Salivary cortisol for monitoring adrenal activity during marathon runs. *Hormone Research,* **25,** 18–23.

Cooley, C.H. (1902, Revised edn, 1922). *Human Nature and the Social Order.* New York: Scribner's.

Cooper, J.L., Morrison, T.L., Bigman, O.L., Abramowitz, S.I., Levin, S. & Krener, P. (1988). Mood changes and affective disorder in the bulimic binge-purge cycle. *International Journal of Eating Disorders,* **7,** 4, 469–74.

Cooper, P.J. & Fairburn, C.G. (1986). The depressive symptoms of bulimia nervosa. *British Journal of Psychiatry,* **148,** 268–274.

Copeland, J.R.M., Kelleher, M.J., Kellett, J.M., Gourlay, A.J., Gurland, B.J., Fleiss, J.L. & Sharpe, L. (1976). A semi-structured clinical interview for the assessment of diagnosis and mental state in the elderly. The Geriatric Mental State Schedule 1. Development and reliability. *Psychological Medicine,* **6,** 439–449.

Copeland, J.R.M., Davidson, I.A., Dewey, M.E., Saunders, P.A., Sharma, V., Sullivan, C. & McWilliam, C. (in press). Dementia, depression, pseudodementia and the neuroses: Prevalence, incidence and three year outcome in Liverpool: GMS-HAS AGECAT.

Coryell, W. (1983). Multiple personality disorder and primary affective disorder. *Journal of Nervous and Mental Disease*, **171**, 388–90.

Costello, E.J., Edelbrock, C. & Costello, A.J. (1985). Validity of the NIMH Diagnostic Interview Schedule for Children: A comparison between psychiatric and pediatric referrals. *Journal of Abnormal and Child Psychology*, **13**, 579–95.

Coyne, J.C. (1976). Toward an interactional description of depression. *Psychiatry*, **39**, 28–40.

Coyne, J.C. (1985). Studying depressed persons interactions with strangers and spouses. *Journal of Abnormal Psychology*, **94**, 2, 231–2.

Creason, C. & Goldman, M. (1981). Varying levels of marijuana use by adolescents and the amotivation syndrome. *Psychological Reports*, **48**, 447–54.

Crisp, A.H., Queen, M. & d'Souza, M. (1984). Myocardial infarction and the emotional climate. *The Lancet*, **17**, 616–19.

Crow, T.J. (1980). Molecular pathology of schizophrenia: More than one disease process? *British Medical Journal*, **280**, 66–8.

Crow, T.J. (1982). Schizophrenia deterioration. *British Journal of Psychiatry*, **143**, 80–3.

Crowe, R.R., Pauls, D.L., Slymen, D.J. & Noyes, K. (1980). A family study of anxiety neurosis. *Archives of General Psychiatry*, **37**, 77–9.

Csikszentmihalyi, M. (1975). *Beyond Boredom and Anxiety*. San Francisco: Jossey-Bass.

Csikszentmihalyi, M. (1978). Intrinsic rewards and emerging motivation. In: M.R. Lepper & D. Greene (eds.), *The Hidden Costs of Reward*, pp. 205–16. New York: Erlbaum.

Csikszentmihalyi, M. (1982). Toward a psychology of optimal experience. In: L. Wheeler (ed.), *Review of Personality and Social Psychology*, vol. 2. Beverly Hills, CA: Sage.

Csikszentmihalyi, M. (1985). Emergent motivation and the evolution of the self. In: D. Kleiber & M.H. Maher (eds.), *Motivation in Adulthood*. Greenwich C.T: Jai Press.

Csikszentmihalyi, M. (1986). Lo studio dell'esperienza quotidiana. In: F. Massimini & P. Inghilleri (eds.), *L'Esperienza Quotidiana. Teoria e Metodo d'Analisi*. Milano: Franco Angeli.

Csikszentmihalyi, M., Larson, R. & Prescott, S. (1977). The ecology of adolescent activity and experience. *Journal of Youth and Adolescence*, **6**, 281–94.

Csikszentmihalyi, M. & Beattie, O. (1979). Life theme: A theoretical and empirical exploration of the origin and effects. *Journal of Humanistic Psychology*, **19**, 1.

Csikszentmihalyi, M. & Graef, R. (1980). The experience of freedom in everyday life. *American Journal of Community Psychology*, **18**, 402–14.

Csikszentmihalyi, M. & Kubey, J. (1981). Television and the rest of life: A systematic comparison of subjective experience. *Public Opinion Quarterly*, **4**, 3, 317–28.

Csikszentmihalyi, M. & Rochberg-Halton, E. (1981). *The Meaning of Things: Domestic Symbols and the Self*. New York: Cambridge University Press.

Csikszentmihalyi, M. & Figurski, T.J. (1982). Self-awareness and aversive experience in everyday life. *Journal of Personality*, **50**, 14–26.

Csikszentmihalyi, M. & Larson, R. (1984). *Being Adolescent: Conflict and Growth in the Teenage Years*. New York: Basic Books.

Csikszentmihalyi, M. & Massimini, F. (1985). On the psychological selection of bio-cultural information. *New Ideas in Psychology*, **3**, 115–38.

Csikszentmihalyi, M. & Larson, R. (1987). Validity and reliability of the Experience Sampling Method. *Journal of Nervous and Mental Disease*, **175**, 526–36.

Csikszentmihalyi, M. & LeFevre, J. (1987). Optimal Experience in Work and Leisure. Paper presented at the 5th Canadian Leisure Research Conference, Halifax, N. S., May.

Csikszentmihalyi, M. & Csikszentmihalyi, I. (eds.) (1988). *Optimal Experience. Psychological Studies of Flow in Consciousness*. Cambridge, UK: Cambridge University Press.

Cullen, I.G. & Godson, V. (1975). *Urban Networks: The Structure of Activity Patterns*. Oxford: Pergamon.

Custance, J. (1952). *Wisdom, Madness and Folly*. New York: Farrar, Straus & Cudahy, Inc.

Daan, S. & Gwinner, E. (1989). *Biological Clocks and Environmental Time. Proceedings of a Symposium in Honour of Prof. Dr. Jürgen Aschoff*. New York: Guilford Press.

Da Costa, J.M. (1871). On irritable heart: A clinical form of functional cardiac disorder and its consequences. *American Journal of Medical Science*, **61**, 17–52.

Davis, R., Freeman, R.J. & Solyom, L. (1985). Mood and food: An analysis of bulimic episodes. *Journal of Psychiatric Research*, **19**, 2/3, 331–5.

Davis, R., Freeman, R.J. & Garner, D.M. (1988). A naturalistic investigation of eating behavior in bulimia nervosa. *Journal of Consulting and Clinical Psychology*, **56**, 2, 273–9.

De Swaan, A. (1981). The politics of agoraphobia: On changes in emotional and relational management. *Theory and Society*, **10**, 337–58.

Delahunt, J.W. & Mellsop, G. (1987). Hormone changes in stress. *Stress Medicine*, **3**, 123–34.

Delespaul, P.A.E.G. & deVries, M.W. (1987). The daily life of ambulatory chronic mental patients. *Journal of Nervous and Mental Disease*, **175**, 537–44.

Delle Fave, A. & Massimini, F. (1988). Modernization and changing contexts of flow in work and leisure. In: M. Csikszentmihalyi & I. Csikszentmihalyi (eds.), *Optimal Experience. Psychological Studies in Flow in Consciousness*. New York: Cambridge University Press.

Dembo, R., Schmeidler, J. & Koval, M. (1976). Demographic, value and behavioral correlates of marijuana use among middle-class youth. *Journal of Health and Social Behavior*, **17**, 177–87.

Derogatis, L.R., Lipman, R.S. & Covi, L. (1973). The SCL-90: an outpatient psychiatric rating scale. *Psychopharmacology Bulletin*, **9**, 13–28.

Devereux, R.B., Pickering, T.G., Harshfield, G.A., Keinert, H.D., Denby, L., Clark, L., Pregibon, D., Jason, M., Kleiner, B., Borer, J.S. & Laragh, J.H. (1983). Left ventricular hypertrophy in patients with hypertension: Importance of blood pressure response to regularly recurring stress. *Circulation*, **68**, 3, 470–6.

deVries, M.W. (1983). Temporal patterning of psychiatric symptoms. *World Psychiatric Association Congress*, Vienna, Abstract.

deVries, M.W. (1985). Anorexia nervosa and affective disorders. *American Journal of Psychiatry*, **142**, 1, 140–1.

deVries, M.W. (1987). Investigating mental disorders in their natural settings. *Journal of Nervous and Mental Disease*, **175**, 509–13.

deVries, M.W., Delespaul, P.A.E.G. & Theunissen, J. (1984). Diurnal variations in the conscious experience of schizophrenics. *Symposium on Development of Schizophrenia*. WPA Congress, Helsinki, Abstract.

deVries, M.W. & Delespaul, P.A.E.G. (1985). Affect and daily life in disordered and non-disordered persons. *WPA Regional Symposium on Affective Disorders*, Greece.

deVries, M.W., Delespaul, P.A.E.G., Dijkman, C.I.M. & Theunissen, J. (1986). Advance in understanding temporal and setting aspects of schizophrenic disorders. In: F. Massimini & P. Inghilleri (eds.), *L'Esperienza quotidiana*, pp. 477–93. Milano: Franco Angeli.

deVries, M.W., Delespaul, P.A.E.G. & Dijkman, C.I.M. (1987). Affect and anxiety in daily life. In: G. Racagni (ed.), *Anxious Depression: Assessment and Treatment*. New York: Raven Press.

deVries, M.W. & Delespaul, P.A.E.G. (1988). *Persons in the Schizophrenic's Environment. Influence on Mental State*. R.U. Limburg, Maastricht: Mimeo Department of Social Psychiatry.

deVries, M.W. & Delespaul, P.A.E.G. (1989). Time, context and subjective experience in schizophrenia. *Schizophrenia Bulletin*, **15**, 2, 233–44.

deVries, M.W., Dijkman-Caes, C.I.M. & Delespaul, P.A.E.G. (1988). De ontbrekende schakel: diagnostiek in de natuurlijke omgeving. *Nederlands Tijdschrift voor Psychiatrie*, **2**, 20, 94–114.

deVries, M.W., Dijkman-Caes, C.I.M. & Delespaul, P.A.E.G. (1990). The sampling of experience: A method of measuring the co-occurrence of anxiety and depression in daily life. In: J.D. Maser & C.R. Cloninger (eds.), *Comorbidity of Anxiety and Mood Disorders*. Washington DC.: American Psychiatric Press.

Diekstra, R.F., Engels, G.I. & Methorst, B.J. (1988). Cognitive therapy for depression: A means of crisis intervention. *Crisis*, **9**, 1, 32–44.

Diener, E., Larson, R.J. & Emmons, R.A. (1984). Person × situation interactions: Choices of situations and congruence response models. *Journal of Personality and Social Psychology*, **47**, 580–92.

Dijkman, C.I.M. & deVries, M.W. (1987). The social ecology of anxiety. Theoretical and quantitative perspectives. *Journal of Nervous and Mental Disease*, **175**, 9, 550–7.

Dijkstra, P. (1974). De zelfboerdelingsschaal voor depressie van Zung. In: H.M. van Praag & H.G.M. Rooymans (eds.), *Stemming en Ontstemming*. Amsterdam: De Erven Bohn.

Dimsdale, J.F. (1984). Generalizing from laboratory to field studies of human stress physiology. *Psychosomatic Medicine*, **46**, 463–9.

Dimsdale, J.E. & Moss, J. (1980). Short-term catecholamine response to psychological stress. *Psychosomatic Medicine*, **42**, 493–7.

Divilbiss, J. & Self, P. (1978). Work analysis by random sampling. *Bulletin of the Medical Library Association*, **66**, 19–32.

Dobson, K.S. (1985). An analysis of anxiety and depression scales. *Journal of Personality Assessment*, **49**, 5, 522–7.

Docherty, J.P., Van Kammen, D.P., Siris, S.G. & Marder, S.R. (1978). Stages of onset schizophrenic psychosis. *American Journal of Psychiatry*, **135**, 4, 420–6.

Dohrenwend, B.S. & Dohrenwend, B.P. (ed.) (1974). *Stressful Life Events: Their Nature and Effects*. New York: Wiley.

Dohrenwend, B.P. & Shrout, P.E. (1985). 'Hassles' in the conceptualization and measurement of life stress varaibles. *American Psychologist*, **40**, 7, 780–5.

Donlon, P. & Blaker, K. (1973). Stages of schizophrenic decompensation and reintegration. *Journal of Nervous and Mental Disease*, **157**, 200–8.

Donlon, P. & Blaker, K. (1975). Clinical recognition of early schizophrenic decompensation. *Diseases of the Nervous System*, **36**, 323–30.

Donner, E. (1985). ESM and Heart Rate Monitoring. Paper presented at the ESM Workshop, University of Chicago.

Donner, E. (1989). *The Contributions of Mood and Arousal to Health and Illness*. University of Chicago: Dissertation, Department of Psychology, December.

Donner, E., Nash, K., Csikszentmihalyi, M. & Chalip, L. (1983). Interpersonal influence in dyadic relations. Paper presented at the Annual Meeting of the Society for Experimental Social Psychology, Nashville, Tennesee; November.

Donner, E., Csikszentmihalyi, M. & Schneider, C. (1987). Toward a holistic model of achievement. Paper presented at the Annual Meeting of the American Psychological Association, New York City, August.

Draper, N. & Smith, H. (1981). *Applied Regression Analysis*. New York: Wiley.

DSP (Department of Social Psychiatry) (1986). *Cross-Classification Analysis*. *Experience Sampling Symposium*. University of Limburg, 13 pp.

Duval, S. & Wicklund, R.A. (1972). *A Theory of Objective Self-awareness*. New York: Academic Press.

Duval, S. & Wicklund, R.A. (1973). Effects of objective self-awareness on attribution of causality. *Journal of Experimental Social Psychology*, **9**, 17–31.

Eaton, W.W. & Ritter, C. (1988). Distinguishing anxiety and depression field survey data. *Psychological Medicine*, **18**, 155–66.

Edwards, G. & Gross, M.M. (1976). Alcohol dependence: Provisional description of the clinical syndrome. *British Medical Journal*, **1**, 1058–61.

Edwards, G., Arif, A. & Hodgson, R. (1981). Nomenclature and classification of drug and alcohol-related problems: A shortened version of a WHO memorandum. *British Journal of Addiction*, **77**, 3–20.

Ehlers, C.L., Frank, E. & Kupfer, D.J. (1988). Social Zeitgebers and biological rhythms: a unified approach to understanding the etiology of depression. *Archives of General Psychiatry*, **45**, 948–52.

Eichberg, R. (1975). Some words of caution on subjective concepts. In: J. Elinson & D. Nurco (eds.), *Operational Definitions on Sociobehavioral Drug Use Research*. National Institute of Drug Abuse.

Elliot, D.H. & Clark, S. (1978). The spatial context of urban activities. In: W. Michelson (ed.), *Public Policy in Temporal Perspective*. The Hague: Mouton.

Ellis, A. (1962). *Reason and Emotion in Psychotherapy*. New York: Lyle Stuart.

Ellis, A. (1973). *Humanistic Psychotherapy: The Rational Emotive Approach*. New York: McGraw-Hill.

Emmelkamp, P.M.G. (1982). *Phobic and Obsessive-compulsive Disorder: Theory, Research and Practice*. New York: Plenum.

Endler, N.S. (1983). Interactionism: A personality model, but not yet a theory. In: M.M. Page (ed.), *Nebraska Symposium on Motivation 1982: Personality – Current Theory and Research*. Lincoln: University of Nebraska Press.

Endler, N.S. & Magnusson, D. (eds.) (1976). *Interactional Psychology and Personality*. New York: Wiley.

Engel, G. (1977). The need for a new medical model: A challenge for biomedicine. *Science*, **196**, 129.

Engelsman, E.L. (1989) Dutch policy on the management of drug related problems. *British Journal of Addiction*, **84**, 211–18.

Epstein, S. (1983). Aggregation and beyond: Some basic issues on the prediction of behavior. *Journal of Personality*, **51**, 360–92.

Ericsson, A.K. & Simon, H.A. (1980). Verbal reports as data. *Psychology Review*, **87**, 215–51.

Ericsson, A.K. & Simon, H.A. (1984). *Protocol Analysis: Verbal Reports as Data*. Cambridge, MA: MIT Press.

Falger, P.R.J. (1989). *Life-span Development and Myocardial Infarction: an Epidemiological Study*. PhD Thesis, Maastricht, the Netherlands.

Falloon, I.R.M. (1985). Behavioral family therapy: A problem-solving approach to family coping. In: L. Leff & C. Vaughn (eds.), *Expressed Functions in Families*. London: Guilford.

Falloon, I.R.M., Boyd, J.L. & McGill, C. (1984). *Family Care of Schizophrenia*, pp. 150–74. London: Guilford.

Faugeron, C. & van Meter, K.M. (1987). *Analysis of deviance and of social classes: The impact of methodological research*. Annual Meeting of the American Sociological Association, 17–20 August, Chicago.

Fenigstein, A., Scheier, M.F. & Buss, A.H. (1975). Public and private self-consciousness: Assessment and theory. *Journal of Consulting and Clinical Psychology*, **43**, 522–7.

Fennel, M.J., Teasdale, J.D., Jones, S. & Damle, A. (1987). Distractions in neurotic and endogenous depression: An investigation of negative thinking in major depressive disorder. *Psychological Medicine*, **17**, 2, 441–52.

Ferguson, G.A. (1959). *Statistical Analysis in Psychology & Education*. Tokyo: McGraw-Hill Kogakusha Ltd.

Figurski, T.J. (1985). *Self and Others: Person-awareness in Everyday Life*. Unpublished doctoral dissertation, The University of Chicago.

Figurski, T.J. (1987a). Self-awareness and other-awareness: The use of perspective in everyday life. In: K. Yardley & T. Honess (eds.), *Self and Identity: Psychosocial Perspectives*, pp. 197–210. Chichester, England: Wiley & Sons.

Figurski, T.J. (1987b). The emotional contingencies of self-awareness in everyday life. In: M.C. Hoover (Chair), *What People Think About*. Symposium conducted at the 95th Annual Convention of the American Psychological Association, New York.

Filstead, W., Reich, W., Parrella, D. & Rossi, J. (1985). Using electronic pagers to monitor the process of recovery in alcoholics and drug abusers. Paper presented at the 34th International Congress on Alcohol, Drug Abuse and Tobacco, Calgary, Alberta, Canada.

Fink, W.L. (1986). Microcomputers and phylogenetic analysis. *Science*, **734**, 1133–9.

Fiske, D. (1971). *Measuring the Concept of Personality*. Chicago: Aldine.

Flavell, J. (1968). *The Development of Role-taking and Communication Skills in Children*. New York: Wiley & Sons.

Folkard, S. (1976). Diurnal variations and individual differences in the perception of intractable pain. *Journal of Psychosomatic Research*, **20**, 289–301.

Folkman, S. & Lazarus, R.S. (1980). An analysis of coping in a middle-aged community sample. *Journal of Health and Social Behavior*, **21**, 219–39.

Folkman, S. & Lazarus, R.S. (1985). If it changes it must be a process: study of emotion and coping during three stages of a college examination. *Journal of Personality & Social Psychology*, **48**, 150–70.

Folkman, S., Lazarus, R.S., Gruen, R.J. *et al.* (1986). Appraisal, coping, health status, and psychological symptoms. *Journal of Personality and Social Psychology*, **50**, 3, 571–9.

Forslund, M. (1978). Functions of drinking for native American and white youth. *Journal of Youth and Adolescence*, **7**, 327.

Forsman, L. & Lundberg, U. (1982). Consistency in catecholamine and cortisol excretion in males and females. *Pharmacology, Biochemistry & Behavior*, **17**, 555–62.

Fortes, M. (1958). Introduction. In: J. Goody (ed.), *The Developmental Cycle in Domestic Groups*. New York: Cambridge University Press.

Frances, A.J., Widiger, T.A. & Pincus, H.A. (1989). The development of DSM-IV. *Archives of General Psychiatry*, **46**, 373–5.

Frankenhaeuser, M. (1980). Psychoneuroendocrine approaches to the study of stressful person-environment transactions. *Selye's Guide to Stress Research*, **1**, 46–70.

Frankenhaeuser, M. (1986). A psychobiological framework for research on human stress and coping. In: M. Appley & R. Trumbull (eds.), *Dynamics of Stress*, pp. 101–16. New York: Plenum.

Franzoi, S.L. & Brewer, L.C. (1984). The experience of self-awareness and its relation to level of self-consciousness: An experiential sampling study. *Journal of Research in Personality*, **18**, 522–40.

Frecska, E., Lukčcs, H., Aratù, M., Mùd, L., AlfÜldi, A. & Magyar, I. (1988). Dexamethasone suppression test and coping behavior in psychosocial stress. *Psychiatry Research*, **23**, 137–45.

Frederikson, M., Sundin, O. & Frankenhaeuser, M. (1985). Cortisol excretion during the defense reaction in humans. *Psychosomatic Medicine*, **47**, 313–19.

Freedman, R.R., Ianni, P., Ettedgui, E. & Puthezhath, N. (1985). Ambulatory monitoring of panic disorder. *Archives of General Psychiatry*, **42**, 244–8.

Freeman, M., Csikszentmihalyi, M. & Larson, R. (1986). Adolescence and its recollection: Toward an interpretive model of development. *Merrill-Palmer Quarterly*, **32**, 167–85.

Freud, S. (1924). The justification for detaching from neurasthenia a particular syndrome: The anxiety neurosis. In: J. Riviere, (ed.), *Collected Papers*, vol. 1. New York: International Psychoanalytic Press.

Freud, S. (1961). The psychopathology of everyday life. In: J. Strachey (ed. &

transl.) *The Standard Edition of the Complete Psychological Works of Sigmund Freud*, vol. VI. London: Hogarth Press. (Originally published in 1901.)

Garety, P. (1985). Delusions: Problems in definition and measurement. *British Journal of Medical Psychology*, **58**, 25–34.

Garfinkel, P.E., Moldofsky, H. & Garner, D.M. (1980). The heterogeneity of anorexia nervosa. *Archives of General Psychiatry*, **37**, 1036–40.

Garner, D., Garfinkel, P.E. & O'Shaunnessy, M. (1985). The validity of the distinction between bulimia with and without anorexia nervosa. *American Journal of Psychiatry*, **142**, 581–7.

Gauthier, J., Pellerin, D. & Renaud, P. (1983). The enhancement of self-esteem: a comparison of two cognitive strategies. *Cognitive Therapy and Research*, **7**, 5, 389–98.

Gawin, F.H. & Kleber, H.D. (1986). Abstinence, symptomatology and psychiatric diagnosis in cocaine abusers: Clinical observations. *Archives of General Psychiatry*, **43**, 107.

Gendlin, E.T. (1973). Experiential psychotherapy. In: R. Corsins (ed.), *Current Psychotherapies*. Itasca, Il.

Gergen, K.J. (1982). *Toward Transformation in Social Knowledge*. New York: Springer-Verlag.

Giannino, S., Graef, R. & Csikszentmihalyi, M. (1979). Well-being and the perceived balance between opportunities and capabilities. Paper presented at the 87th Convention of the American Psychiatric Association, New York, New York.

Glad, W. & Adesso, V.J. (1976). The relative importance of socially induced tension and behavioral contagion for smoking behavior. *Journal of Abnormal Psychology*, **85**, 119–21.

Glassman, A.H., Jackson, W.K., Walsh, B.T. & Roose, S.P. (1984). Cigarette craving, smoking withdrawal, and clonidine. *Science*, **226**, 864–6.

Goffman, E. (1959). *The Presentation of Self in Everyday Life*. New York: Doubleday.

Goffman, E. (1963). *Behavior in Public Places*. New York: Free Press.

Goldberg, D. & Huxley, P. (1980). *Mental Illness in the Community. The Pathway to Psychiatric Care*. London: Tavistock.

Good, B.J. & Kleinman, A.M. (1984). *Culture and Anxiety: Cross-cultural Evidence for the Patterning of Anxiety Disorders*. Bethesda, M.D.: National Institute of Mental Health.

Goodstadt, M., Cook, G. & Gruson, V. (1978). The validity of reported drug use: The randomized response technique. *International Journal of Addiction*, **13**, 359–67.

Gorsuch, R. & Butler, M. (1976). Initial drug abuse: A review of predisposing social-psychological factors. *Psychology Bulletin*, **83**, 120–37.

Gottman, J.M. (1981). *Time Series Analysis. A Comprehensive Introduction for Social Scientists*. Cambridge, UK: Cambridge University Press.

Graef, R., Csikszentmihalyi, M. & Giffin, P. (1978). Flow and work satisfaction. Unpublished manuscript.

Graef, R., Gianinno, S. & Csikszentmihalyi, M. (1981). Energy consumption in leisure and perceived happiness. In: J. Claxton, C.D. Anderson,

REFERENCES

J.R.B. Ritchie & G. McDougall (eds.), *Consumers and Energy Conservation: International Perspectives on Research and Policy Options.* New York: Praeger.

Graef, R., Csikszentmihalyi, M. & Giannino, S. (1983). Measuring intrinsic motivation in everyday life. *Leisure Studies,* 155–68.

Green, H. (1970). *I Never Promised You a Rose Garden.* New York: New American Library.

Greenberg, M.S. & Beck, A.T. (1989). Depression versus anxiety: A test of the content-specificity hypothesis. *Journal of Abnormal Psychology,* **98,** 1, 9–12.

Greene, A. (1985). Self-concept and life transitions in early adolescence. Paper presented at the biannual meeting of the Society for Research on Child Development, Toronto, Ontario, Canada.

Griez, E. & van den Hout, M. (1983a). Treatment of phobophobia by exposure to CO_2 induced anxiety symptoms. *Journal of Nervous and Mental Disease,* **171,** 8, 506–8.

Griez, E. & van den Hout, M. (1983b). Carbon dioxide and anxiety: Cardiovascular effects of a single inhalation. *Journal of Behavioral Therapy and Experimental Psychiatry,* **14,** 297–301.

Grinspoon, L. (1977). *Marijuana Reconsidered.* Cambridge, MA: Harvard University Press.

Gross, D.R. (1984). Time allocation: A tool for the study of cultural behavior. *American Review of Anthropology,* **13,** 519–58.

Gruenberg, E.M. (1967). The social breakdown syndrome – some origins. *American Journal of Psychiatry,* **123,** 1481–9.

Guechot, J., Passa, P., Villette, J.M., Gourmel, B., Tabuteau, F., Cathelineau, G. & Dreux, C. (1982). Physiological and pathological variations in saliva cortisol. *Hormone Research,* **16,** 357–64.

Guidano, V.F. & Liotti, G. (1983). *Cognitive Processes and Emotional Disorders: A Structural Approach to Psychotherapy.* New York: Guilford.

Gunderson, J.G. (1984). *Borderline Personality Disorder.* Washington, DC: American Psychiatric Association.

Gurin, G., Veroff, J. & Field, S. (1960). *Americans View Their Mental Health.* New York: Basic.

Gurney, C., Roth, M., Garside, R.F., Kerr, T.A. & Shapira, K. (1972). Studies in the classification of affective disorders. The relationship between anxiety states and depressive illness. II. *British Journal of Psychiatry,* **121,** 162–6.

Guttman, L. (1954). The principle components of scalable attitudes. In: P.F. Lazarsfeld (ed.), *Mathematical Thinking in the Social Sciences,* pp. 224–46. New York: Free Press.

Guttman, L. (1984). What is not what in statistics. Statistical inference revisited. *Bulletin de Méthodologie Sociologique,* **4,** 3–35.

Gwirtsman, H.E., Roy-Byrne, P., Yager, J. & Gerner, R.H. (1983). Neuroendocrine abnormalities in bulimia. *American Journal of Psychiatry,* **140,** 5, 559–63.

Hall, E.T. (1959). *The Silent Language.* New York: Doubleday.

Halmi, K.A. (1985). Relationship of eating disorders to depression: Biological similarities and differences. *International Journal of Eating Disorders,* **4,** 4, 667–80.

Hamilton, J.A., Haier, R.J. & Buchsbaum, M.S. (1984). Intrinsic enjoyment and boredom coping scales: Validation with personality, evoked potential and attention measures. *Personality and Individual Differences*, **5**, 183–93.

Hamilton, J.A., Alagna, S.W. & Pinkel, S. (1984). Gender differences in anti-depressant and activating drug effects on self-perception. *Journal of Affective Disorders*, **7**, 235–43.

Hamilton, J.A., Parry, B.L., Blumenthal, S., Alagna, A. & Herz, E. (1984). Premenstrual changes: A guide to evaluation and treatment. *Psychiatry Annals*.

Hamilton, N.G., Ponzoha, C.A., Cutler, D.L. & Weigel, R.M. (1989). Social networks and negative versus positive symptoms of schizophrenia. *Schizophrenia Bulletin*, **15**, 4, 625–33.

Hamilton, M. (1960). A rating scale for depression. *Journal of Neurology and Neurosurgical Psychiatry*, **23**, 56–62.

Hamilton, M. (1982). Symptoms and assessment of depression. In: E.S. Paykel (ed.), *Handbook of Affective Disorders*, pp. 3–11. Edinburgh: Churchill Livingstone.

Harré, R. & Secord, P.F. (1972). *The Explanation of Social Behavior*. Oxford, UK: Blackwell.

Harrow, M. & Marengo, J. (1986). Schizophrenic thought disorder at follow-up: Its persistence and prognostic significance. *Schizophrenia Bulletin*, **12**, 373–93.

Harvey, A.S. (1978). The role of time budgets in national and regional economic accounting. In: W. Michelson (ed.), *Public Policy in Temporal Perspective*. The Hague: Mouton.

Hatsukami, D., Eckert, E., Mitchell, J.E. & Pyle, R. (1984). Affective disorder and substance abuse in women with bulimia. *Psychological Medicine*, **14**, 701–4.

Hays, W.L. (1973). *Statistics for the Social Sciences*, 2nd edn. London: Holt, Rinehart & Winston.

Hedlund, J.L. & Vieweg, B.W. (1980). The Brief Psychiatric Rating Scale (BPRS): A comprehensive review. *Journal of Operational Psychiatry*, **11**, 1, 47–65.

Heinrichs, D.W. & Carpenter, W.T. (1985). Prospective study of prodromal symptoms in schizophrenic relapse. *American Journal of Psychiatry*, **142**, 3, 371–3.

Hellhammer, D.H., Heib, C., Hubert, W. & Rolf, L. (1985). Relationships between salivary cortisol release and behavioral coping under examination stress. *IRCS Medical Sciences*, **13**, 1179–80.

Hellhammer, D.H., Kirschbaum, C. & Belkien, L. (1987). Measurement of salivary cortisol under psychological stimulation. In: J. Hingtgen, D. Hellhammer & G. Huppmann (eds.), *Advanced Methods in Psychobiology*, pp. 281–9. Toronto: C.J. Hogrefe Inc.

Hennessey, J. & Levine, S. (1979). Stress, arousal and the pituitary adrenal system: a psychoendocrine hypothesis. *Progress in Psychobiology and Physiological Psychology*, **8**, 133–78.

Herbert, J., Moore, G.F., de la Riva, C. & Watts, F.N. (1986). Endocrine responses and examination anxiety. *Biological Psychology*, **22**, 215–26.

Herzog, D.B. (1982). Bulimia in the adolescent. *American Journal of Diseases of Children*, **136**, 985–9.

Herzog, D.B. (1984). Are anorexic and bulimic patients depressed? *American Journal of Psychiatry*, **141**, 12, 1594–7.

Hesselbrock, M.N., Meyer, R.E. & Keener, J.J. (1985). Psychopathology in hospitalized alcoholics. *Archives of General Psychiatry*, **42**, 1050–5.

Hibbert, G.A. (1984). Ideational components of anxiety: Their origin and context. *British Journal of Psychiatry*, **144**, 618–24.

Hinde, R.A. (1976). The use of differences and similarities in comparative psychopathology. In: G. Serban & A. Kling (eds.), *Animal Models in Human Psychobiology*.

Hinz, L.D. & Williamson, D.A. (1987). Bulimia and depression: A review of the affective variant hypothesis. *Psychological Bulletin*, **102**, 1, 150–8.

Hochhauser, M. (1979). Bias in drug abuse survey research. *International Journal of Addiction*, **14**, 675–87.

Holahan, C.J. & Moos, R.H. (1987). Personal and contextual determinants of coping strategies. *Journal of Personality and Social Psychology*, **52**, 5, 946–55.

Hood, J. & Garner, D. (1982). Locus of control as a measure of ineffectiveness in anorexia nervosa. *Journal of Consulting and Clinical Psychology*, **50**, 3–13.

Hoover, M.D. (1983). *Individual Differences in the Relation of Heart Rate to Self-reports*. Doctoral dissertation, The University of Chicago.

Hoover, M. (1984). *An Exploration of the Relationships Among Moods, Activities, Heart Rate, and Gross Motor Activity in the Daily Lives of Eight People*. PhD dissertation, University of Chicago.

Horevitz, R.P. & Braun, B.G. (1984). Are multiple personalities borderline? *Psychiatric Clinics of North America*, **7**, 69–89.

Hormuth, S.E. (1983). Ortwechsel als Gelegenheit zur Anderung des Selbst. (Relocation as an opportunity for self-concept change.) Report and continuation proposal to the German Science Foundation (DFG). University of Heidelberg, Psychological Institute.

Hormuth, S.E. (1984). Transitions in commitments to roles and self-concept change: Recreation as a paradigm. In: V.L. Allen & E. van de Vliert (eds.), *Role Transitions: Explorations and Explanations*. New York: Plenum.

Hormuth, S.E. (1985). *Methoden für psychologische Forschung im Feld (Diskussionspapier Nr. 43)*. Heidelberg: Psychologischen Institut der Universität Heidelberg.

Hormuth, S.E. (1986). The sampling of experiences in situ. *Journal of Personality*, **54**, 262–93.

Hormuth, S.E. (1990). *The Ecology of the Self. Relocation and Self-concept Change*. Cambridge, UK: Cambridge University Press.

van den Hout, M. & Griez, E. (1984a). Validity and utility of the present state examination in assessing neurosis. *Journal of Psychiatric Research*, **18**, 161–72.

van den Hout, M. & Griez, E. (1984b). Panic symptoms after inhalation of carbon dioxide. *British Journal of Psychiatry*, **144**, 503–7.

Hudson, J.I., Pope, J.H. Jr., Jonas, J.M. *et al.* (1983). Family history study of anorexia nervosa and bulimia. *British Journal of Psychiatry*, **142**, 133–8.

Hughes, J.R. (1987). Craving as a psychological construct. *British Journal of Addiction*, **82**, 38–9.

Hughes, P.L., Wells, L.A., Cunningham, C.J. & Ilstrup, D.M. (1986). Treating bulimia with desipramine: A double-blind, placebo-controlled study. *Archives of General Psychiatry*, **43**, 182–6.

Hurlburt, R.T. (1979). Random sampling of cognitions and behavior. *Journal of Research in Personality*, **13**, 103–11.

Hurlburt, R.T. (1980). Validation and correlation of thought sampling with retrospective measures. *Cognitive Therapy and Research*, **4**, 235–8.

Hurlburt, R.T. (1990). *Sampling Normal and Schizophrenic Inner Experience*. New York: Plenum Press.

Hurlburt, R.T. & Sipprelle, C.R. (1978). Random sampling of cognitions in alleviating anxiety attacks. *Cognitive Therapy and Research*, **2**, 165–9.

Hurlburt, R. & Melancon, M.A. (1987a). Single case study, 'Goofed-Up' images. Thought sampling with a schizophrenic woman. *Journal of Nervous and Mental Disease*, **175**, 9, 575–8.

Hurlburt, R.T. & Melancon, S.M. (1987b). P-technique factor analyses of individuals' thought and mood sampling data. *Cognitive Therapy and Research*, **11**, 4, 487–500.

Hurlburt, R.T., Lech, B.C. & Saltman, S. (1984). Random sampling of thought and mood. *Cognitive Therapy and Research*, **8**, 263–75.

Ickes, W.J., Wicklund, R.A. & Ferris, C.B. (1973). Objective self-awareness and self-esteem. *Journal of Experimental Social Psychology*, **9**, 202–19.

Ikard, F.F., Green, D. & Horn, D. (1969). A scale to differentiate between types of smoking as related to the management of affect. *International Journal of the Addictions*, **4**, 649–59.

Ingraham, L.H. (1974). 'The Nam' and 'The World': Heroin use by U.S. army enlisted men serving in Vietnam. *Psychiatry*, **37**, 114–28.

Istvan, J. & Matarazzo, J.D. (1984). Tobacco, alcohol, and caffein use: A review of their interrelationships. *Psychological Bulletin*, **95**, 301–26.

Izard, C.E. (1972). *Patterns of Emotions*. New York: Academic Press.

Jaffe, J.H. (1984). Evaluating drug abuse treatment: A comment on the state of the art. In: F.M. Tims & J.P. Ludford (eds.), *Drug Abuse Treatment Evaluation: Strategies, Progress, and Prospects*, (NIDA Research Monograph 51), Rockville, Maryland, pp. 13–28.

James, W. (1890). *The Principles of Psychology*. New York: Henry Holt.

Jarret, R.B. & Nelson, R.O. (1987). Mechanisms of change in cognitive therapy of depression. *Behavior Therapy*, **18**, 3, 227–41.

Jellinek, E.M. (1960). *The Disease Concept of Alcoholism*. New Haven: Hillhouse Press.

Jessor, R., Jessor, S. & Finney, J. (1973). A social psychology of marijuana use: Longitudinal studies of high school and college youth. *Journal of Personality and Social Psychology*, **26**, 1–15.

Joffe, R., Lowe, M.R. & Fisher, E.B. (1981). A validity test of the Reasons for Smoking test. *Addictive Behaviors*, **6**, 41–5.

Johnson, A. (1973). Time allocation in a Machiquenga community. *Ethology*, **14**, 301–10.

Johnson, C. & Larson, R. (1982). Bulimia: An analysis of moods and behavior. *Psychosomatic Medicine*, **44**, 341–51.

Johnson, C. & Connors, M.E. (1987). *The Etiology and Treatment of Bulimia Nervosa: A Biopsychosocial Perspective*. New York: Basic Books.

Jones, D.M. (1985). Bulimia: A false self identity. *Clinical Social Work Journal*, **13**, 4, 305–16.

Jones, K.V., Copolov, D.L. & Outch, K.H. (1986). Type A, test performance and salivary cortisol. *Journal of Psychosomatic Research*, **30**, 699–707.

Jones, R. (1971a). Marijuana-induced 'high': Influences of expectation, setting and previous drug experience. *Pharmacological Review*, **23**, 359–67.

Jones, R. (1971b). Tetrahydrocannabinol and the marijuana-induced social 'high', or the effects on the mind of marijuana. *Annals of the New York Academy of Science*, **191**, 155–65.

Junginger, J. & Frame, C.L. (1985). Self-report of the frequency and phenomenology of verbal hallucinations. *Journal of Nervous and Mental Disease*, **173**, 3, 149–55.

Juster, F.T. (1975). *The Investment of Time by U.S. Household: An Initial View*. Ann Arbor: Time Use Workshop.

Juster, F.T. (1985). The validity and quality of Time Use Estimates obtained from Recall Diaries. In: F.T. Juster & F.P. Stafford (eds.), *Time, Goods, and Well-Being*. Ann Arbor: Institute for Social Research, The University of Michigan.

Juster, F.T., Courant, P.N. & Dow, G.K. (1979). Social Acounting and Social Indicators: A Framework for the Analysis of Well Being. Ann Arbor: Working Paper Series, Survey Research Center.

Kahlbaum, K.L. (1863). *Gruppierung der Psychischen Krankheiten*. Danzig: Kafemann.

Kahn, J.P., Michaud, C., Gross, M.J., Burlet, C., Mejean, L. & Laxenaire, M. (1991). Applications of salivary cortisol determinations of psychiatric and stress research. In: C. Kirschbaum, D. Hellhammer & G.F. Read (eds.), *Assessment of Hormones and Drugs in Saliva in Biobehavioral Research*. Bern: Hans Huber.

Kandel, D. (1973). Adolescent marijuana use: Role of parents and peers. *Science*, **181**, 1067–70.

Kandel, D. (1978). *Longitudinal Research on Drug Use; Empirical Findings and Methodological Issues*. Somerset, NJ: Halsted.

Kanner, A.D., Coyne, J.C., Schaefer, C. & Lazarus, R.S. (1981). Comparison of two modes of stress measurement: Daily hassles and uplifts versus major life events. *Journal of Behavioral Medicine*, **4**, 1, 1–39.

Kaplan, B. (1964). *The Inner World of Mental Illness*. New York: Grune & Stratton.

Kaplan, C.D. (1977). The heroin system: A general economy of crime and addiction. *Crime et/and Justice*, **5**, 179–96.

Kaplan, C.D. & Wogan, M. (1978). The psychoanalytic theory of addiction: A reevaluation by use of a statistical model. *American Journal of Psychoanalysis*, **38**, 317–26.

Kaplan, C.D., van Meter, K.M. & Korezak, D. (1985). *Estimating Cocaine Prevalence and Incidence in Three European Community Cities*. Commission of the European Community (CEC), Luxemburg, 19 September.

398

Kaplan, C.D., Korf, D. & Sterk, C. (1987). Temporal and social contexts of heroin-using populations. An illustration of the snowball sampling technique. *Journal of Nervous and Mental Disease*, **175**, 9, 566–74.

Kathol, R.G., Noyes, R. & Lopez, A. (1988). Similarities in hypothalamic-pituitary-adrenal axis activity between patients with panic disorder and those experiencing external stress. *Psychiatric Clinics of North America*, **11**, 335–48.

Keller, K.E. (1983). Dysfunctional attitudes and the cognitive therapy for depression. *Cognitive Therapy and Research*, **7**, 5, 437–44.

Kelly, G. (1955). *The Psychology of Personal Constructs*. New York: Norton.

Kendall, P.C. (1986). Cognitive processes and procedures in behavior therapy. *Annual Review of Behavior Therapy Theory and Practice*, **9**, 132–79.

Kendler, K.S., Gruenberg, A.M. & Tsuang, M.T. (1985). Subtype stability in schizophrenia. *American Journal of Psychiatry*, **142**, 7, 827–32.

Khantzian, E.J. (1985). The self-medication hypothesis of addictive disorders: Focus on heroin and cocaine dependence. *The American Journal of Psychiatry*, **142**, 1259–64.

Khantzian, E.J. & Treece, C. (1985). DSM-III psychiatric diagnosis of narcotic addicts. *Archives of general Psychiatry*, **42**, 1067–71.

Kirchler, E. (1984). Das Befinden von Wehrpflichtigen in Abhängigkeit von personehen und situativen Gegebenheiten. *Psychologie und Praxis: Zeitschrift für Arbeits- und Organisationspsychologie*, **28**, 16–25.

Kirschbaum, C. & Hellhammer, D.H. (1989). Salivary cortisol in psychobiological research: An overview. *Neuropsychobiology*, **22**, 150–69.

Kirschbaum, C. & Hellhammer, D. (1991). Cortisol and behavior: Methodological considerations and practical implications of the measurement of cortisol in saliva. In: C. Kirschbaum, D. Hellhammer & G.F. Read (eds.), *Assessment of Hormones and Drugs in Saliva in Biobehavioral Research*. Bern: Hans Huber.

Klein, D.F. & Rabkin, J.G. (eds.) (1981). *Anxiety: New Research Concepts and Current Concepts*. New York: Raven Press.

Kleitman, N. (1963). *Sleep and Wakefulness*, 2nd edn. Chicago: University of Chicago Press.

Klerman, G.L. (1984). The advantages of DSM-III. *American Journal of Psychiatry*, **14**, 4, 539–42.

Klerman, G.L. (1986). Current trends in clinical research on panic attacks, agoraphobia and related anxiety disorders. *Journal of Clinical Psychiatry* (supplement), **47**, 6, 37–9.

Klinger, E. (1984). A consciousness-sampling analysis of test anxiety and performance. *Journal of Personality and Social Psychology*, **47**, 1376–90.

Klinger, E., Barta, S. & Maxeimer, M. (1980). Motivational correlates of thought content frequency and commitment. *Journal of Personality and Social Psychology*, **39**, 1222–37.

Kluft, R.P. (1984a). Introduction to multiple personality disorder. *Psychiatry Annals*, **14**, 51–5.

Kluft, R.P. (1984b). Treatment of multiple personality disorder. *Psychiatric Clinics of North America*, **7**, 9–31.

Kluft, R.P. (ed.) (1985). *Childhood Antecedents of Multiple Personality*. Washington, DC: American Psychiatric Press.

Kohut, H. (1971). *The Analysis of the Self.* New York: International Universities Press.

Kosten, T.R., Rounsaville, B.J., Babor, T.F., Spitzer, R.L. & Willians, J.B.W. (1987a). Substance use disorders in DSM III-R: The dependence syndrome across different psychoactive substances. *British Journal of Psychiatry,* **151,** 834–43.

Kosten, T.R., Rounsaville, B.J., Babor, T.F., Spitzer, R.L. & Williams, J.B.W. (1987b). The dependence syndrome across different psychoactive substances: Revised DSM-III. In: L.S. Harris (ed.), *Problems of Drug Dependence, 1986,* pp. 36–9. Rockville, Maryland: National Institute on Drug Abuse.

Kovacs, M. (1985). Rating scales to assess depression in school-aged children. *Acta Paedopsychiatrica,* **46,** 305–15.

Kozlowski, L.T. & Wilkinson, D.A. (1987). Use and misuse of the concept of craving by alcohol, tobacco, and drug researchers. *British Journal of Addiction,* **82,** 31–6.

Kraepelin, E. (1896). *Psychiatrie, ein Lehrbuch für Studierende und Arzte.* Leipzig, J.A. Barth.

Kripke, D.F. (1983). Phase advance theories for affective illnesses. In: F. Goodwin & T. Wehr (eds.), *Circadian Rhythms in Psychiatry: Basic and Clinical Studies.* California: Boxwood Press.

Kubey, R. & Csikszentmihalyi, M. (1990). *Television and the Quality of Life: How Viewing Shapes Everyday Experience.* Hillsdale, New Jersey: Lawrence Erlbaum Associates, Publishers.

Lader, M., Lang, R.A. & Wilson, G.D. (1987). Patterns of improvement in depressed inpatients. *Maudsley Monographs,* 30.

Laessle, R.G., Kittl, S., Fichter, M.M., Wittchen, H. & Pirke, K.M. (1987). Major affective disorder in anorexia nervosa and bulimia: A descriptive diagnostic study. *British Journal of Psychiatry,* **151,** 785–9.

Lamiell, J.T. (1981). Toward an idiothetic psychology of personality. *American Psychologist,* **36,** 3, 276–89.

Larmore, K., Ludwig, A.M. & Cain, R.L. (1977). Multiple personality – an objective case study. *British Journal of Psychiatry,* **31,** 35–40.

Larsen, R.J. (1987). The stability of mood variability: a spectral analytic approach to daily mood assessments. *Journal of Personality and Social Psychology,* **52,** 1195–204.

Larson, R. (1979). *The Significance of Time Alone in Adolescents' Lives.* Doctoral dissertation, The University of Chicago.

Larson, R. (1983). Adolescents' daily experience with family and friends: Contrasting opportunity systems. *Journal of Marriage and the Family,* **45,** 739–50.

Larson, R. (1987). On the independence of positive and negative affect within hour-to-hour experience. *Motivation and Emotion,* **11,** 145–56.

Larson, R. (1989). Beeping children and adolescents: A method for studying time use and daily experience. *Journal of Youth and Adolescence,* in press.

Larson, R. (1990). The solitary side of life: An examination of the time people spend alone from childhood to old age. *Developmental Review,* in press.

Larson, R. (1989). Is feeling 'in control', related to happiness in daily life? *Psychological Reports,* **64,** 775–84.

Larson, R. & Csikszentmihalyi, M. (1978). Experiential correlates of time alone in adolescence. *Journal of Personality*, **46**, 677–93.

Larson, R., Csikszentmihalyi, M. & Graef, R. (1980). Mood variability and the psycho-social adjustment of adolescents. *Journal of Youth and Adolescence*, **9**, 469–90.

Larson, R. & Johnson, C. (1981). Anorexia nervosa in the context of daily experience. *Journal of Youth and Adolescence*, **10**, 455–71.

Larson, R., Csikszentmihalyi, M. & Graef, R. (1982). Time alone in daily experience: Loneliness or renewal? In: L.A. Peplau & D. Perlman (eds.), *Loneliness: A Sourcebook of Current Theory, Research and Therapy*. New York: Wiley.

Larson, R. & Csikszentmihalyi, M. (1983). The experience sampling method. In: H. Reis (ed.), *New Directions for Naturalistic Methods in the Behavioral Sciences*. San Francisco: Jossey-Bass.

Larson, R., Csikszentmihalyi, M. & Freeman, M. (1984). Alcohol and marijuana use in adolescents' lives: A random sample of experiences. *International Journal of Addictions*, **19**, 367–81.

Larson, R. & Johnson, C. (1985). Bulimia: Disturbed patterns of solitude. *Addictive Behaviors*, **10**, 281–90.

Larson, R. & Lampman-Petraitis, C. (1989). Daily emotional states as reported by children and adolescents. *Child Development*, **60**, 1250–60.

Larson, R. & Richards, M. (eds.) (1989). The changing life space of early adolescence. Special issue of the *Journal of Youth and Adolescence*, **18**, 6, 501–626.

Larson, R. & Delespaul, P.A.E.G. (1990). Analysing Experience Sampling data. A Guidebook for the Perplexed. (This volume).

Larson, R., Raffaelli, M., Richards, M.H., Ham, M. & Jewell, L. (1990). The ecology of depression in childhood and early adolescence: A profile of daily psychological states. *Journal of Abnormal Psychology*, **99**, 1.

Lazarus, R.S. (1984). Puzzles in the study of daily hassles. *Journal of Behavioral Medicine*, **7**, 4, 375–89.

Lazarus, R.S. & Folkman, S. (1984). *Stress, Appraisal, and Coping*. New York: Springer.

LeFevre, J., Hendricks, C., Church, R. & McClintock, M. (1985). Psychological and social behavior in couples over menstrual cycle: 'On-the-spot' sampling from everyday life. Paper presented at the 6th Conference of the Society for Menstrual Cycle Research, Galveston.

Leff, J.P. (1978). Psychiatrists' versus patients' concepts of unpleasant emotions. *British Journal of Psychiatry*, **133**, 306–13.

Leff, J. & Vaughn, C. (1985). *Expressed Emotion in Families*. New York: The Guilford Press.

Lerman, I.C. (1981). *Classification et Analyse Ordinale des Données*. Paris: Dunod.

Leventhal, H. & Avis, N. (1976). Pleasure, addiction, and habit: Factors in verbal report of factors in smoking behavior? *Journal of Abnormal Psychology*, **5**, 478–88.

Levine, J.H. (1988). The methodology of the Atlas of Corporate Interlocks. *Bulletin de Méthodologie Sociologique*, **17**, 20–58.

Lewin, K. (1936). *Principles of Topological Psychology*. New York: McGraw-Hill.

Lewin, K. (1943). Defining the 'field at a given time'. *Psychological Review*, **50**, 292–310.

Ley, R. (1985). Agoraphobia, the panic attack and the hyperventilation syndrome. *Behavior Research & Therapy*, **23**, 79–81.

Liberman, R.P. (ed.) (1988) *Psychiatric Rehabilitation of Chronic Mental Patients*. Washington: American Psychiatric Press, Inc.

Lichtenstein, E. & Brown, R.A. (1982). Current trends in the modification of cigarette dependence. In: A. Bellack, M. Hersen & A.E. Kazdin (eds.), *International Handbook of Behavior Modification and Therapy* (vol. 22). New York, NY: Academic Press.

van Limbeek, J., Schalben, H.F.A., Geerlings, P.K., Wouters, L., de Groot, P.A., Sijblings, G. & Beelen, W. (1986). Het gebruik van het Diagnostisch Interview Schema (DIS) bij het vaststellen van psychopathologie bij alcohol- en drugverslaafden. *Tijdschrift voor Psychiatrie*, **28**, 459–74.

Lin, N., Woelfel, M.W. & Light, S.C. (1985). The buffering effect of social support subsequent to an important life event. *Journal of Health and Social Behavior*, **26**, 247–63.

Lindesmith, A. (1968). *Addiction and Opiates*. Chicago: Aldine.

Lindesmith, A. (1975). A reply to McAuliffe and Gordon's. A test of Lindesmith's theory of addiction. *American Journal of Sociology*, **81**, 147–53.

Loewenstein, R.J., Hamilton, J., Alagna, S., Reid, N. & deVries, M.W. (1987). Experiental sampling in the study of multiple personality disorder. *American Journal of Psychiatry*, **144**, 19–24.

Ludwig, A.M., Brandsma, J.M., Wilbur, C.B. *et al.* (1972). The objective study of multiple personality or are four heads better than one? *Archives of General Psychiatry*, **26**, 298–310.

Ludwig, A.M. Wikler, A. & Stark, L.H. (1974). The first drink. *Archives of General Psychiatry*, **30**, 539–47.

Lundberg, U. & Frankenhaeuser, M. (1980). Pituitary-adrenal and sympathetic-adrenal correlates of distress and effort. *Journal of Psychosomatic Research*, **24**, 125–30.

Maddi, S.R., Kobasa, S.C. & Hoover, M. (1979). An alienation test. *Journal of Human Psychology*, **19**, 73–6.

Magnusson, D. & Endler, N.S. (1977). Interactional psychology: Present status and future prospects. In: D. Magnusson & N.S. Endler (eds.), *Personality at the Crossroads: Current Issues in Interactional Psychology*. Hillside, NJ: Erlbaum.

Malinowski, B. (1927). *Sex and Repression in Savage Society*. London: Rontledge & Kegan P. Ltd.

Malinowski, B. (1935). *Coral Gardens and Their Magic. Soil Tilling and Agricultural Rites* (vol. 1). Bloomington: Indiana University Press.

Margraf, J., Taylor, C.B., Ehlers, A., Roth, W.T. & Agras, W.S. (1987). Panic attacks in the natural environment. *Journal of Nervous and Mental Disease*, **175**, 9, 558–65.

Marks, I.M. & Herst, E.R. (1970). A survey of 1200 agoraphobics in Britain. *Social Psychiatry*, **5**, 16–24.

Marks. I.M. & Matthews, A.M. (1979). Brief standard self-rating for phobic patients. *Behavior Research and Therapy*, **17**, 263–7.

Marlatt, G.A. (1987). Craving notes. *British Journal of Addiction*, **82**, 42–3.

Marengo, J. & Harrow, M. (1986). Schizophrenic thought disorder at follow-up: A persistent or episodic course? *Archives of General Psychiatry*, **44**, 651–9.

Marschall, P. (1987). Physical complaints, anxiety and its body outcomes: a psychophysiological field study. *Journal of Psychopathology and Behavioral Assessment*, **9**, 353–67.

Marshall, T. & Mazie, A.S. (1987). A cognitive approach to treating depression. *Social Casework*, **68**, 9, 540–5.

Mason, J.C., Lauks, J. & Bachus, F. (1985). Patient predicted length of stay and diagnosis-related-groups. *American Journal of Psychiatry*, **142**, 369–71.

Mason, J.W. (1968). A review of psychoendocrine research on the pituitary-adrenal cortical system. *Psychosomatic Medicine*, **30**, 576–607.

Mason, J.W. (1975). Psychologic stress and endocrine function. In: E. Sachar (ed.), *Topics in Psychoendocrinology*, pp. 1–18. New York: Grune & Stratton.

Mason, J.W., Giller, E.L., Kosten, T.R., Ostroff, R.B. & Podd, L. (1986). Urinary free-cortisol levels in posttraumatic stress disorder patients. *Journal of Nervous and Mental Disease*, **174**, 145–9.

Massimini, F. & Inghilleri, P. (eds.) (1986). *L'Esperienza Quotidiana: Teoria e Metodo d'Analisi*. Milan: Franco Angeli.

Massimini, F., Csikszentmihalyi, M. & Delle Fave, A. (1986). Selezione psicologica e flusso di coscienza. In: F. Massimini & P. Inghilleri (eds.), *L'Esperienza Quotidiana. Teoria e Metodo d'Analisi*. Milano: Franco Angeli.

Massimini, F., Csikszentmihalyi, M. & Carli, M. (1987). Optimal experience: A tool for psychiatric rehabilitation. *Journal of Nervous and Mental Disease*, **175**, 9, 545–50.

Massimini, F. & Carli, M. (1988). The systematic assessment of flow in daily experience. In: M. Csikszentmihalyi & I. Csikszentmihalyi (eds.) *Optimal Experience. Psychological Studies of Flow in Consciousness*. Cambridge, UK: Cambridge University Press.

Massimini, F., Csikszentmihalyi, M. & Delle Fave, A. (1988). Flow and bio-cultural evolution. In: M. Csikszentmihalyi & I. Csikszentmihalyi (eds.), *Optimal Experience. Psychological Studies of Flow in Consciousness*. Cambridge, UK: Cambridge University Press.

Massimini, F. & Delle Fave, A. (1988). Experience Sampling Method and the adolescents' daily life: A cross-national analysis. In: A. Fusco, F.M. Battisti & R. Tomassoni (eds.), *Issues in Cognition and Social Representation*. Milano: Franco Angeli.

Mayer, E. (1974). Behavior programs and evolutionary strategies. *American Scientist*, **62**, 650–9.

Mayer, J.M. (1977). Assessment of depression. In: P.M. Reynolds (ed.), *Advances in Psychological Assessment*, vol. 4, pp. 358–425. San Francisco: Jossey-Bass.

Mayers, P. (1978). *Flow in Adolescence and Its Relation to School Experience*. Ph.D. Dissertation, The University of Chicago.

McAdams, D. & Constantian, C.A. (1983). Intimacy and affiliation motives in daily living: An experience sampling analysis. *Journal of Personality and Social Psychology*, **45**, 851–61.

McAuliffe, W.E. & Gordon, R.A. (1974). A test of Lindesmith's theory of addiction: The frequency of euphoria among long-term addicts. *American Journal of Sociology*, **79**, 795–840.

McAuliffe, W.E. & Gordon, R.A. (1975). Issues in testing Lindesmith's theory. *American Journal of Sociology*, **81**, 154–63.

McAuliffe, W.E. & Gordon, R.A. (1980). Reinforcement and the combination of effects: Summary of a theory of opiate addiction. In: D.J. Lettieri, M. Sayers & H. Wallenstein Pearson (eds.), *Theories on Drug Abuse: Selected Contemporary Perspectives*. (NIDA Research Monograph 30), pp. 137–41. Rockville, MD: NIDA.

McGuire, M.T. & Fairbanks, L.A. (1977). Ethology: psychiatry's bridge to behavior. In: M.T. McGuire & L.A. Fairbanks (eds.), *Ethological Psychiatry: Psychopathology in the Context of Evolution Biology*, pp. 1–40. New York: Grune & Straton.

McGuire, M.T. & Polsky, R.H. (1979). Behavioral changes in hospitalized acute schizophrenics. An ethological perspective. *Journal of Nervous and Mental Disease*, **167**, 11, 651–7.

McKennel, A.C. (1970). Smoking motivation factors. *British Journal of Social and Clinical Psychology*, **9**, 8–22.

McLellan, A.T., Luborsky, L., Woody, G.E. & O'Brien, C.P. (1980). An improved diagnostic evaluation instrument for substance abuse patients. The Addiction Seventy Index. *Journal of Nervous and Mental Disease*, **168**, 26–33.

McLellan, A.T., Luborsky, L., Woody, G.E., O'Brien, C.P.O. & Druley, K.A. (1983). Increased effectiveness of substance abuse treatment: A prospective study of patient-treatment 'matching'. *Journal of Nervous and Mental Disease*, **171**, 597–605.

McNair, D.M., Lorr, M. & Dropplemen, L.F. (1971). *Manual for the Profile of Mood States. Educational and Industrial Testing Service*. San Diego, California 92107.

McSweeney, B. (1979). *Negative Impact of Development on Women Reconsidered*. Doctoral Thesis, Medford, MA: Fletcher School of Diplomacy.

Mead, G.H. (1934). *Mind, Self, and Society*. Chicago: University of Chicago Press.

Mehan, H. & Wood, H. (1975). *The Reality of Ethnomethodology*. New York: John Wiley.

Meldrum, S.J. (1988a). Ambulatory monitoring: A bibliography of techniques and technology published in the World Literature in 1985. *Journal of Ambulatory Monitoring*, **1**, 4, 329–32.

Meldrum, S.J. (1988b). Ambulatory monitoring: A bibliography of techniques and technology published in the World Literature in the Third quarter of 1988. *Journal of Ambulatory Monitoring*, **1**, 4, 333–4.

Merrick, W. (1988). Dysphoric moods in normal and depressed adolescents. Unpublished PhD dissertation, University of Chicago. Chicago, Illinois.

Metropolitan Life Insurance Company: *How You Can Control Your Weight*. Pamphlet available from Metropolitan Life, One Madison Avenue, New York, NY 10010 (originally published, 1959).

Meyer, R.E. & Mirin, S.M. (1979). *The Heroin Stimulus: Implications for a Theory of Addiction*. New York: Plenum Press.

Michelson, W. (ed.) (1978). *Public Policy in Temporal Perspective*. The Hague: Mouton.

Miller, J.G. (1970). *Living System*. New York: Miller.

Miller, N.S. & Gold, M.S. (1990). The disease and adaptive models of addiction: A reevaluation. *Journal of Drug Issues*, **20**, 1, 29–35.

Miller, P.M., Fredericksen, L.W. & Hosford, R.L. (1979). Social interaction and smoking topography in heavy and light smokers. *Addictive Behaviors*, **4**, 147–53.

Minge-Klevana, W. (1980). Does labor time decrease with industrialization? *Current Anthropology*, **21**, 278–87.

Minors, D.S. & Waterhouse, J.M. (1981). *Circadian Rhythms and the Human*. Bristol: J. Wright & Sons Ltd., Stonebridge Press.

Mischel, W. (1968). *Personality and Assessment*. New York: Wiley.

Mischel, W. (1981). A cognitive-social learning approach to assessment. In: T. Merluzzi, C. Glass & M. Genest (eds.), *Cognitive Assessment*. New York: Guilford.

Monk, T.H., Flaherty, J.F., Frank, E., Hoskinson, K. & Kupfer, D.J. (1990). The Social Rhythm Metric: an instrument to quantify the daily rhythms of life. *Journal of Nervous and Mental Disease*, **178**, 2, 120–6.

Monroe, S.M. (1983). Major and minor life events as predictors of psychological distress: further issues and findings. *Journal of Behavioral Medicine*, **6**, 2, 189–205.

Mott, R., Small, I. & Anderson, J. (1965). Comparative study of hallucinations. *Archives of General Psychiatry*, **12**, 595–601.

Mullaney, J. (1987). Measurement of anxiety and depression. In: G. Racagni, & E. Smeraldi (eds.), *Anxious Depression, Assessment and Treatment*. New York: Raven Press.

Munroe, R.H. & Munroe, R.L. (1971a). Household density and infant care in an East African society. *Journal of Social Psychology*, **83**, 9–13.

Munroe, R.H. & Munroe, R.L. (1971b). Effect of environnmental experience on spatiability in an East African society. *Journal of Social Psychology*, **83**, 15–22.

Murphy, E. (1982). Social origins of depression in old age. *British Journal of Psychiatry*, **141**, 135–42.

Murphy, E. (1983). The prognosis of depression in old age. *British Journal of Psychiatry*, **142**, 111–19.

Murray, H.A. (1938). *Explorations in Personality*. New York: Oxford University Press.

Nelson, R.O. (1977). Assessments and therapeutic functions of self-monitoring. In: M. Hersen, R.M. Eisler & P. Miller (eds.), *Progress in Behavior Modification* (vol. 5). New York: Academic Press.

Nesse, R.M., Curtis, G., Thyer, B., McCann, D., Huber-Smith, M. & Knopf, R. (1985). Endocrine and cardiovascular responses during phobic anxiety. *Psychosomatic Medicine*, **47**, 320–32.

Newcomb, M.D. & Harlow, L.L. (1986). Life events and substance use among adolescents: Mediating effects of perceived loss of control and meaninglessness in life. *Journal of Personality and Social Psychology*, **51**, 564–77.

Niaura, R.S., Rohsenow, D.J., Binkoff, J.A., Monti, P.M., Pedraza, M. & Abrams, D.B. (1988). Relevance of cue reactivity to understanding alcohol and smoking relapse. *Journal of Abnormal Psychology*, **97**, 133–52.

Nicolson, N.A., van Poll, R. & deVries, M. (1991). Ambulatory monitoring of salivary cortisol and stress in daily life. In: C. Kirschbaum, D. Hellhammer & G.F. Read (eds.), *Assessment of Hormones and Drugs in Saliva in Biobehavioral Research*. Bern: Hans Huber.

Norman, W.R. (1967). On estimating psychological relationships: Social desirability and self-report. *Psychological Bulletin*, **63**, 129.

O'Brien, R.G. & Kister Kaiser, M. (1985). MANOVA method for analyzing repeated measures designs: An extensive primer. *Psychological Bulletin*, **97**, 316–33.

Offer, D. & Sabshin, M. (1967). Research alliance versus therapeutic alliance: A comparison. *American Journal of Psychiatry*, **123**, 1519–26.

Orcutt, J. (1972). Toward a sociological theory of drug effects: A comparison of marijuana and alcohol. *Sociological and Social Research*, **56**, 242–53.

Overall, J.E. (1974). The Brief Psychiatric Rating Scale in psychopharmacology research. In: P. Pichot (ed.), *Psychological Measurements in Psychopharmacology. Modern Problems in Pharmacopsychiatry*, **7**, 67–78.

Pao, P.N. (1979). *Schizophrenic Disorders. Theory and Treatment from a Psychodynamic Point of View*. New York: International University Press.

Parsons, J.B., Burns, D.D. & Perloff, J.M. (1988). Predictions of dropout and outcome in cognitive therapy for depression. *Cognitive Therapy and Research*, **12**, 6, 557–75.

Paton, S., Kessler, R. & Kandel, D. (1977). Depressive mood and adolescent illicit drug use: A longitudinal analysis. *Journal of Genetic Psychology*, **131**, 267–89.

Pawlik, K. & Buse, L. (1982). Rechnergestützte Verhaltensregistrierung im Feld: Beschreibung und erste psychometrische Uberprüfung einer neuen Erhebungsmethode. *Zeitschrift für Differentielle und Diagnostische Psychologie*, **3**, 101–18.

Paykel, E.S., Prusoff, B.A., Klerman, G.L. & DiMascio, A. (1973). Self-report and clinical interview ratings in depression. *Journal of Nervous and Mental Disease*, **156**, 3, 166–82.

PCOC (President's Commission on Organized Crime) (1986). In: *America's Habit: Drug Abuse, Drug Trafficking and Organized crime*. Washington, DC: US Government Printing Office.

Pennebaker, J.W., Gonder-Frederick, L., Cox, D.J. & Hoover, C.W. (1985). The perception of general vs. specific visceral activity and the regulation of health-related behavior. *Advances in Behavioral Medicine*, **1**, 165–98.

Perloff, D. & Sokolow, M. (1978). The representative blood pressure: Usefulness of office, basal, home and ambulatory readings. *Cardiovascular Medicine*, **3**, 655–68.

Perloff, D., Sokolow, M. & Cowan, R. (1983). The prognostic value of ambulatory blood pressure. *JAMA*, **249**, 2793–8.

406

Pervin, L.A. (1985). Personality: Current controversies, issues, and directions. *Annual Review of Psychology*, **36**, 83–114.

Peterson, C. & Seligman, M.E.P. (1984). Causal explanations as a risk factor for depression: theory and evidence. *Psychological Review*, **91**, 3, 347–74.

Pickering, T.G., Harshfield, G.A., Kleinert, H.D., Blank, S. & Laragh, J.H. (1982). Blood pressure during normal daily activities, sleep, and exercise. *JAMA*, **247**, 992–6.

Pickering, T.S., Harshfield, G.A., Devereux, R.B. & Laragh, J.H. (1985). What is the role of ambulatory blood pressure monitoring in the management of hypertensive patients? *Hypertension*, **7**, 171–7.

Pincomb, G.A., Lovallo, W.R., Passey, R.B., Brackett, D.J. & Wilson, M.F. (1987). Caffeine enhances the physiological response to occupational stress in medical students. *Health Psychology*, **6**, 101–12.

Pitts, F.N. (1971). Biochemical factors in anxiety neurosis. *Behavioral Science*, **16**, 82–91.

Pitts, F.N. & McClure, J.M. (1967). Lactate metabolism in anxiety neurosis. *New England Journal of Medicine*, **277**, 1329–36.

van de Ploeg, H.M., Defares, P. & Spielberger, C. (1979). *Handleiding bij de Zelfbeoordelingsvragenlijst (ZBV): Een Nederlandstalige Bewerking van de Spielberger State-Trait Anxiety Inventory (STAI-DY)*. Lisse, Holland: Swets & Zeitlinger.

van de Ploeg, H.M. (1988). *Examen/Toets Attitude Vragenlijst* (Dutch version of the Test Anxiety Inventory). Lisse, Holland: Swets & Zeitlinger.

Plutchik, R. & van Praag, H.M. (1987). Interconvertibility of five self-report measures of depression. *Psychiatry Research*, **22**, 243–56.

van Poll, R., Nicolson, N. & Sulon, J. (1991). Diurnal variation in salivary cortisol in oral contraceptive users. In: C. Kirschbaum, D. Hellhammer & G.F. Read (eds.), *Assessment of Hormones and Drugs in Saliva in Biobehavioral Research*. Bern: Hans Huber.

Pomerleau, O.F. & Pomerleau, C.S. (1984). Neuroregulators and the reinforcement of smoking: Towards a biobehavioral explanation. *Neuroscience and Biobehavioral Reviews*, **8**, 502–13.

Pomerlau, O.F., Turk, D. & Fertig, J.B. (1984). The effects of cigarette smoking on pain and anxiety. *Addictive Behaviors*, **9**, 265–71.

Pope, H.G., Hudson, J.I., Jonas, J.M. & Yurgelum-Todd, D. (1983). Bulimia treated with imipramine: A placebo-controlled, double-blind study. *American Journal of Psychiatry*, **140**, 5, 554–8.

Portegijs, P. (1988). Wanneer heeft de acute rugpijnpatiënt rugpijn? Mimeo, Department of Social Psychiatry, University of Limburg, Maastricht.

Poznanski, E.O., Freeman, L. & Mokros, H. (1983). Children's Depression Rating Scale – Revised. *Psychopharmacology Bulletin*, **21**, 979–89.

Preble, E. & Casey, J.J. Jr. (1969). Taking care of business – the heroin user's life on the street. *International Journal of Addictions*, **4**, 1–24.

Prod'homme, A., Breton, L. & Guenneguez, L. (1983). Note méthodologique sur l'utilisation de l'algorithme de vraisemblance de liens en sciences humaines. *Actes des Journées de Classification*, pp. 367–83. Bruxelles: Société francophone de classification.

Puig-Antich, J., Blau, S., Marx, N., Greenhill, L.L. & Chambers, W. (1978). Prepubertal major depressive disorder: A pilot study. *Journal of the American Academy of Child Psychiatry*, **17**, 695–707.

Putnam, F.W. (1984). The psychophysiologic investigation of multiple personality disorder. *Psychiatric Clinics of North America*, **7**, 31–41.

Putnam, F.W. Jr., Post, R.M., Guroff, J.J. *et al.* (1983). 100 Cases of multiple personality disorder. *New Research Abstracts of the 136th Annual Meeting of the American Psychiatric Association*. Washington, DC: APA.

Putnam, F.W., Loewenstein, R.J., Silberman, E. *et al.* (1984). Multiple personality disorder in a hospital setting. *Journal of Clinical Psychiatry*, **45**, 172–5.

Pyle, R.L., Mitchell, J.E. & Eckert, E.D. (1981). Bulimia: A report of 34 cases. *Journal of Clinical Psychiatry*, **42**, 2, 60–4.

Pyszczynski, T. & Greenberg, J. (1985). Depression and preference for self-focusing stimuli after success and failure. *Journal of Personality and Social Psychology*, **49**, 1066–75.

Pyszczynski, T. & Greenberg, J. (1986). Evidence for a depressive self-focusing style. *Journal of Research in Personality*, **20**, 95–106.

Pyszczynski, T. & Greenberg, J. (1987). The role of self-focused attention in the development, maintenance, and exacerbation of depression. In: K. Yardley & T. Honess (eds.), *Self and Identity: Psychological Perspectives*, pp. 307–22. Chichester, England: Wiley & Sons.

Quigley, M.E. & Yen, S.S.C. (1979). A midday surge in cortisol levels. *Journal of Clinical Endocrinology and Metabolism*, **49**, 945–7.

Rabin, A.I., Doneson, S.L. & Jentons, R.L. (1979). Studies of psychological functions in schizophrenia. In: L. Bellak (ed.), *Disorders of the Schizophrenic Syndrome*, pp. 181–231. New York: Basic Books.

Raffaelli, M. & Duckett, E. (1989). 'We were just talking. . .': Conversations in early adolescence. *Journal of Youth and Adolescence*, **18**, 6, 567–82.

Rahe, R.H., Karson, S., Howard, N.S., Jr., Rubin, R.T. & Poland, R.E. (1990). Psychological assessments on American hostages freed from captivity in Iran. *Psychosomatic Medicine*, **52**, 1–16.

Rankin, H., Hodgson, R. & Stockwell, T. (1979). The concept of craving and its measurement. *Behavioral Research and Therapy*, **17**, 389–96.

Reis, H.T., Wheeler, L., Spiegel, N. *et al.* (1982). Physical attractiveness in social interaction: II. Why does appearance affect social experience? *Journal of Personality and Social Psychology*, **43**, 979–96.

Reynolds, T.D. (1965). Fluctuations in schizophrenic behavior. *Medical Annals of the District of Columbia*, **34**, 11, 520–49.

Reynolds, T.D. (1976). Quantitative studies of schizophrenic behavior. *Behavioural Processes*, **1**, 347–72.

Rizzuto, A.M. (1985). Eating and monsters: A psychodynamic view of bulimarexia, In: S.W. Emmett (ed.), *Theory and Treatment of Anorexia Nervosa and Bulimia: Biomedical, Sociocultural, and Psychological Perspectives*, pp. 194–210. New York: Brunner/Mazel.

Robins, L.N., Davis, D.H. & Goodwin, D.W. (1974). Drug use in the U.S. army enlisted men in Vietnam: A follow-up on their return home. *American Journal of Epidemiology*, **99**, 235–49.

Robins, L.N., Helzer, J.E., Weissman, M.M. *et al.* (1984). Lifetime prevalence of specific psychiatric disorders in three sites. *Archives of General Psychiatry*, **41**, 949–58.

Robinson, J. (1976). *Changes in Americans' Use of Time; 1965–1975*. Cleveland, Ohio: Cleveland State University Communication Research Center.

Robinson, J. (1977). *How Americans Use Time: A Social-Psychological Analysis of Everyday Behavior*. New York: Praeger. (Further analyses were published in *How Americans Used Time in 1965–66*. Ann Arbor: University Microfilms, Monograph Series 1977.)

Robinson, J. (1985). Testing the validity and reliability of diaries versus alternative time use measures. In: F. Juster & F. Stafford (eds.), *Time, Goods, and Well-Being*. Ann Arbor: Institute for Social Research, The University of Michigan.

Roffe, D.J., Bertram, C.D. & Hunyor, S.N. (1985). Real time detection of significant blood pressure events in ambulant subjects. *Clinical Experience in Hypertension*, **A7** (2&3), 299–307.

Rogers, C.R. (1961). *On Becoming a Person: A Therapist's View of Psychotherapy*. Boston: Houghton Mifflin.

Rogers, H. & Layton, B. (1979). Two methods of predicting drug taking. *International Journal of Addiction*, **14**, 299–310.

Rogoff, B. (1978). Spot observation: An introduction and examination. *Quarterly Newsletter of the Institute for Comparative Human Development, Rockfeller University*, **2**, 21–6.

Romme, M.A.J. (ed.) (1978). *Voorzieningen in de Geestelijke Gezondheidszorg. Een Gids voor Consumenten en Hulpverleners*. Alphen a/d Rijn: Samson.

Rorer, L.G. (1965). The great response-style myth. *Psychological Bulletin*, **63**, 129.

Rose, J., Ananda, R. & Jarvik, M.E. (1983). Cigarette smoking during anxiety-provoking and monotonous tasks. *Addictive Behaviors*, **8**, 353–9.

Rose, R.M. (1984). Overview of endocrinology of stress. In: G.M. Brown, S.H. Koslow & S. Reichlin (eds.), *Neuroendocrinology and Psychiatric Disorder*, pp. 95–122. New York: Raven Press.

Rose, R.M. (1987). Endocrine abnormalities in depression and stress - An overview. In: U. Halbreich (ed.), *Hormones and Depression*, pp. 31–47. New York: Raven Press.

Rosen, J.C., Leitenberg, H., Fischer, C. & Khazam, C. (1986). Binge-eating episodes in bulimia nervosa: The amount and type of food consumed. *International Journal of Eating Disorders*, **5**, 2, 255–67.

Roth, M. & Mountjoy, C.Q. (1981). The distinction between anxiety states and depressive disorders. In: E.S. Paykel (ed.), *Handbook of Affective Disorders*, pp. 6, 48, 49, 54, 499, 707. New York: Guilford.

Roth, D., Rehm, L.P. & Rozensky, R.H. (1980). Self-reward, self-punishment and depression. *Psychological Reports*, **47**, 3–7.

Rounsaville, B.J., Weissman, M.W., Kleber, H.D. & Wilber, C. (1982). Heterogeneity of psychiatric diagnosis in treated opiate addicts. *Archives of General Psychiatry*, **39**, 161–6.

Rounsaville, B.J. & Kleber, H. (1985). Untreated opiate addicts: How do they differ from those seeking treatment? *Archives of General Psychiatry*, **42**, 1072–7.

Rounsaville, B.J., Kosten, T.R., Weissman, M.W. & Kleber, H.D. (1986). Prognostic significance of psychopathology in untreated opiate addicts. *Archives of General Psychiatry*, **43**, 739–45.

Rounsaville, B.J., Kosten, T.R., Williams, J.B.W. & Spitzer, R.L. (1987). A field trial of DSM-III-R psychoactive substance dependence disorders. *American Journal of Psychiatry*, **144**, 3, 351–4.

Rouse, B.A., Kozel, N.J. & Richards, L.G. (1985). *Self-report Methods of Estimating Drug Use: Meeting Current Challenges to Validity*, NIDA Research Monograph 57. Rockville, Maryland: NIDA.

Runyan, W.M. (1983). Idiographic goals and methods in the study of lives. *Journal of Personality*, **51**, 413–37.

Rupp, A.H., Steinwachs, D.M. & Salkever, D.S. (1984). The effect of hospital payment methods on the pattern and cost of mental health care. *Hospital & Community Psychiatry*, **35**, 456–9.

Russell, G. (1979). Bulimia nervosa: An ominous variant of anorexia nervosa. *Psychology Medicine*, **9**, 429–48.

Russell, M.A.H. (1976). Smoking and nicotine dependence. In: R.J. Gibbins, Y. Israel, H. Kalant, R.I. Popham, W. Schmidt & R.G. Smart (eds.), *Research Advances in Alcohol and Drug Problems*, vol. 3. New York: John Wiley.

Russell, M.A.H. & Feyerabend, C. (1978). Cigarette smoking: A dependence on high-nicotine boli. *Drug Metabolism Reviews*, **8**, 29–57.

Ryback, R.S., Longabaugh, R. & Fowler, D.R. (1981). *The Problem Oriented Record in Psychiatry and Mental Health Care – Revised Edition*. New York: Grune & Stratton.

Sachar, E.J., Mason, J.W., Kolmer, H.S., Jr. & Artiss, K.L. (1963). Psychoendocrine aspects of acute schizophrenic reactions. *Psychosomatic Medicine*, **25**, 510.

Sachar, E.J., Mackenzie, J.M. & Binstock, W.A. (1967). Corticosteroid responses to psychotherapy of depression: I. Evaluations during confrontation of loss. *Archives of General Psychiatry*, **16**, 461.

Sameroff, A., Seifer, C. & Zax, M. (1982). Early development of children at risk for emotional disorders. *Monographs of Social Research in Child Development*, **47**, 7.

Sapir, E. (1921). *Language: An Introduction to the Study of Speech*. New York: Harvest Book, Harcourt, Brace & World, Inc.

SAS (1985). *User's Guide Statistics*, Version 5 edn. Cary, NC: SAS Institute, Inc.

Saunders, R. (1985). Bulimia: An expanded definition. *Social Casework*, **66**, 603–10.

Savin-Williams, R.C. & Demo, D.H. (1983). Situational and transituational determinants of adolescent self-feelings. *Journal of Personality and Social Psychology*, **44**, 824–33.

Schachter, S. (1978). Pharmacological and psychological determinants of smoking. *Annals of Internal Medicine*, **88**, 104–14.

Schaeffer, M.A. & Baum, A. (1984). Adrenal cortisol response to stress at Three Mill Island. *Psychosomatic Medicine*, **46**, 227–37.

Schmitt, J.P. (1983). Focus of attention in the treatment of depression. *Psychotherapy Research*, **20**, 4, 457–63.

Schreurs, P.J.G. & van de Willige, G. (1988). *De Utrechtse Copinglijst (UCL)*. Lisse, the Netherlands: Swets & Zeitlinger.

Schuster, S.O., Murrell, S.A. & Cook, W.A. (1980). Person, setting, and interaction contributions to nursery school social behavior patterns. *Journal of Personality*, **48**, 24–37.

Sechehaye, M. (1951). *Autobiography of a Schizophrenic Girl*. New York: Grune & Stratton.

Shaffer, H.J. & Zinberg, N.E. (1985). The social psychology of intoxicant use: The natural history of social settings and social control. *Bulletin of the Society of Psychologists in the Addictive Behaviors*, **4**, 49–55.

Shaffer, H.J. & Jones, S.B. (1989). *Quitting Cocaine: The Struggle Against Impulse*. Lexington, Mass.: Lexington Books.

Sheehan, D.V. (1982). Panic attacks and phobias. *New England Journal of Medicine*, **307**, 156–8.

Sheehan, D.V., Sheehan, K.E. & Minichiello, W.E. (1981). Age of onset of phobic disorders: a reevaluation. *Comprehensive Psychiatry*, **22**, 544–53.

Shick, J. & Freedman, D. (1975). Research in nonnarcotic drug abuse. In: S. Arieti (ed.), *American Handbook of Psychiatry*, 2nd edn, vol. 6. New York: Basic Books.

Shick, J., Dorux, W. & Hughes, P. (1978). Adolescent drug using groups in Chicago parks. *Drug and Alcohol Dependence*, **3**, 199–210.

Shiffman, S. (1982). Relapse following smoking cessation: A situational analysis. *Journal of Consulting and Clinical Psychology*, **50**, 71–86.

Shiffman, S., Read, L., Maltese, J., Rapkin, D. & Jarvik, M.E. (1985). Preventing relapse in exsmokers. In: G.A. Marlatt & J.R. Gordon (eds.), *Relapse Prevention: Maintenance Strategies in the Treatment of Addictive Behaviors*. New York: Guilford Press.

Shiffman, S. & Prange, M. (1988). Self-reported and self-monitored smoking patterns. *Addictive Behaviors*, **13**, 201–4.

Siegel, S. (1979). The role of conditioning in drug tolerance and addiction. In: J.D. Kechen (ed.), *Psychopathology in Animals: Research and Treatment Implications*. New York: Academic Press.

Simon, H.A. (1969). *Sciences of the Artificial*. Boston: MIT Press.

Sinclair, E. & Alexon, J. (1985). Creating diagnostic related groups: A manageable way to deal with DSM-III. *American Journal of Orthopsychiatry*, **55**, 3, 426–33.

Singer, J.L. (1975). Navigating the stream of consciousness: Research in daydreaming and related inner experience. *American Psychologist*, **30**, 727–38.

Skinner, B.F. (1953). *Science and Human Behavior*. New York: MacMillan.

Skinner, H.A. & Goldberg, A.E. (1986). Evidence for a drug dependence syndrome among narcotic users. *British Journal of Addiction*, **81**, 479–84.

Snyder, M. (1981). On the influence of individuals on situations. In: N. Cantor & J.F. Kihlstrom (eds.), *Personality, Cognition, and Social Interaction*. Hillsdale, NJ: Erlbaum.

Solomon, R.L. (1977). An opponent-process theory of acquired motivation: IV.

REFERENCES

The affective dynamics of addiction. In: J. Maseer & M.E.P. Seligman (eds.), *Psychopathological Experimental Models*. San Francisco: W.H. Freeman.

Sorokin, P. & Berger, C. (1939). *Time Budgets and Human Behavior*. Cambridge, MA: Harvard University Press.

Spencer, C. (1971). Random time sampling with self-observation for library cost studies: Unit costs of interlibrary loans and photocopies at a regional medical library. *Journal of American Social and Information Sciences*, **32**, 153–60.

Spielberger, C.D., Gorsuch, R.L. & Lushiene, R.E. (1970). *STAI Manual for the State-Trait Anxiety Inventory*. Palo Alto, California: Consulting Psychologist Press.

Spitzer, R.L., Endicott, J. & Robins, E. (1978). Research diagnostic criteria. *Archives of General Psychiatry*, **35**, 773–82.

Spitzer, R.L. & Williams, J.B. (1984). Diagnostic dilemmas. *Psychosomatics*, **25**(supplement), 16–20.

Spradley, J.P. (1979). *The Ethnographic Interview*. New York: Holt, Rinehart & Winston.

Stavrakaki, C. & Vargo, B. (1986). The relationship of anxiety and depression: A review of the literature. *British Journal of Psychiatry*, **149**, 7–16.

Steiner, H. & Levine, S. (1988). Acute stress response in anorexia nervosa: A pilot study. *Child Psychiatry and Human Development*, **18**, 208–18.

Stern, W. (1921). *Die differentielle Psychologie in ihren methodischen Grundlagen*. (Differential psychology in its methodological foundations.) Leipzig: Barth.

Stern, S.L., Dixon, K.N., Nemzer, E., Lake, M.D., Sansone, R.A., Smeltzer, D.J., Lantz, S. & Schrier, S.S. (1984). Affective disorder in the families of women with normal weight bulimia. *American Journal of Psychiatry*, **141**, 10, 1224–7.

Stoffelmayr, B.E., Benishek, L.A., Humphreys, K., Lee, J.A. & Mavis, B. (1989). Substance abuse prognosis with an additional psychiatric diagnosis. *Journal of Psychoactive Drugs*, **21**, 145–52.

Stokman, F.N. & van Schuur, W.H. (1980). Basic scaling. *Quality and Quantity*, **14**, 1, 5–30.

Stone, P.J. (1972). The analysis of time-budget data. In: A. Szalai *et al.* (eds.), *The Use of Time*. The Hague: Mouton.

Stone, P.J. (1978). Women's time patterns in eleven countries. In: W. Michelson (ed.), *Public Policy in Temporal Perspective*. The Hague: Mouton.

Stone, P.J. & Nicolson, N. (1987). Infrequently occurring activities and contexts in time use data. *Journal of Nervous and Mental Disease*, **175**, 9, 519–25.

Strauss, J.S. (1989). Mediating processes in schizophrenia. *British Journal of Psychiatry*, **155**, 9–14.

Strauss, J.S., Bartko, J.J. & Carpenter, W.T. (1981). New directions in diagnosis: The longitudinal processes of schizophrenia. *American Journal of Psychiatry*, **138**, 7, 954–8.

Strauss, J.S. & Carpenter, W.T. Jr. (1981). *Schizophrenia*. New York & London: Plenum Medical Books Company.

Strauss, J.S., Hafez, H., Lieberman, P. & Harding, C.M. (1985) The course of psychiatric disorder, III: Longitudinal principles. *American Journal of Psychiatry*, **142**, 3, 289–96.

Stravynski, A. & Greenberg, D. (1987). Cognitive therapies with neurotic disorders: Clinical utility and related issues. *Comprehensive Psychiatry*, **28**, 2, 141–50.

Strober, M. (1981). The significance of bulimia in juvenile anorexia nervosa: An exploration of possible etiologic factors. *International Journal of Eating Disorders*, **1**, 28–43.

de Swaan, A. (1981). The politics of agoraphobia: on changes in emotional and relational management. *Theory and Society*, **10**, 337–58.

Szalai, A., Converse, P., Feldheim, P. *et al.* (1972). *The Use of Time*. The Hague: Mouton.

Szymanski, H.V., Simon, J.C. & Gutterman, N. (1983). Recovery from schizophrenic psychosis. *American Journal of Psychiatry*, **140**, 3, 335–8.

Tamarin, J., Weiner, S. & Mendelson, J. (1970). Alcoholics' expectancies and recall of experiences during intoxication. *American Journal of Psychiatry*, **126**, 1697–704.

Tart, C. (1971). *On Being Stoned: A Psychological Study of Marijuana Intoxication*. Palo Alto, Ca.: Science and Behavior Books.

Tarter, R.E., Alterman, A.I. & Edwards, K.L. (1985). Vulnerability to alcoholism in men: A behavior-genetic perspective. *Journal of Studies of Alcohol*, **46**, 329–56.

Taylor, C.B., Sheikh, J., Agras, W.S. *et al.* (1986). Ambulatory heart rate changes in patients with panic attacks. *American Journal of Psychiatry*, **143**, 478–82.

Teasdale, J.D., Fennell, M.J., Hibbert, G.A. & Amies, P. (1984). Cognitive therapy for major depressive disorder in primary care. *British Journal of Psychiatry*, **144**, 400–6.

Teasdale, J.D. & Fennell, M.J. (1988). Immediate affects on depression of cognitive therapy. *Cognitive Therapy and Research*, **6**, 3, 343–52.

Tennen, H., Herzberger, S., Nelson, H. *et al.* (1987). Depressive attributional style: The role of self-esteem. *Journal of Personality*, **55**, 4, 631–61.

Thakor, N.V., Yang, M., Ameresan, M., Reiter, E., Hoehn-Saric, R. & McLeod, D.R. (1989). Micro-computer-based ambulatory monitor for vital signs in anxiety disorders. *Journal of Ambulatory Monitoring*, **2**, 4, 377–94.

Thomas, D. & Diener, E. (1989). Memory accuracy in the recall of emotions. Unpublished manuscript, University of Illinois.

Thorndike, E.L. (1937). How we spend our time and what we spend it for. *Scientific Monthly*.

Tinbergen, N. (1963). On the aims and methods of ethology. *Zeitschrift für Tierpsychology*, **20**, 410–33.

Tomkins, S. (1966). Psychological model for smoking behavior. *American Journal of Public Health*, **56**, 17–20.

Tseng, W.S. & McDermott, J.F. Jr. (1981). *Culture, Mind and Therapy: An Introduction to Cultural Psychiatry*. New York: Brunner, Mazel.

U.S. Department of Health and Human Services (1982). *The Health Consequences of Smoking: Cancer. A Report of the Surgeon General*. U.S. Department of Health and Human Services, Public Health Office. Office of Smoking and Health. DHHS Publication No. (PHS) 82-50179.

U.S. Department of Health and Human Services (1983). *The Health Consequences of Smoking: Cardiovascular Disease. A Report of the Surgeon General*. U.S. Department of Health and Human Services, Public Health Office. Office of Smoking and Health. DHHS Publication No. (PHS) 84-5020.

U.S. Department of Health and Human Services (1984). *The Health Consequences of Smoking: Chronic Obstructive Lung Disease. A Report of the Surgeon General*. U.S. Department of Health and Human Services, Public Health Office. Office of Smoking and Health. DHHS Publication No. (PHS) 82-5020.

Ursin, H. & Murison, R.C.C. (1984). Classification and description of stress. In: G.M. Brown, S.H. Koslow & S. Reichlin (eds.), *Neuroendocrinology and Psychiatric Disorder*, pp. 123–31. New York: Raven.

Vaillant, G. (1983). *The Natural History of Alcoholism: Cause, Pattern and Paths to Recovery*. Boston: Harvard University Press.

Vallacher, R.R. & Wegner, D.M. (1987). *A Theory of Action Identification*. Hillsdale, NJ: Erlbaum.

Van Egeren, L.F. & Madarasmi, S. (1988). A computer-assisted diary (CAD) for ambulatory blood pressure monitoring. *American Journal of Hypertension*, **1**, 179S–185S.

Van Meter, K.M. (1985). Block-modelling and cross-classification techniques for estimating population parameters from network data. *Workshop on the Methodology of Applied Drug Research*. Luxembourg: European Community Health Directorate.

Van Meter, K.M. (1986). Basic typology and multimethod analysis in the social sciences. *XIth World Congress of the International Sociological Association. New Delhi, India, 18-22 August*; & *International Review of Sociology*.

Van Valkenburg, C., Akiskal, H.S., Puzantian, V.R. & Rosenthal, T.L. (1984). Clinical, family history, and naturalistic outcome – Comparison with panic and major depressive disorders. *Journal of Affective Disorders*, **6**, 67–82.

Vanek, J. (1974). Time spent in housework. *Scientific American*, **231**, 116–220.

Vickers, R.R. (1988). Effectiveness of defenses: A significant predictor of cortisol excretion under stress. *Journal of Psychosomatic Research*, **32**, 21–9.

Vining, R.F., McGinley, R.A., Maksvytis, J.J. & Ho, K.Y. (1983). Salivary cortisol: A better measure of adrenal cortical function than serum cortisol. *Annals of Clinical Biochemistry*, **20**, 329–35.

Vining, R.F. & McGinley, R.A. (1986). Hormones in saliva. *CRC Critical Reviews in Clinical Laboratory Sciences*, **23**, 95–145.

Wada, T. (1922). An experimental study of hunger and its relation to activity. *Archives of Psychological Monographs*, **8**, 1–65.

Wald, F.D.M. & Mellenbergh, G.J. (1990). The short version of the Dutch translation of the Profile of Mood States (POMS). *Nederlands Tijdschrift voor Psychologie*, **45**, 86–90.

Walker, K. (1982). The potential for measurement of nonmarket household production with time-use data. In: Z. Staikov (ed.), *It's About Time*. Sophia, Bulgaria: Institute of Sociology at the Bulgarian Academy of Sciences.

Wallace, J.M., Thornton, W.E., Kennedy, H.L., Pickering, T.G., Harshfield, G.A., Frohlich, E.D., Messerli, F.H., Gifford, R.W. & Bolen, K. (1984). Ambulatory blood pressure in 199 normal subjects, a collaborative study. In: M.A. Weber, & J.M. Drayer (eds.), *Ambulatory Blood Pressure Monitoring*, pp. 117–28. Darmstadt: Steinkopf.

Wallace, J. & Zweben, J.E. (1989). Editor's introduction. *Journal of Psychoactive Drugs*, **21**, 135–7.

Walsh, B.T., Stewart, J.W., Roose, S.P., Gladis, M. & Glassman, A.H. (1984). Treatment of bulimia with phenelzine: A double-blind, placebo-controlled study. *Archives of General Psychiatry*, **41**, 1105–9.

Watkins, J.T. & Rush, A.J. (1988) Cognitive response test. *Cognitive Therapy and Research*, **7**, 5, 425–35.

Watson, D. & Tellegen, A. (1985). Toward a consensual structure of mood. *Psychological Bulletin*, **98**, 219–35.

Watts, F.N. & Bennett, D.H. (1983). *Theory and Practice of Psychiatric Rehabilitation*. Chichester: John Wiley & Sons.

Weber, M. (1947a). *The Theory of Social and Economic Organization*. New York: Free Press.

Weber, M. (1947b). *The Methodology of the Social Sciences*. New York: Free Press.

Weber, M.A. & Drayer, J.M. (1984). *Ambulatory Blood Pressure Monitoring*. Darmstadt: Steinkopf.

Wegner, D.M. & Vallacher, R.R. (1977). *Implicit Psychology: An Introduction to Social Cognition*. New York: Oxford University Press.

Wegner, D.M. & Vallacher, R.R. (1980). *The Self in Social Psychology*. New York: Oxford University Press.

Weil, A. (1972). *The Natural Mind*. Boston: Houghton Mifflin.

Weil, A., Zinberg, N. & Nelson, J. (1968). Clinical and psychological effects of marijuana in man. *Science*, **162**, 1234–42.

Weiner, M. (1983). The ego activation method: An in vivo cognitive therapy integrating behavioral and psychodynamic approaches. *Cognitive Therapy and Research*, **7**, 1, 11–18.

Weiner, H. (1985). The psychobiology and pathophysiology of anxiety and fear. In: A.H. Tuma & J.D. Mazer (eds.), *Anxiety & the Anxiety Disorders*, pp. 333–54. Hillsdale, NJ: Lawrence Erlbaum Assoc.

Wells, A. (1985). *Variations in Self-esteem in the Daily Life of Mothers*. Doctoral dissertation, The University of Chicago.

Wender, P.H. & Klein, D.F. (1981). *Mind, Mood and Medicine*. New York: Farrar, Straus, Giroux.

Whitehead, C.C., Polsky, R.H., Crookshank, C. & Fik, E. (1984). Objective and subjective evaluation of psychiatric ward redesign. *American Journal of Psychiatry*, **141**, 5, 639–44.

Whiting, B. (1977). Changing lifestyles in Kenya. *Daedelus*, **106**, 2.

Whiting, B. & Whiting, J.W.M. (1975). *Children of Six Cultures*. Cambridge, Massachusetts: Harvard University Press.

WHO Expert Committee on Mental Health (1955). The 'craving' for alcohol. *Quarterly Journal of Studies on Alcohol*, **16**, 33–60.

WHO (1981). WHO Nomenclature and Classification of Drug and Alcohol Related Problems: A WHO Memorandum. *Bulletin WHO*, **59**, 2, 225–42.

Wicker, A.W. (1979). *An Introduction to Ecological Psychology*. Cambridge, U.K.: Cambridge University Press.

Wicklund, R.A. (1975). Objective self-awareness. In: L. Berkowitz (ed.), *Advances in Experimental Social Psychology*, vol. 8, pp. 233–75. New York: Academic Press.

Widem, P., Pincus, H.A., Goldman, H.H. *et al.* (1984). Prospective payment for psychiatric hospitalization: context and background. *Hospital & Community Psychiatry*, **35**, 447–51.

Wiggins, J.S. (1964). Convergence among stylistic response measures from objective personality tests. *Educational and Psychological Measures*, **24**, 551–62.

Wikler, A. (1973). Dynamics of drug dependence: Implications of a conditioning theory for research and treatment. *Archives of General Psychiatry*, **28**, 611–16.

Wilkinson, I.M. & Blackburn, I.M. (1981). Cognitive style in depressed and recovered patients. *British Journal of Clinical Psychology*, **20**, 283–92.

Willems, E. (1969). Planning a rationale for naturalistic research. In: E. Willems & H. Rausch (eds.) *Naturalistic Viewpoints in Psychological Research*. New York: Holt, Reinhart & Winston.

Wilson, M.H. (1951). *Good Company: A Study of Nyakyusa Age Villages*. London: Oxford University Press.

Wilson, T.P. (1986). Qualitative 'versus' quantitative methods in social research. *Bulletin de Méthodologie Sociologique*, **10**, 25–51.

Winnicott, D.W. (1958). The capacity to be alone. *International Journal of Psychoanalysis*, **39**, 416–20.

Wishnie, H.A. (1975). Inpatient therapy with borderline patients. In: J.E. Mack (ed.), *Borderline States in Psychiatry*. New York: Grune & Stratton.

Wittersheim, G., Brandenberger, G. & Follenius, M. (1985). Mental task-induced strain and its after-effect assessed through variations in plasma cortisol levels. *Biological Psychology*, **21**, 123–32.

Wolf, E.S. (1987). Some comments on the self-object concept. In: K. Yardley & T. Honess (eds.), *Self and Identity: Psychological Perspectives*, pp. 259–72. Chichester, England: Wiley & Sons.

Wolff, C.T., Friedman, S.B., Hofer, M.A. & Mason, J.W. (1964). Relationship between psychological defenses and mean urinary 17-hydroxicorticosteroid excretion rates. *Psychosomatic Medicine*, **26**, 576–609.

Wolpe, J. (1958). *Psychotherapy by Reciprocal Inhibition*. Stanford: Stanford University Press.

Wolpe, J. (1969). *The Practice of Behavior Therapy*. New York: Pergamon.

Woodbury, M.A., Clive, J.A. & Garson, A. (1978). Mathematical typology: A grade of membership technique for obtaining disease definition. *Comparative Biological Research*, **11**, 277–98.

Wright, J. & Beck, A. (1983). Cognitive therapy of depression: Theory and practice. *Hospital and Community Psychiatry*, **34**, 12, 1119–27.

Wüst, S., Kirschbaum, C. & Hellhammer, D. (1991). Smoking increases salivary cortisol. In: C. Kirschbaum, D. Hellhammer & G.F. Read (eds.), *Assessment of Hormones and Drugs in Saliva in Biobehavioral Research*. Bern: Hans Huber.

Wynne, L.C., Cromwell, R.L. & Matthysse (eds.) (1978). *The Nature of Schizophrenia: New Approaches to Research and Treatment*. New York: John Willey and Sons.

Yarmey, D. (1979). *The Psychology of Eyewitness Testimony*. New York: Free Press.

Zautra, A.J., Guarnaccia, C.A. & Dohrenwend, B.P. (1986). Measuring small life events. *American Journal of Community Psychology*, **14**, 6, 629–55.

Zautra, A.J., Guarnaccia, C.A., Reich, J.W. *et al.* (1988). The contribution of small events to stress and distress. In: L.H. Cohen (ed.), *Life Events and Psychological Functioning*. pp. 123–48. Newbury Park: Sage.

von Zerssen, D., Doerr, P., Emrich, H.M., Lund, R. & Pirke, K.M. (1987). Diurnal variation of mood and the cortisol rhythm in depression and normal states of mind. *European Archives of Psychiatry & Neurological Sciences*, **237**, 36–45.

Zettle, R.D. & Hayes, S.C. (1987). Component and process analysis of cognitive therapy. *Psychological Reports*, **61**, 3, 939–53.

Zinberg, N.E. (1984). *Drug, Set, and Setting: The Basis for Controlled Intoxicant Use*. New Haven: Yale University Press.

Zinberg, N.E. & Shaffer, H.J. (1985). The social psychology of intoxicant use: The interaction of personality and social setting. In: H.B. Milkman & H.J. Shaffer (eds.), *The Addictions. Multidisciplinary Perspectives and Treatments*, pp. 57–74. Massachusetts: Lexington Books.

Zitrin, C.M., Klein, D.F. & Woerner, M.G. (1978). Behavior therapy, supportive psychotherapy, imipramine and phobias. *Archives of General Psychiatry*, **35**, 307–16.

Zubin, J. (1989). Suiting therapeutic interventions to the scientific models of aethology. *British Journal of Psychiatry*, **155**, 9–14.

Zubin, J., Steinhauer, S.R., Day, R. & Van Kammen, D.P. (1985). Schizophrenia at the crossroads: A blueprint for the 80s. *Comprehensive Psychiatry*, **26**, 3, 217–40.

Zung, W.W.K. & Durhan, N.C. (1965). A self-rating depression scale. *Archives of General Psychiatry*, **12**, 63–70.

van Zuuren, F.J. (1982). *Fobie, Situatie en Identiteit: Een Studie over de Situatievermijding en Identiteitsproblematiek van Twee Soorten Fobici*. Published thesis, University of Amsterdam.

Zuzanek, J. (1980). *Work and Leisure in the Soviet Union: A Time Budget Analysis*. New York: Praeger.

List of contributors

Alagna, S. – Ph.D.
Medical Psychology
Uniformed Services University of
  Health Sciences
Jones Bridge Road
Bethesda, Md., U.S.A.

Asmussen, L. – M.A.
1105 West Nevada Street
University of Illinois
Champagne, Illinois 61801, U.S.A.

Carli, M. – M.D.
Istituto di Psicologia della Facolta
  Medica
dell'Universita degli Studi di Milano
via Francesco Sforza 23
20122 Milano, Italy

Copeland, J.R.M. – M.D.
Department of Psychogeriatrics
Royal Liverpool Hospital
Prescot Street
Liverpool L7 8XP, U.K.

Csikszentmihalyi, M. – Ph.D.
Department of Behavioral Sciences
University of Chicago
5848 S. University Av.
Chicago, Illinois 60637, U.S.A.

Delespaul, P.A.E.G. – M.A.
Department of Social Psychiatry
University of Limburg
P.O. Box 616
6200 MD Maastricht, The Netherlands

Delle Fave, A. – M.D.
Istituto di Psicologia della Facolta
  Medica
dell'Universita degli studi di Milano
via Francesco Sforza 23
20122 Milano, Italy

deVries, M.W. – M.D.
Department of Social Psychiatry
University of Limburg
P.O. Box 616
6200 MD Maastricht, The Netherlands

van Diest, R. – M.A.
Department of Clinical Psychiatry
University of Limburg
P.O. Box 616
6200 MD Maastricht, The Netherlands

Dijkman-Caes, C.I.M. – M.A.
Department of Social Psychiatry
University of Limburg
P.O. Box 616
6200 MD Maastricht, The Netherlands

Donner, E. – Ph.D.
Committee on Human Development
University of Chicago
5441 S. Kenwood
Chicago, Illinois, U.S.A.

Figurski, T.J. – Ph.D.
Wayne State University
Detroit, Michigan 48202, U.S.A.

Freeman, M. – Ph.D.
Department of Behavioral Sciences
University of Chicago
5848 S. University Av.
Chicago, Illinois 60637, U.S.A.

Hamilton, J. – M.D.
Biology of Depression Research Unit
Center for Studies of Affective
  Disorders
The National Institute of Mental
  Health (NIMH)
Rm. 10-C-26, Parklawn Blgd.
Rockville, Md. 20857, U.S.A.

Hilwig, M. – M.D.
Department of Social Psychiatry
University of Limburg
P.O. Box 616
6200 MD Maastricht,The Netherlands

Hopkins, R. – M.D.
Department of Psychogeriatrics
Royal Liverpool Hospital
Prescot Street
Liverpool L7 8XP, U.K.

Hormuth, S.E. – M.D.
Psychology Institute
University of Heidelberg
Hauptstrasse 47-51
D-6900 Heidelberg, Germany

Hurlburt, R.T. – Ph.D.
Department of Psychology
University of Nevada
4505 South Maryland Parkway
Las Vegas, Nevada 89154, U.S.A.

Kaplan, C.D. – Ph.D.
IPSER
P.O. Box 214
6200 AE Maastricht,
The Netherlands

Kassel, J. – M.A.
Department of Psychology
University of Pittsburgh
Pittsburgh, PA 15260, U.S.A.

Kraan, H. – M.D., Ph.D.
Department of Social Psychiatry
University of Limburg
P.O. Box 616
6200 MD Maastricht,
The Netherlands

Larson, R. – Ph.D.
1105 West Nevada Street
University of Illinois
Champagne, Illinois 61801, U.S.A.

Loewenstein, R.J. – M.D.
Department of Psychiatry
UCLA
Veteran's Administration
Wadsworth Medical Center
Wilshire and Sawtelle Blvds
Los Angeles, CA 90073, U.S.A.

Madarasmi, S. – M.D.
Department of Psychiatry
Michigan State University
East Lansing, Michigan 48824,
U.S.A.

Massimini, F. – M.D., Ph.D.
Istituto di Psicologia della Facolta
   Medica
dell'Universita degli Studi di Milano
via Francesco Sforza 23
20122 Milano, Italy

Meertens, H. – M.D.
Department of Social Psychiatry
University of Limburg
P.O. Box 616
6200 MD Maastricht, The Netherlands

Melancon, S.M. – M.A.
Department of Psychology
University of Nevada
4505 South Maryland Parkway
Las Vegas, Nevada 89154, U.S.A.

Merrick, W.A. – Ph.D.
Clinical/Forensic Neuropsychology
Whiting Forensic Institute
Middletown, CT, U.S.A.

Nicolson, N. – Ph.D.
Department of Neuropsychology and
   Psychobiology
University of Limburg
P.O. Box 616
6200 MD Maastricht, The Netherlands

Paty, J. – M.A.
Department of Psychology
University of Pittsburgh
Pittsburgh, PA 15260, U.S.A.

van der Poel, E. – M.A.
Department of Social Psychiatry
University of Limburg
P.O. Box 616
6200 MD Maastricht, The Netherlands

Portegijs, P. – M.D.
Department of Social Psychiatry
University of Limburg
P.O. Box 616,
6200 MD Maastricht, The Netherlands

Reid, N. – R.N.
Clinical Neuropharmacology Branch
NIMH, NIH Clinical Center
Ward 6D
Bethesda, Md. 20205, U.S.A.

Robinson, J.P. – Ph.D.
Department of Sociology
Survey Research Center
College Park
Maryland 20742, U.S.A.

Shiffman, S. – Ph.D.
Department of Psychology
University of Pittsburgh
Pittsburgh, PA 15260, U.S.A.

Stone, P.J. – Ph.D.
Department of Psychology and Social
   Relations
William James Hall
Harvard University
Cambridge
Massachusetts 02138, U.S.A.

Van Egeren, L.F. – M.D.
Department of Psychiatry
Michigan State University
East Lansing, Michigan 48824,
U.S.A.

Van Meter, K.M. – Ph.D.
LISH CNRS
54, bd. Raspail
F-75006 Paris, France

Volovics, L. – Ph.D.
Medical Information and Statistics
University of Limburg
P.O. Box 616
6200 MD Maastricht,The Netherlands

Wilson, K.C.M. – M.D.
Department of Psychogeriatrics
Royal Liverpool Hospital
Prescot Street
Liverpool L7 8XP, U.K.

Index